CLINICAL PRACTICE
OF PEDIATRIC PSYCHOLOGY

CLINICAL PRACTICE OF PEDIATRIC PSYCHOLOGY

Edited by

Michael C. Roberts
Brandon S. Aylward
Yelena P. Wu

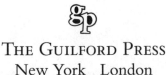

THE GUILFORD PRESS
New York London

© 2014 The Guilford Press
A Division of Guilford Publications, Inc.
72 Spring Street, New York, NY 10012
www.guilford.com

Printed in the United States of America

This book is printed on acid-free paper.

Last digit is print number: 9   8   7   6   5   4   3   2   1

The authors have checked with sources believed to be reliable in their efforts to
provide information that is complete and generally in accord with the standards
of practice that are accepted at the time of publication. However, in view of the
possibility of human error or changes in behavioral, mental health, or medical
sciences, neither the authors, nor the editors and publisher, nor any other party
who has been involved in the preparation or publication of this work warrants
that the information contained herein is in every respect accurate or complete,
and they are not responsible for any errors or omissions or the results obtained
from the use of such information. Readers are encouraged to confirm the information contained in this book with other sources.

Library of Congress Cataloging-in-Publication Data

Clinical practice of pediatric psychology / edited by Michael C. Roberts,
Brandon S. Aylward, Yelena P. Wu.
    p. ; cm.
  Includes bibliographical references and index.
  ISBN 978-1-4625-1411-3 (alk. paper)
  I. Roberts, Michael C., editor of compilation.   II. Aylward, Brandon S., editor of
compilation.   III. Wu, Yelena P., editor of compilation.
  [DNLM: 1. Child Psychology.   2. Pediatrics.   WS 105]
  RJ499.3
  618.92′89—dc23
                                                                2014000722

About the Editors

Michael C. Roberts, PhD, ABPP, is Professor and former Director of the Clinical Child Psychology Program and Dean of Graduate Studies at the University of Kansas. He has published close to 200 journal articles and book chapters related to understanding and influencing children's physical and mental health. Dr. Roberts has authored or coedited 18 books, including *Handbook of Pediatric Psychology, Fourth Edition,* and and is currently the Editor of *Training and Education in Professional Psychology.* He is a recipient of the Award for Distinguished Contributions to Education and Training from the American Psychological Association and the Martin P. Levin Mentorship Award from the Society of Pediatric Psychology.

Brandon S. Aylward, PhD, is Assistant Professor of Pediatrics at Emory University School of Medicine and a researcher in the Sibley Heart Center Cardiology and Division of Pediatric Neurology at Children's Healthcare of Atlanta. Dr. Aylward has published journal articles and book chapters in the areas of pediatric psychology, analytic methods, and health technology, and serves on the editorial boards of several journals. He is engaged in multidisciplinary clinics focusing on pediatric cardiology, neurodevelopmental outcomes, and self-management/adherence. He is a recipient of the C. Eugene Walker Education Award from the Society of Pediatric Psychology.

Yelena P. Wu, PhD, is Assistant Professor in the Department of Family and Preventive Medicine and the Huntsman Cancer Institute at the University of Utah. Her research interests include identifying risk and protective factors influencing pediatric medical regimen adherence and health outcomes, and dissemination of empirically based assessments and interventions for adherence. Dr. Wu has published numerous articles and book chapters on psychosocial and health outcomes among individuals with chronic conditions across the lifespan. She is a recipient of the C. Eugene Walker Education Award from the Society of Pediatric Psychology.

Contributors

Melissa A. Alderfer, PhD, Center for Healthcare Delivery Science, Nemours/Alfred I. duPont Hospital for Children, Wilmington, Delaware

Brandon S. Aylward, PhD, Department of Pediatrics, Emory University School of Medicine, and Divisions of Pediatric Neurology and Sibley Heart Center Cardiology, Children's Health Care of Atlanta, Atlanta, Georgia

Glen P. Aylward, PhD, ABPP, Division of Developmental–Behavioral Pediatrics/Psychology, Southern Illinois University School of Medicine, Springfield, Illinois

Lamia P. Barakat, PhD, Division of Oncology, The Children's Hospital of Philadelphia, and Perelman School of Medicine, University of Pennsylvania, Philadelphia, Pennsylvania

Martha U. Barnard, PhD, Department of Pediatrics/Behavioral Pediatrics, University of Kansas Medical Center, Kansas City, Kansas

Kelsey Borner, BA, Clinical Child Psychology Program, University of Kansas, Lawrence, Kansas

Cindy L. Buchanan, PhD, Department of Psychiatry, University of Colorado, Anschutz Medical Campus, and Department of Child Psychiatry and Behavioral Sciences, Children's Hospital Colorado, Aurora, Colorado

Lisa M. Buckloh, PhD, Division of Psychology and Psychiatry, Nemours Children's Clinic, Jacksonville, Florida

Catherine Butz, PhD, Division of Pediatric Psychology and Neuropsychology, Nationwide Children's Hospital, and Department of Pediatrics, The Ohio State University, Columbus, Ohio

Bryan D. Carter, PhD, Department of Pediatrics, Division of Child and Adolescent Psychiatry and Psychology, University of Louisville School of Medicine, Louisville, Kentucky

Caitlin Conroy, PsyD, Mayo Family Pediatric Pain Rehabilitation Center, Boston
Children's Hospital, and Department of Psychiatry, Harvard Medical School,
Waltham, Massachusetts

Valerie McLaughlin Crabtree, PhD, Department of Psychology, St. Jude Children's
Research Hospital, Memphis, Tennessee

Christopher C. Cushing, PhD, Department of Psychology, Oklahoma State
University, Stillwater, Oklahoma

Lauren C. Daniel, PhD, Division of Oncology, The Children's Hospital of
Philadelphia, Philadelphia, Pennsylvania

Allison G. Dempsey, PhD, Center for Clinical Research and Evidence-Based
Medicine, Department of Pediatrics, University of Texas Health Science
Center at Houston, Houston, Texas

Christina L. Duncan, PhD, Department of Psychology, West Virginia University,
Morgantown, West Virginia

David A. Fedele, PhD, Department of Clinical and Health Psychology, University
of Florida, Gainesville, Florida

Cynthia A. Gerhardt, PhD, Center for Biobehavioral Health, The Research
Institute at Nationwide Children's Hospital, and Department of Pediatrics
and Psychology, The Ohio State University, Columbus, Ohio

Joanne M. Gillespie, PhD, Pediatric Health Psychology Service, IWK Health
Centre, and Department of Psychology, Dalhousie University, Halifax,
Nova Scotia, Canada

Shanna M. Guilfoyle, PhD, Division of Behavioral Medicine and Clinical
Psychology, Cincinnati Children's Hospital Medical Center, University of
Cincinnati College of Medicine, Cincinnati, Ohio

Linda A. Hawkins, PhD, Division of Adolescent Medicine, The Children's Hospital
of Philadelphia, Philadelphia, Pennsylvania

Matthew C. Hocking, PhD, Division of Oncology, The Children's Hospital of
Philadelphia, Philadelphia, Pennsylvania

Barbara Jandasek, PhD, Bradly Hasbro Children's Research Center, Rhode Island
Hospital, and Alpert Medical School of Brown University, Providence,
Rhode Island

Rebecca J. Johnson, PhD, Division of Developmental and Behavioral Sciences,
Department of Pediatrics, Children's Mercy Hospitals and Clinics, University
of Missouri–Kansas City School of Medicine, Kansas City, Missouri

Bryan T. Karazsia, PhD, Department of Psychology, The College of Wooster,
Wooster, Ohio

Keri J. Brown Kirschman, PhD, Department of Psychology, University of Dayton,
Dayton, Ohio

Stephen Lassen, PhD, Department of Pediatrics, University of Kansas Medical
Center, Kansas City, Kansas

Kathleen Lemanek, PhD, Division of Pediatric Psychology and Neuropsychology,

Nationwide Children's Hospital, and Department of Pediatrics, The Ohio State University, Columbus, Ohio

Deirdre E. Logan, PhD, Division of Pain Medicine, Department of Anesthesiology, Perioperative and Pain Medicine, Boston Children's Hospital, and Department of Psychiatry, Harvard Medical School, Boston, Massachusetts

Anne M. Lynch-Jordan, PhD, Department of Pediatrics, Division of Behavioral Medicine and Clinical Psychology, Cincinnati Children's Hospital Medical Center, University of Cincinnati College of Medicine, Cincinnati, Ohio

Loretta A. Martin-Halpine, PsyD, Department of Child and Adolescent Psychiatry and Behavioral Sciences, Pediatric Feeding and Swallowing Center, The Children's Hospital of Philadelphia, Philadelphia, Pennsylvania

Elizabeth N. McLaughlin, PhD, Pediatric Health Psychology Service, IWK Health Centre, and Department of Psychology, Dalhousie University, Halifax, Nova Scotia, Canada

Lisa J. Meltzer, PhD, Department of Pediatrics, National Jewish Health, Denver, Colorado

Jodi A. Mindell, PhD, Department of Psychology, Saint Joseph's University, and Sleep Center, The Children's Hospital of Philadelphia, Philadelphia, Pennsylvania

Avani C. Modi, PhD, Division of Behavioral Medicine and Clinical Psychology, Center for Treatment Adherence and Self-Management, Cincinnati Children's Hospital Medical Center, University of Cincinnati College of Medicine, Cincinnati, Ohio

Timothy D. Nelson, PhD, Department of Psychology, University of Nebraska–Lincoln, Lincoln, Nebraska

Susana R. Patton, PhD, Department of Pediatrics/Behavioral Pediatrics, University of Kansas Medical Center, Kansas City, Kansas

Sean Phipps, PhD, Department of Psychology, St. Jude Children's Research Hospital, Memphis, Tennessee

Jerilynn Radcliffe, PhD, ABPP, Department of Pediatrics, Division of Developmental and Behavioral Pediatrics, The Children's Hospital of Philadelphia, and Perelman School of Medicine, University of Pennsylvania, Philadelphia, Pennsylvania

Lisa Y. Ramirez, PhD, Department of Child and Adolescent Psychiatry and Psychology, MetroHealth Medical Center, Cleveland, Ohio

Michael C. Roberts, PhD, ABPP, Clinical Child Psychology Program, University of Kansas, Lawrence, Kansas

Mary T. Rourke, PhD, Institute for Graduate Clinical Psychology, Widener University, Chester, Pennsylvania

Terry Stancin, PhD, Department of Psychiatry, MetroHealth Medical Center, Case Western Reserve University, Cleveland, Ohio

Ric G. Steele, PhD, ABPP, Clinical Child Psychology Program, University of Kansas, Lawrence, Kansas

Lynne Sturm, PhD, Department of Pediatrics, Riley Hospital for Children, Indiana School of Medicine, Indianapolis, Indiana

Aimee N. Thompson, PsyD, Division of Behavioral Medicine and Clinical Psychology, Cancer and Blood Diseases Institute, Cincinnati Children's Hospital Medical Center, Cincinnati, Ohio

Suzanne M. Thompson, PhD, Pediatric Psychology, St. Louis Children's Hospital, St. Louis, Missouri

Shari L. Wade, PhD, Division of Physical Medicine and Rehabilitation, Cincinnati Children's Hospital Medical Center, University of Cincinnati College of Medicine, Cincinnati, Ohio

Victoria W. Willard, PhD, Department of Psychology, St. Jude Children's Research Hospital, Memphis, Tennessee

Yelena P. Wu, PhD, Department of Family and Preventive Medicine and Huntsman Cancer Institute, University of Utah School of Medicine, Salt Lake City, Utah

Preface

Increasingly, psychologists, counselors, social workers, and other behavioral specialists who work with children and their families find themselves working in medical contexts that focus on patient problems regarding management of chronic illness, recovery from injury or surgery, and maintenance of health-promoting lifestyles. We developed this book to support practitioners seeking reliable approaches and tools in their work with the range of problems presenting in pediatric settings. We sought to provide a clinically focused pediatric psychology resource for professionals, one that could also be used as a text in undergraduate and graduate level courses. Although other texts, such as the *Handbook of Pediatric Psychology*, appropriately emphasize more of the research base for the field, clinical applications need greater elaboration for the variety of presenting issues that pediatric psychologists encounter across practice settings. This volume provides an overview to the field of pediatric psychology with a focus on clinical applications grounded in evidence-based practice. It presents examples of the clinical problems seen in pediatric situations that interact with both medical and psychosocial issues.

The first section of the book offers a broad perspective on the field of practice in pediatric and child health psychology, briefly describing the research and evidence base for clinical practice, and demonstrates the varied clinical roles that psychologists working with pediatric populations may hold. The next two sections focus on the clinical treatment of children with specific pediatric illnesses or health concerns, and the psychological factors associated with them.

The chapters provide descriptions of psychological practice, assessment and intervention strategies, and the decision-making processes that occur in the course of clinical practice within pediatric psychology. They also illuminate the range and complexity of clinical cases presenting in different settings of pediatric psychology. The authors include one or more clinical case examples in their chapters, describing how the psychologist addresses the presenting issues using the research evidence base in case conceptualization and clinical decision making. We asked the authors to comment on their clinical cases by explaining decision points and highlighting important learning and teaching considerations. The case examples are accompanied by the authors' commentaries to highlight the psychologist's roles, multidisciplinary collaboration, and key issues in their work. The cases reported in the chapters are based on patients with real presenting problems; however, all authors have affirmed that they have disguised information that might identify the patients, their families, or situations.

In organizing the book and editing the chapters, we became ever more mindful of the complexity of situations and problems at the interface of pediatric medicine and psychology. The authors who have contributed to this book present the issues in clinical practice involving multiple perspectives and approaches, explicate conceptual and theoretical considerations, incorporate the empirical evidence base into practice, and integrate clinical cases illustrating a pediatric psychologist's activities. In preparing this book to be an informational resource for the vibrant field of pediatric psychology, we and the chapter authors hope to benefit clinicians, trainees, and their future patients and families.

MICHAEL C. ROBERTS
BRANDON S. AYLWARD
YELENA P. WU

Contents

PART III. PEDIATRIC CONDITIONS
AND THE ROLE OF THE PSYCHOLOGIST

PART I

OVERVIEW AND FOUNDATIONS OF PEDIATRIC PSYCHOLOGY

CHAPTER 1

Overview of the Field of Pediatric Psychology

MICHAEL C. ROBERTS
BRANDON S. AYLWARD
YELENA P. WU

As the phrase implies, "pediatric psychology" is an amalgam of clinical applications and psychological science with the medical and health problems of children, adolescents, and their families, all within the context of collaborations with health care providers. The practice specialty of pediatric psychology developed primarily to fill unmet needs that became increasingly apparent and noticed by medical professionals. Pediatric and family physicians were and are confronted with a range of health and behavioral problems that require an integrated medical–psychological approach to treat comprehensively and effectively (Roberts, 1986). This chapter provides an overview of clinical practice within pediatric psychology, including a brief history, important theoretical models used in practice, main features of practice, innovations, and training issues.

HISTORY OF PEDIATRIC PSYCHOLOGY

Considerable changes in pediatric practice were associated with the decline of infectious diseases that had often resulted in impairment and death in the 1950s and 1960s. Improvements in mortality and morbidity were achieved

3

through advances in immunization, improved sanitation, and disease control. In addition, improved medical treatments dramatically increased survival for life-threatening illnesses. Thus, as the types of patient cases presenting in pediatric practice changed, medical services and hospital-based policies correspondingly changed to accommodate the new needs. Specifically, professionals increasingly recognized that their patients were more often presenting with emotional and psychological problems in both outpatient and inpatient settings.

Historically, pediatricians and professional psychologists in independent practice settings could not fully meet the needs of children and their families within their traditional frameworks, experiences, and training backgrounds. Importantly, the health care professional usually had inadequate training to competently manage these issues and insufficient time in daily practice to devote proper attention to them. These psychological, developmental, behavioral, educational, and child management issues challenged physicians and nurses both to identify and then to treat them, with a lack of adequate referral and follow-through to psychological practitioners. However, when children and families were referred out of the medical practice and served in more traditional mental health clinics, such as child guidance clinics or outpatient psychiatric clinics, the patients would have been altered, with changes in perceptions, behavior, responses, and motivation, in the process of being interviewed, diagnosed, and referred to another agency or professional (Roberts, 1986; Walker, 1979). Pediatricians needed direct access for their patients to psychological services; psychologists sought to provide more accessible and effective services for children, adolescents, and their families.

In an evolution during the 1960s, a "new marriage" was proposed for psychology and pediatrics (Kagan, 1965), which was eventually strengthened over time based on mutually beneficial interactions developing through both individual collaborations and systemic relationships. The "marriage" of pediatrics and psychology is now not so new; nonetheless, as a field of integrated practice, this relationship retains some of the vibrancy of its development and creative concepts, with a continual growing together as the "marital" arrangement matures.

Logan Wright, one of the recognized founders of pediatric psychology, defined the field as dealing "primarily with children in a medical setting which is nonpsychiatric in nature" (1967, p. 323). A closely related definition in the *Journal of Pediatric Psychology (JPP)* masthead indicated:

> The field and the contents of this Journal are defined by the interests and concerns of psychologists who work in interdisciplinary settings such as children's hospitals, developmental clinics, and pediatric or medical group practices.

A more comprehensive articulation was described in a revised mast-head statement of *JPP* in 1988 that moved beyond the setting-based defini-tion to advance the field to include a more expansive range of issues and activities:

> Pediatric psychology is an interdisciplinary field addressing the full range of physical and mental development, health, and illness issues affecting children, adolescents, and families . . . wide range of topics exploring the relationship between psychological and physical well-being of children and adolescents including: understanding, assessment, and intervention with developmental disorders; evaluation and treatment of behavioral and emotional problems and concomitants of disease and illness; the role of psychology in pediatric medicine; the promotion of health and development; and the prevention of illness and injury among children and youth.

As currently conceptualized, pediatric psychology integrates the traditional bases of scientific foundations and applied practice of psy-chology with the issues and settings of pediatric health. As such, profes-sionals utilize evidence-based methods that have been developed within a scientist-practitioner orientation to enhance health and development of children and adolescents. Areas of its clinical science and applica-tions include the assessment of and intervention for (1) psychological and developmental conditions that influence the occurrence of and recovery from pediatric medical disorders and (2) the behavioral and emotional concomitants of injury, disease, and developmental disorders. The field of pediatric psychology encompasses a multitude of activities that pro-mote health and prevent or control disease and injury. Parts of pediat-ric psychologists' activities are oriented not only toward the education and nurturing of psychologist trainees but also toward training other health care providers and professionals. In addition to advocating for and working with patients to improve their health behaviors, pediatric psychologists advocate for the improvement of health care systems, such as enhancement of the organization and delivery of services for children and for changes in societal conditions that impede the fulfillment of chil-dren's development.

The Society of Pediatric Psychology (SPP) recently formulated a more concise "mission statement" to capture the purposes of the organization and its members:

> SPP aims to promote the health and psychological well-being of chil-dren, youth and their families through science and an evidence-based approach to practice, education, training, advocacy, and consultation. (Palermo, 2012, p. 1)

An even more concise "vision statement" for the organization called for "healthier children, youth, and families" (Palermo, 2012, p. 1). Although these statements do not define the field per se, they do convey the focal points of the practice of pediatric psychology and its health-oriented scientific approaches and move away from the earlier setting-based definitions offered in the *JPP* masthead statements.

Formal definitions of the field notwithstanding, what really defines a field are the activities of those who work as practitioners and clinical investigators: "Despite all the verbiage that can be written defining pediatric psychology practice, one characteristic more than anything else defines the field—the types of cases evaluated and treated by the pediatric psychologist" (Roberts, 1986, p. 19). As is shown in the cases presented in later chapters of this book, pediatric psychologists provide (1) psychosocial services for issues related to pediatric health conditions (e.g., fostering coping and adjustment to the diagnosis of a chronic illness, improving adherence to a medical treatment regimen, pain management, school reintegration); (2) psychological services for mental health problems appearing in medical settings along with a pediatric problem (e.g., behavioral disobedience after hospitalization); (3) assessment and treatment for psychological problems presenting in a medical setting without a concomitant medical condition (e.g., through primary care referrals for attention-deficit/hyperactivity disorder [ADHD]); (4) programs for health promotion, disease and injury prevention, and early intervention; (5) assessment, intervention, and programming to improve functioning for children and adolescents with intellectual and developmental disabilities; and (6) advocacy for public policy supporting children and families and promoting public health advancements. There are two conceptual frameworks that commonly inform and drive pediatric psychology clinical practice.

CONCEPTUAL FRAMEWORKS

Developmental Perspective

Given the focus on children and adolescents, pediatric psychologists apply a developmental perspective to their work and must recognize the rapidity and extensiveness of the changes occurring in children in terms of their physical, cognitive, psychological/emotional, and social abilities and functioning. This developmental orientation helps to determine (1) changes to expect over time and as comparison for tracking when development goes awry; (2) intervention and prevention services that might be most needed and for certain presenting problems; and (3) psychological services that might be offered to maximize appropriate return to functioning (Jackson, Wu, Aylward, & Roberts, 2012; Roberts, 1986; Spirito et al., 2003).

Biopsychosocial Model

Many pediatric psychologists explicitly orient toward the biopsychosocial model built on the social ecology model of Bronfenbrenner (1979; see also Spirito & Kazak, 2006, and Wu, Aylward, & Roberts, Chapter 3, this volume). This model considers the multiple elements that influence child development in general and that specifically affect how the child and family might adapt to changes in psychological and physical conditions. For example, if a child has a chronic illness, this social ecological model articulates the numerous systems surrounding the child depicted in a series of concentric rings surrounding the individual child or adolescent. The microsystem, closest to the child, would include the illness, parents, and other family members. Expanding outward, the mesosystem includes peers, schools, and the medical settings and staff. The exosystem involves the parents' social networks, culture and social class, religious institutions, and social services (see Figure 43.1 in Steele & Aylward, 2009). This model indicates points at which psychosocial interventions might be made for children with pediatric conditions at multiple levels within the multiple systems. A biopsychosocial perspective enhances the pediatric psychologist's recognition of the systemic influences and complexity of factors surrounding a child who is learning to live with and manage a medical condition.

As a corollary to this model, over the years, several changes may be observed in the practice aspects of the pediatric psychology field. These include movement from an orientation that assumed that a child with a chronic medical condition would have, or would be at high risk for, deficits in psychosocial functioning to a model that focuses more on strengths and resilience in finding how children and their families cope and adjust and how to help those who are experiencing difficulty move to improved functioning.

PEDIATRIC PSYCHOLOGY SETTINGS FOR PRACTICE

The settings in which pediatric psychologists conduct these activities are similarly diverse, including (1) medical outpatient clinics with pediatricians or family medicine physicians in primary care, such as private practices and clinics attached to medical centers and children's hospitals (these could include general pediatrics practice); (2) inpatient units in children's hospitals for initial diagnosis and intensive treatment (these could be specialty units for cancer treatment or a general ward); (3) psychology or interdisciplinary outpatient clinics and child guidance clinics (e.g., for emotional and behavior problems associated with medical conditions or independently presenting in primary care, services for children with developmental disabilities); (4) specialty facilities, clinics, and centers for specified conditions (e.g., intellectual disabilities, epilepsy); and (5) community support agencies and groups (e.g., summer camps for children with specific conditions, such as cancer, sickle cell disease, and diabetes). The various types of settings of pediatric psychology practice are illustrated in the different case descriptions throughout the book (see especially Lassen, Wu, & Roberts, Chapter 2, this volume).

CHARACTERISTICS OF
PEDIATRIC PSYCHOLOGY PRACTICE

The greatest number of pediatric psychologists practice in hospitals or medical institutions, even though more pediatric patients are seen for general health care in outpatient or primary care settings. This is likely a result of available financial reimbursement practices for psychologists in institutions. Across settings, factors influencing psychologists' practice include the nature of pediatric practice in offices and hospitals and differences in training, orientation to diagnosis, and terminology between medical and psychology providers (Roberts, 1986). Other chapters in this volume illustrate the practice setting differences, for example, Chapters 2 (Lassen et al., on common concerns and settings); 5 (Carter, Thompson, & Thompson, on pediatric consultation–liaison in the children's hospital); 6 (Stancin, Sturm, & Ramirez, on primary care practice); and 7 (Conroy & Logan, on multidisciplinary and interdisciplinary teams). All of the chapters in this volume concerning clinical problems and the case examples similarly describe the various practice parameters. For example, whether in outpatient or inpatient settings, medical practice is more fast paced than many traditional professional psychologists are accustomed to experiencing, and it influences the nature of pediatric psychology practice (Roberts, 1986). For example, there are increasing requirements that, for financial reasons, physicians and other medical providers see larger numbers of patients in a day, often with limited time per patient. Further, an office-based practitioner may see a diversity of presenting problems, including well-child visits, visits for episodic illnesses, follow-up care for a chronic illness, and visits focused on child behavior concerns. In addition, medical providers and psychologists differ in the training they receive. For instance, broadly speaking, whereas medical providers receive extensive training on understanding and diagnosing the medical and biological underpinnings of presenting problems, along with their associated medical diagnoses, psychologists receive extensive training on understanding the psychosocial influences on presenting problems along with the associated psychological diagnoses. In addition, psychologists typically receive more training than their medical colleagues on managing the interpersonal and psychosocial challenges with which children and their families present.

The pediatric psychologist often must adapt to fit the medical practice model through brief interventions with child and caregiver. Psychological assessment and interactions with patients and the physician correspondingly need to be economical and time efficient. Consultations with the health care provider are typically brief and targeted to the most important considerations. Extensive diagnostic workups are therefore not as valued in pediatric practice. Targeted and to-the-point psychological reports are more likely to be read and utilized than are lengthy, esoteric reports presenting large amounts of psychological jargon. Pediatric psychology reports typically are action-based communications about what was found in the consultation and recommendations for parents, for the physician, and for the psychologist about addressing the referred issues. Any reports by necessity indicate the problem and the referral question, with a brief exposition of what was assessed and the results, and they place the greatest emphasis on what is recommended. Consequently, the quick-paced nature of medically related work requires modifying well-trained assessment and psychological report-writing skills. In addition, successful partnerships between medical professionals and pediatric psychologists often require both sides to be willing to accept and endorse a biopsychosocial approach to assessment, case conceptualization, and treatment.

In response to the demands for efficient and effective interventions, particularly in medical settings, the pediatric psychologist also likely employs briefer interventions. Behavioral and cognitive-behavioral strategies are frequently implemented. These interventions typically have a stronger evidence base, are more demonstrably effective, can be targeted to specific clinical problems, and can be implemented by a variety of caregivers than more traditional psychiatric or psychological therapies. Beyond the interventions themselves, pediatric psychologists must use a variety of necessary clinical skills, including establishing rapport and providing support and empathy.

A variety of theoretical approaches are being developed to meet the needs of the pediatric psychologist's patient population, including with motivational interviewing (Hilliard, Ramey, Rohan, Drotar, & Cortina, 2011; Jensen et al., 2011) and acceptance and commitment therapy (Masuda, Cohen, Wicksell, Kemani, & Johnson, 2011). Often, the application of existing therapy techniques to a pediatric psychology population is made in the context of clinical case studies that might later be developed through more systematic evaluations of effectiveness. Historically, pediatric psychologists have demonstrated a pragmatic eclecticism that invokes innovation and an attitude of "if it works, use it."

Evidence-based practice in pediatric psychology clearly relies on clinician judgment about the applicability of empirically supported treatments and careful observations of effectiveness applied to individual patients. Psychologists are expected to solve problems, as do most medical professionals, with an emphasis placed on observable or measurable outcomes, not ill-defined or nebulous results. Indeed, in many situations, successful outcomes are readily observable. For example, a child with a feeding disorder starts eating and gaining weight, a child with encopresis gains continence and decreases frequency of soiling, a child with diabetes learns to increasingly monitor exercise and nutrition to improve in adherence to the medical regimen, or a reduction in pain symptoms occurs for a child with sickle cell disease after a psychological intervention. In pediatrics and, concomitantly, in pediatric psychology, there is an emphasis on demonstrable effectiveness and an orientation to practical interventions and accountability for results. Duncan and Dempsey (Chapter 4, this volume) provide more information on financial issues and outcomes for reimbursement.

ADVANCES AND INNOVATIONS

Early research in the field described the types of presenting problems, the characteristics of children and families with different medical conditions, and the psychological sequelae to these conditions. For example, Wright described the intellectual sequelae of meningitis and Rocky Mountain spotted fever (Wright, 1972; Wright & Jimmerson, 1971). Lee Salk, another founder of the field, described the psychological impact of hemophilia on pediatric patients and their families (Salk, Hilgartner, & Granich, 1972). Similarly, much of the research published in *JPP* would be categorized as primarily descriptive or "explicative" (Roberts, 1992; Roberts, McNeal, Randall, & Roberts, 1996). Explicative research includes examinations of relationships among the various measures of psychological and pediatric variables in order to produce a comprehensive view of the factors related to medical or psychological conditions. Studies with an explicative purpose, for example, have considered the relationship of coping responses of children with pediatric conditions (e.g., sickle cell disease, cancer, diabetes, spina bifida) and family members' adjustment to having a child who has a chronic illness. A few of these descriptive studies have directly led to clinical interventions for the pediatric psychologist or medical staff to implement. However, Tercyak et al. (2006) indicated that this descriptive work serves as early-phase research, with later phases making the application for clinical practice. *JPP*, published by the SPP, is a significant resource in terms of the scientific base for knowledge in the field; the SPP has now embarked on a new publication, *Clinical Practice of Pediatric Psychology*, published in conjunction with the American Psychological Association, to fulfill the practice needs of professional pediatric psychologists with attention to applications in the various types of practices and settings.

The founders of the field created many new treatments and evaluated these innovative interventions because they were often faced with challenging cases that presented in pediatric settings. For example, as a pioneer in practice and in documenting what was effective in pediatric psychology, Logan Wright described devising a successful intervention for helping wean children off of their "addiction" to breathing through tracheotomy cannula, a situation that previously produced a high mortality rate (Wright, Nunnery, Eichel, & Scott, 1968, 1969). He also developed and evaluated treatment for children's refusals to swallow liquids or solids (Wright, 1971), for a child's self-induced seizure (Wright, 1973a), and for encopresis that had been ineffectively treated to that time (Wright, 1973b, 1975; Wright & Walker, 1976). Many treatments have become well established with empirical research and clinical applications.

Innovation is still important and necessary today in pediatric psychology practice. Currently, for instance, interventions such as using telehealth and technology devices are being developed and tested. As examples of these developments, a CD-ROM has been used to present an intervention for recurrent pediatric headaches (Connelly, Rapoff, Thompson, & Connelly, 2006). A Web-based program for HIV-positive youth has been found to enhance adherence to antiretroviral therapy (Shegog, Markham, Leonard, Bui, & Paul, 2012). Electronic monitoring of medication adherence through recording chips on medicine bottle caps has been used in multiple applications (Maikranz, Steele, Dreyer, Stratman, & Bovaird, 2007). Smartphones and other electronic devices now provide the technology to engage pediatric patients by prompting and recording behavior, to implement psychosocial and educational interventions, and to provide feedback on performance (e.g., Hilliard et al., 2011; McClellan, Schatz, Puffer, Sanchez, Stancil, & Roberts, 2009). Thus, consistent with the innovative foundations of pediatric psychology, the field continually advances.

EDUCATION AND TRAINING
FOR PEDIATRIC PSYCHOLOGY

No single path of preparation seems to have defined the pediatric psychologist in the United States in the past. Increasingly, however, the emerging model seems to be one of education and training in professional psychology within the specialty of clinical child and adolescent psychology focusing on pediatric psychology. There are no accreditation requirements or legal restrictions for practice in pediatric psychology other than the license for practice in psychology and, in some settings, gaining hospital privileges. Some hospitals also require that staff psychologists obtain board certification (viz., through the American Board of Clinical Child and Adolescent Psychology; Finch, Lochman, Nelson, & Roberts, 2012).

Nonetheless, recognizing the special expertise (knowledge, attitudes, and skills) that is required of the pediatric psychologist, the SPP formed a task force to articulate the training domains for the field. The 12 domains outlined by Spirito et al. (2003, Table 1) for the specific field of pediatric psychology were adapted from the categories of preparation and training presented by Roberts et al. (1998) for psychologists working with children and adolescents. These pediatric psychology domains are (1) lifespan developmental psychology; (2) lifespan developmental psychopathology; (3) child, adolescent, and family assessment; (4) intervention strategies; (5) research methods and systems evaluations; (6) professional, ethical, and legal issues; (7) diversity; (8) the role of multiple disciplines in service delivery systems; (9) prevention, family support, and health promotion; (10) social issues affecting children, adolescents, and families; (11) consultation and liaison roles; and (12) disease process and medical management (Spirito et al., 2003, p. 92).

Spirito et al. (2003) elaborated these domains to include children's development and the process of disease and effects of medical treatments, applications of psychological principles, and empirically supported assessments and treatments in child health psychology in medical settings. The report outlined the need for specialized scientific strategies as applied to pediatric psychology topics, such as through the psychologists' involvement in clinical trials for medical concerns, research into health services delivery systems such as multidisciplinary teams, consultation–liaison, and primary care. The pediatric psychology trainee at multiple levels of preparation also needs to gain an understanding of both healthy and atypical development, risky health activities, diseases and medical treatment regimens, and biopsychosocial interventions that can prevent problems that may carry over into the child's adulthood. These types of issues are illustrated throughout the following chapters in this book and the cases described. The American Academy of Pediatrics (1992) advocated (and continues to do so) for the development of a medical home for the child patient and family in which the "medical care of infants, children, and adolescents ideally should be accessible, continuous, comprehensive, family-centered, coordinated, and compassionate" (p. 774). The pediatric medical home also incorporates the concept that both medical and nonmedical needs of the child and family are given attention. The concept of a pediatric medical home is inherently part of the integrated health care movement within current health care reform, which has called for patient-centered medical homes (Long, Bauchner, Sege, Cabral, & Garg, 2012; see also Lassen et al., Chapter 2, this volume). These concepts, when implemented correctly, can lead to improved quality and coordinated care (Beacham, Kinman, Harris, & Masters, 2012; Kleinsorge, Roberts, Roy, & Rapoff, 2010; Long et al., 2012; Pidano, Kimmelblatt, & Neace, 2011).

Importantly, the pediatric psychologist has (and will have) a significant role in the implementation of medical home and integrated care concepts. As can be seen in these domains and medical concepts, there is an inherent focus on the systemic issues in the biopsychosocial model, with attention to the special situations posed in pediatric settings presenting with patients with medical conditions. The trainee preparing for a career in pediatric psychology needs to develop a specialized knowledge base, skill set, and professional functioning. Health care reform (as represented by the Affordable Care Act) will influence future developments in pediatric psychology (Rozensky, 2011; Rozensky & Janicke, 2012; Roberts, Canter, & Odar, 2012). The encompassing concepts and definition of "health service psychology" will be inclusive of all specialties and subfields, importantly including pediatric psychology, with implications for training, professional functions, and reimbursement (Health Service Psychology Education Collaborative, 2013).

CONCLUDING REMARKS

The field of pediatric psychology has not just survived through the years but has thrived. Starting with an initial set of 75 psychologist members, the SPP now has approximately 1,600 members with very active scientist-practitioners in a range of settings from university research and training settings to children's hospitals and major medical centers to independent and group practice with pediatricians and family medicine physicians. The maintenance and growth of this field in a relatively short period of time can be traced to the value attributed to the concepts and psychological applications in meeting the multiple needs of children in the medical setting with a set of complex problems requiring interdisciplinary collaborations. The expansion of pediatric psychology practitioners and scientists throughout the United States and internationally has been propelled by the well-received effectiveness of pediatric psychologists as individual practitioners interacting with patients and medical personnel and of pediatric psychology as an integrative field collectively demonstrating the worth of its practitioners' knowledge and skills.

REFERENCES

American Academy of Pediatrics Task Force on the Definition of the Medical Home. (1992). The medical home. *Pediatrics, 90*, 774.

Beacham, A. O., Kinman, C., Harris, J. G., & Masters, K. S. (2012). The patient-centered medical home: Unprecedented workforce growth potential for professional psychology. *Professional Psychology: Research and Practice, 43*, 17–23.

Bronfenbrenner, U. (1979). *The ecology of human development.* Cambridge, MA: Harvard University Press.

Connelly, M., Rapoff, M. A., Thompson, N., & Connelly, W. (2006). Headstrong: A pilot study of a CD-ROM intervention for recurrent pediatric headache. *Journal of Pediatric Psychology, 31*(7), 737–747.

Finch, A. J., Lochman, J. E., Nelson, W. M., & Roberts, M. C. (2012). *Specialty competencies in clinical child and adolescent psychology.* Oxford, UK: Oxford University Press.

Health Service Psychology Education Collaborative. (2013). Professional psychology in health care services: A blueprint for education and training. *American Psychologist, 68*, 411–426.

Hilliard, M. E., Ramey, C., Rohan, J. M., Drotar, D., & Cortina, S. (2011). Electronic monitoring feedback to promote adherence in an adolescent with fanconi anemia. *Health Psychology, 30*(5), 503–509.

Jackson, Y., Wu, Y. P., Aylward, B. S., & Roberts, M. C. (2012). Application of the competency cube model to clinical child psychology. *Professional Psychology: Research and Practice, 43*(5), 432–441.

Jensen, C. D., Cushing, C. C., Aylward, B. S., Craig, J. T., Sorell, D. M., & Steele, R. G. (2011). Effectiveness of motivational interviewing interventions for adolescent substance use behavior change: A meta-analytic review. *Journal of Consulting and Clinical Psychology, 79*, 433–440.

Kagan, J. (1965). The new marriage: Pediatrics and psychology. *American Journal of Diseases of Childhood, 110*, 272–278.

Kleinsorge, C. A., Roberts, M. C., Roy, K. M., & Rapoff, M. A. (2010). The program evaluation of services in a primary care clinic: Attaining a medical home. *Clinical Pediatrics, 49*(6), 548–559.

Long, W. E., Bauchner, H., Sege, R. D., Cabral, H. J., & Garg, A. (2012). The value of the medical home for children without special health care needs. *Pediatrics,129*, 87–98.

Maikranz, J. M., Steele, R. G., Dreyer, M. L., Stratman, A. C., & Bovaird, J. A. (2007). The relationship of hope and illness-related uncertainty to emotional adjustment and adherence among pediatric renal and liver transplant recipients. *Journal of Pediatric Psychology, 32*(5), 571–581.

Masuda, A., Cohen, L. L., Wicksell, R. K., Kemani, M. K., & Johnson, A. (2011). A case study: Acceptance and commitment therapy for pediatric sickle cell disease. *Journal of Pediatric Psychology, 36*(4), 398–408.

McClellan, C. B., Schatz, J. C., Puffer, E., Sanchez, C. E., Stancil, M. T., & Roberts, C. W. (2009). Use of handheld wireless technology for a home-based sickle cell pain management protocol. *Journal of Pediatric Psychology, 34*(5), 564–573.

Palermo, T. (2012, October). The president's message. *Society of Pediatric Psychology Progress Notes, 36*(3), 1–2.

Pidano, A. E., Kimmelblatt, C. A., & Neace, W. P. (2011). Behavioral health in the pediatric primary care setting: Needs, barriers, and implications for psychologists. *Psychological Services, 8*(3), 151–165.

Roberts, M. C. (1986). *Pediatric psychology: Psychological interventions and strategies for pediatric problems.* New York: Pergamon Press.

Roberts, M. C. (1992). Vale dictum: An editor's view of the field of pediatric psychology and its journal. *Journal of Pediatric Psychology, 17*, 785–805.

Roberts, M. C., Canter, K. S., & Odar, C. C. (2012). Commentary: A call to action to secure the future of pediatric psychology: Resonating to the points of Rozensky and Janicke (2012). *Journal of Pediatric Psychology, 37*(4), 369–375.

Roberts, M. C., Carlson, C. I., Erickson, M. T., Friedman, R. M., La Greca, A. M., Lemanek, K. L., et al. (1998). A model for training psychologists to provide services for children and adolescents. *Professional Psychology: Research and Practice, 29*, 293–299.

Roberts, M. C., McNeal, R. E., Randall, C. J., & Roberts, J. C. (1996). A necessary reemphasis on integrating explicative research with the pragmatics of pediatric psychology. *Journal of Pediatric Psychology, 21*(1), 107–114.

Rozensky, R. H. (2011). The institution of the institutional practice of psychology: Health care reform and psychology's future workforce. *American Psychologist, 66*, 794–808.

Rozensky, R. H., & Janicke, D. M. (2012). Commentary: Healthcare reform and psychology's workforce: Preparing for the future of pediatric psychology. *Journal of Pediatric Psychology, 37*(4), 359–368.

Salk, L., Hilgartner, M., & Granich, B. (1972). The psycho-social impact of hemophilia on the patient and his family. *Social Science and Medicine, 6*, 491–505.

Shegog, R., Markham, C. M., Leonard, A. D., Bui, T. C., & Paul, M. E. (2012). "+CLICK": Pilot of a web-based training program to enhance ART adherence among HIV-positive youth. *AIDS Care, 24*(3), 310–318.

Spirito, A., Brown, R. T., D'Angelo, E., Delamater, A., Rodrigue, J., & Siegel, L. (2003). Society of Pediatric Psychology task force report: Recommendations for the training of pediatric psychologists. *Journal of Pediatric Psychology, 28*(2), 85–98.

Spirito, A., & Kazak, A. E. (2006). *Effective and emerging treatments in pediatric psychology.* Oxford, UK: Oxford University Press.

Steele, R. G., & Aylward, B. S. (2009). An overview of systems in pediatric psychology research and practice. In M. C. Roberts & R. G. Steele (Eds.), *Handbook of pediatric psychology* (4th ed., pp. 649–655). New York: Guilford Press.

Tercyak, K. P., Sampilo, M. L., Brancu, M., Beck-Hyman, M., Browne, A., Kitessa, D., et al. (2006). Applying a behavioral epidemiology framework to research phases in child health psychology. *Journal of Clinical Psychology in Medical Settings, 13*(2), 201–205.

Walker, C. E. (1979). Behavioral intervention in a pediatric setting. In J. R. McNamara (Ed.), *Behavioral approaches to medicine: Application and analysis* (pp. 227–266). New York: Plenum.

Wright, L. (1967). The pediatric psychologist: A role model. *American Psychologist, 22*(4), 323–325.

Wright, L. (1971). Conditioning of consummatory responses in young children. *Journal of Clinical Psychology, 27*(3), 416–419.

Wright, L. (1972). Intellectual sequelae of Rocky Mountain spotted fever. *Journal of Abnormal Psychology, 80*(3), 315–316.

Wright, L. (1973a). Aversive conditioning of self-induced seizures. *Behavior Therapy, 4*(5), 712–713.

Wright, L. (1973b). Handling the encopretic child. *Professional Psychology, 4*(2), 137–144.

Wright, L. (1975). Outcome of a standardized program for treating psychogenic encopresis. *Professional Psychology, 6*(4), 453–456.

Wright, L., & Jimmerson, S. (1971). Intellectual sequelae of hemophilus influenzae meningitis. *Journal of Abnormal Psychology, 77*(2), 181–183.

Wright, L., Nunnery, A., Eichel, B., & Scott, R. (1968). Application of conditioning principles to problems of tracheostomy addiction in children. *Journal of Consulting and Clinical Psychology, 32*(1), 603–606.

Wright, L., Nunnery, A., Eichel, B., & Scott, R. (1969). Behavioral tactics for reinstating natural breathing in infants with tracheostomy. *Pediatric Research, 3*(4), 275–278.

Wright, L., & Walker, C. E. (1976). Behavioral treatment of encopresis. *Journal of Pediatric Psychology, 4*(1), 35–37.

CHAPTER 2

Common Presenting Concerns and Settings for Pediatric Psychology Practice

STEPHEN LASSEN
YELENA P. WU
MICHAEL C. ROBERTS

Pediatric psychologists practice at the interface of medicine and psychology, focusing on the utility of behavioral science to childhood health issues. This interface creates opportunities for the pediatric psychologist to appropriately assess, consult, and intervene with considerable effectiveness. The practice of pediatric psychology in a variety of clinical settings represents the excitement of applications of psychological knowledge and techniques in improving the lives of children, adolescents, and their families. These applications are evidenced in different practice settings, in the mixture of problems presented, and in the complexity of experiences in working interprofessionally with practitioners in other disciplines. Problems handled by pediatric psychologists range from developmental concerns presented by a premature infant to chronic illness in an older adolescent who is transitioning to adult medical services, with a multitude of health problems in between. As is discussed in this chapter, pediatric psychologists work in medical centers with inpatient and outpatient units, primary care clinics for pediatrics and family medicine, mental health outpatient clinics, specialty centers for specific problems, and community settings such as camps,

17

groups, and health promotion activities. In these settings and attending to multiple presenting problems, pediatric psychologists work collaboratively with practitioners from other disciplines, such as medicine and its specialties, nursing, social work, dietetics, and speech and language specialists, among others.

Pediatric psychology practitioners, in the nascent stages of the field, did not define themselves by what they specifically did; the definitions of the field they proffered were essentially setting-based. For example, according to Logan Wright (1967), pediatric psychology "deals primarily with children in a medical setting which is nonpsychiatric in nature" (p. 323), whereas the masthead of the inaugural issue of the *Journal of Pediatric Psychology* (*JPP*; 1976) stated:

> The field and the contents of this Journal are defined by the interests and concerns of psychologists who work in interdisciplinary settings such as children's hospitals, developmental clinics, and pediatric or medical group practices.

The earlier practitioners wrote about their applied activities in practice or unit descriptions (e.g., Drotar, 1977; Singer & Drotar, 1989; Magrab & Davitt, 1975; O'Malley & Koocher, 1977). These presentations were useful in illustrating the range of problems, interventions, and settings for the field.

Unfortunately for a more comprehensive summary of what pediatric psychologists do in clinical practice, the field has not benefited from a workforce analysis to describe itself. Although the present volume is illustrative of the clinical practice of pediatric psychology, this could not be a comprehensive volume that portrays all aspects of the field. Nonetheless, as noted by Roberts (1986), "one characteristic more than anything else defines the field—the types of clinical case evaluated and treated by the pediatric psychologist" (p. 19). Based on past literature, Roberts (1986) noted that common referral problems included negative behaviors (e.g., disobedience, tantrums), toileting issues, school-related problems, and adjustment to illness. Later reports included programmatic evaluations of outpatient units in which descriptions of services conveyed the types of problems and interventions taken by the pediatric psychologist (Carter et al., 2003; Charlop, Parrish, Fenton, & Cataldo, 1987; Finney, Riley, & Cataldo, 1991; Gelfand et al., 2004; Krahn, Eisert, & Fifield, 1990; Olson, Holden, Friedman, & Faust, 1988; Rodrigue, Hoffmann, Rayfield, & Lescano, 1995; Sobel, Roberts, Rayfield, Barnard, & Rapoff, 2001; Sobel, Roberts, Rapoff, & Barnard, 2001).

Although there have been descriptive reports on pediatric psychology practices in outpatient/primary care and inpatient consultation–liaison services, there has not been a comprehensive workforce analysis that could answer the general question of how pediatric psychologists work or a demographic picture of who is in the workforce, composition characteristics (e.g., gender, age, salaries, training background and competencies, experience of practitioners), professional functions (e.g., job descriptions, workload, daily and hourly activities, relative value units, reimbursement procedures), and evaluation of clinical services (e.g., program or unit evaluation, individual effectiveness outcomes, perceptions of value to patient care and health care system). An analysis would also have to assess needs for pediatric psychology services, to consider trends in population demographics, to create health and illness projections for the future, and to outline schemes for private and public reimbursement for services and organization of integrated care—all of which would affect future hiring and expansion or cutbacks. Thus the field needs to be strategically prepared to meet current and future needs for services. Such an analysis could also identify potential innovations for services and psychological staff, while pointing out where applied research needs to focus attention to enhance the evidence base for the field. Rozensky and Janicke (2012) and Roberts, Canter, and Odar (2012) called for a comprehensive workforce analysis to meet the field's needs for information (advancing on the survey approach provided by Opipari-Arrigan, Stark, & Drotar, 2006, to "benchmark" performance) in order to focus on the characteristics and activities of pediatric psychology in the changing health care field.

In this chapter, we discuss the activities and functions of pediatric psychologists working in collaborative as well as independent functions in inpatient practice settings, outpatient practice settings, and other types of health care placements.

OUTPATIENT PRACTICE SETTINGS

Hospital-Based Clinics

As pediatric psychologists have become more specialized in their clinical practice and medical subspecialties have recognized the contributions that pediatric psychologists can make to clinical care, the hospital-based clinic has been a common setting in which pediatric psychologists see patients. Within this setting, a pediatric psychologist may meet with a patient and family in a medical clinic before, during, or after the medical visit. Patients may be referred to the psychologist for specific concerns, such as those identified by a medical provider, or the psychologist may meet with all or most patients presenting to the clinic. Session length can vary depending on clinic or patient need but can be shorter than the typical 50-minute therapy session, and the psychologist may meet with the patient and/or family at subsequent clinic visits to monitor intervention outcomes or to provide additional intervention. Typically, information on the psychologist's assessment, conceptualization, and intervention is communicated to the medical team via the medical record or case conferencing, may be incorporated into the patient's overall treatment plan, and may inform future approaches and interventions that team members use with the patient and family.

Common referral questions can differ between hospital-based clinics depending on the populations served (e.g., pain conditions vs. sleep problems) and clinic structure. However, some presenting concerns can arise regardless of medical condition: assessing for and addressing psychosocial factors contributing to the medical condition or its management, difficulty in adjusting to a new medical diagnosis or in continuing to cope with illness, negative impact of illness on the patient's functioning, and nonadherence to the prescribed medical regimen. See Table 2.1 for interventions typically provided in this setting.

Case Example 1: Sally

Sally was a 13-year-old girl who had recently received a kidney transplant, and the medical team was concerned that she was not taking all of her posttransplant medications, which were essential to her survival. When the psychologist on the team met with Sally and her mother to assess factors that might affect Sally's and her family's ability to adhere to the prescribed medication regimen, he learned that Sally was forgetting to take her morning medication dose when her mother was not home to remind her. The psychologist used a problem-solving intervention with Sally and her family to generate a number of potential solutions to her forgetting to take her morning dose and to discuss implementing the agreed-upon solution in the coming weeks.

Specialized Care Settings

Specialized care settings include outpatient psychology or behavioral medicine clinics housed within a larger facility, such as a children's hospital. Families may be referred to these settings by medical providers, or they may self-refer for services, and referral questions may range widely. Pediatric psychologists may offer assessment (e.g., cognitive and academic testing) and treatment (i.e., therapy) services. Most often, patients seen for ongoing treatment in these settings have regularly scheduled (e.g., weekly) appointments.

Common presenting problems in specialized care settings include school issues and behavioral problems such as noncompliance, aggression, and hyperactivity. Other referral questions can include mood concerns and difficulty coping with a medical diagnosis (Charlop et al., 1987; Sobel,

TABLE 2.1. Outpatient Setting Interventions

Hospital-based clinics

- Making broad and targeted assessments of functioning (tailored to referral question)
- Teaching and facilitating use of problem-solving strategies
- Providing psychoeducation on relevant topics—normal development, typical challenges associated with adherence to medical regimen
- Facilitating communication between medical team and patient and family
- Implementating brief cognitive-behavioral or other therapeutic techniques to address the referral question (e.g., providing behavioral activation techniques for a patient with mild depressive symptoms)
- Referring to more intensive services if needed

Specialized care

- Providing psychoeducation on the rationale for recommended interventions
- Teaching families behavioral strategies (e.g., reinforcement, planned ignoring) to address noncompliance and aggression
- Using cognitive-behavioral or other therapeutic strategies to address mood or coping concerns (Charlop et al., 1987; Sobel, Robert, Rayfield, et al., 2002)

Primary care

- Making brief assessment of referral concern
- Providing psychoeducation on child development and/or the referral problem
- Using behavioral strategies, such as for toileting or to address behavior problems
- Initiating problem-solving interventions
- Serving as an advocate for children
- Giving referrals for further evaluations or services

Private practice

- Pediatric psychologists use a variety of assessment and intervention strategies in this setting, which differ depending on the psychologist's theoretical orientations (e.g., cognitive-behavioral, family systems, psychodynamic).
- Because treatment is typically provided on a more frequent basis by pediatric psychologists in private practice than by primary care physicians or in hospital-based clinics, interventions may be implemented over a longer period of time, with numerous opportunities for modifying treatments as patients' needs change.

Roberts, Rayfield, et al., 2001). Because these settings are often situated within the context of a larger medical facility, patients referred to pediatric psychologists frequently have a medical condition that may or may not be directly related to the referral question (e.g., a child whose leukemia is in remission and who presents with significant behavioral problems at home). Interventions used in specialized care settings are guided by the psychologist's assessment of the referred youth's functioning, the severity and nature of the presenting problems, and the presenting problem's impact on the youth's and family's functioning. Although a range of evidence-based interventions are available for common clinical presenting problems in children (*www.effectivechildtherapy.com*), pediatric psychologists can modify treatments to meet the needs of children with health conditions. See Table 2.1 for interventions typically provided in this setting.

Primary Care

Pediatric psychologists may also provide clinical services within a primary care setting, such as in a pediatrician's office. These services could follow varying models of collaboration between the psychologist and the primary care provider and may include screening for behavioral, developmental, emotional, or social problems, providing brief and problem-focused therapy, facilitating referral to further psychological or other services, prevention of psychological concerns, promoting healthy development, and consulting with medical providers (see Stancin, Sturm, & Ramirez, Chapter 6, this volume). Similar to clinical practice within hospital-based clinics, psychologists in the primary care setting also may meet with patients for varying amounts of time, often shorter than in specialized care settings. Follow-up sessions are provided as needed (Drotar, 1995; Stancin, Perrin, & Ramirez, 2009; Schroeder, 2004).

Common presenting problems in pediatric primary care include behavioral and attention problems (e.g., acting out, hyperactivity, inattention); mood concerns; anxiety; toileting; coping with family or developmental transitions, such as divorce, adolescence, or a death in the family; and concerns about child development (Hickson, Altemeier, & O'Connor, 1983; Lavigne et al., 1993). Some of these psychosocial concerns may be less severe than those seen in specialized outpatient settings, given the wide range of families served within pediatric primary care settings. See Table 2.1 for interventions typically provided in this setting. Given the brief nature of primary care appointments and interventions, psychologists may provide additional information in the form of handouts, through scheduled parent groups, or via telephone conversations with families (Schroeder, 2004).

Case Example 2: Diana

Diana was a 3-year-old girl. At her well-child visit with her pediatrician, her mother expressed frustration about Diana's behavior (e.g., noncompliance with parents and babysitter's requests) and concern about how Diana would do in preschool the following year. The pediatric psychologist assessed the frequency and severity of Diana's behavioral problems and information on the context and consequences associated with these behaviors. Based on the information gathered, the psychologist provided the family with education on developmentally expected behavioral problems for children Diana's age and several strategies to manage Diana's behaviors, including attending to positive behaviors, providing differential attention to positive and negative behaviors, and appropriate use of time-out. The psychologist planned to follow up with the family at their next medical appointment and provided her contact information should the family have further questions or want a referral for additional outpatient services.

Private Outpatient

Pediatric psychologists practicing in private practice settings typically see patients in a freestanding clinic or office (i.e., one not attached to a larger facility such as a hospital). Sessions are more similar to those in the specialized care setting, lasting approximately 50–60 minutes. Depending on their interests and training and on the needs of the communities served, pediatric psychologists in private outpatient settings may specialize in treating or providing assessment for certain referral concerns (e.g., anxiety disorders, adjustment issues related to medical problems). Common presenting problems in private outpatient settings include adjustment issues, mood, behavioral, and attention problems, family conflict, coping with acute or ongoing stressors (e.g., medical condition, divorce), and developmental concerns. See Table 2.1 for interventions typically provided in this setting.

Case Example 3: Tonia

Tonia was a 15-year-old girl presenting with irritable mood and high levels of conflict with her mother. After completing a clinical interview with Tonia and her mother, reviewing results of self- and parent-reported forms measuring mood-related concerns, and discussing treatment options with the family, the pediatric psychologist initiated a depression-focused treatment. Over the course of 10 sessions, this treatment consisted of providing Tonia and her family with psychoeducation on depression in adolescents and the rationale for the treatment approach, increasing Tonia's behavioral activation (e.g., increasing engagement in enjoyed activities), teaching problem-solving and communication skills, and modifying inaccurate and maladaptive cognitions or thoughts.

INPATIENT HOSPITAL PRACTICE SETTINGS

Consultation–Liaison

Pediatric psychologists who work in consultation–liaison (C-L) settings within a hospital are typically involved in both assessment of and intervention with children who have been hospitalized medically (consultant role), as well as in activities that are focused on more broad, programmatic, and/or protocol issues, education of the patient's medical team, and collaboration with other health care professionals (liaison role; see Carter, Thompson, & Thompson, Chapter 5, this volume). An important part of the consultation process is communicating specific recommendations and a plan back to the child's medical team.

C-L pediatric psychologists, especially those who work on generalist services within a hospital, are often asked to provide assessment and intervention services in a variety of areas. Common referral questions can be grouped into three broad categories: (1) coping with and adjustment to physical illness and hospitalization, (2) premorbid psychological functioning that is the main reason for the hospital admission or that is interfering with the child's hospitalization (e.g., oppositional behavior present prior to the admission is interfering with medical care), and (3) psychological concerns that are part of the child's physical illness, treatment, or management (e.g., mood disorder due to a general medical condition, delirium secondary to medication). See Table 2.2 for interventions typically used in C-L settings.

Case Example 4: Lauren

Lauren, a 6-year-old girl with cystic fibrosis, was admitted to the hospital for a pulmonary exacerbation. Lauren had a history of poor adherence to her medical regimen, which included multiple daily breathing treatments and medications. The team was also concerned about her poor weight gain. The C-L team was consulted to evaluate her adherence and reasons for her poor weight gain. After meeting with Lauren and her parents, the consulting psychologist discovered that Lauren was frequently noncompliant and oppositional at home with most of the directions given by her parents and other adults. The psychologist introduced and implemented several behavioral strategies with Lauren to improve her overall adherence while in the hospital. This plan was discussed with Lauren's medical team, as well as her parents, who were encouraged to continue using the plan once she was discharged home.

Emergency Room

Many children with mental health emergencies and serious medical events initially present to the emergency department (ED) for assessment, stabilization, and management. Pediatric psychologists may provide clinical services to children in the ED. The pediatric psychologist plays a vital role in

TABLE 2.2. Inpatient Setting Interventions

Consultation–liaison
- Implementing cognitive-behavioral techniques (e.g., relaxation training)
- Providing problem-solving strategies for coping with hospitalization and medical treatment
- Using behavioral strategies for increasing adherence and/or meeting goals of hospitalization
- Facilitating communication between medical team and patient and family
- Assisting medical team in implementing interventions
- Educating medical team about development, adherence barriers, behavioral strategies
- Facilitating disposition planning

Emergency room
- Using relaxation training and other cognitive-behavioral techniques for acute stabilization
- Providing psychoeducation for families and staff on behavioral techniques (e.g., reinforcement, planned ignoring, issuing effective commands) to use with disruptive youth
- Using problem-solving strategies to address presenting problem
- Assisting medical team with disposition planning

Specialized care
- Implementing cognitive-behavioral techniques to manage mood and anxiety concerns
- Educating children about parental illness
- Educating parents and family members on typical childhood reactions to parental illness
- Using behavioral strategies in supporting children during a parent's illness
- Providing problem-solving and educational strategies to help parents to transition to parenthood or to learn to care for a medically fragile infant and cope with a child's hospitalization

the assessment, intervention, and disposition of such emergencies. A pediatric psychologist in the ED will typically work collaboratively with other mental health professionals, such as child psychiatrists, social workers, and psychiatric nurses, to provide these services.

Common presenting problems in the ED setting include suicide attempts or ideation, drug or alcohol abuse, behavioral emergencies (violent/aggressive behavior), child abuse, somatoform disorders, and psychosis. Other referral questions can focus on child and family response to their presenting emergency, be it medical or psychological in nature (e.g., disruptive behaviors in the ED, refusing treatment, coping with a medical trauma). See Table 2.2 for interventions typically used in the emergency room setting.

Case Example 5: Charley

Charley was a 12-year-old boy who presented to the ED after becoming violent and physically aggressive toward his mother at their home. Charley continued to threaten physical harm to his mother and medical staff in the ED but was cooperative in answering questions. The pediatric psychologist suggested that Charley's mother wait outside the room until he was able to calm himself down. An interview with Charley and his mother by the pediatric psychologist revealed a gradual increase in conflict over the past several months. Charley attributed this increased conflict to difficulty in school, a best friend moving away, and parents' limit setting. The psychologist worked with Charley and his mother to generate several preliminary solutions to these concerns, to identify the role of deteriorating mood in the recent conflict, and to gain agreement and motivation for outpatient therapy. The psychologist worked with the ED team to arrange outpatient follow-up for Charley and his parents.

Specialized Inpatient Care Settings

Pediatric psychologists provide a wide range of services in specialized inpatient care settings. These settings are typically housed within a hospital and can include intensive care units (ICU), burn units, and rehabilitation services. Psychologists working in these specialized areas often have additional expertise and training in the area in which they are working. Many of the presenting problems in these types of inpatient settings tend to be similar to those discussed previously with C-L services (e.g., coping with illness/hospitalization, premorbid psychological difficulties complicating medical treatment, psychological sequelae of medical illness). However, important differences exist, especially in settings in which the child is not the patient (e.g., adult medical services) or in cases in which the child is too young or unable to participate in assessment and intervention but in which there are significant psychological needs that affect the child (e.g., in neonatal intensive care units [NICUs]). In settings in which the well child of a chronically or terminally ill parent or caregiver is the focus of the psychological services, referral questions typically involve coping with a parent's or caregiver's illness, acute grief reactions, and educating the child and family unit about how to support the child. When the psychologist is working with the parent, caregiver, or family of an infant or child who cannot participate, common referral questions revolve around the parents' or the family's coping with the child's medical status and/or hospitalization. Concerns about parent–child interactions and lack of parent education are also common reasons for referral. See Table 2.2 for interventions typically used in some specialized care settings.

Case Example 6: Ms. Taylor

Ms. Taylor delivered her first baby at 28 weeks' gestation. Her baby was hospitalized in the NICU and was on a ventilator for respiratory difficulties. Ms. Taylor had difficulty sleeping and eating after the birth. She did not like to come onto the unit to see her baby due to feelings of anxiety and sadness. When she came on the unit to visit, she declined to perform any of the baby's care for fear she would hurt her baby or do something wrong. The psychologist met with Ms. Taylor, normalized many of the reactions she was experiencing, and taught her several relaxation techniques to use as she prepared for and came to the unit for visits. The psychologist also worked with nursing staff and taught them how to model and encourage Ms. Taylor to be more involved in the baby's care.

EMERGING AREAS OF PRACTICE

Primary Care/Integrated Care

As health care reform continues to evolve, the implications for pediatric psychology indicate that a greater role in practice may arise through the concepts of integrated care and primary care (Long, Bauchner, Sege, Cabral, & Garg, 2012). Gröne and Garcia-Barbero (2001), with the World Health Organization, defined integrated care as "a concept bringing together inputs, delivery, management and organization of services related to diagnosis, treatment, care, rehabilitation and health promotion. Integration is a means to improve the services in relation to access, quality, user satisfaction and efficiency" (p. 7). Integrated care involves coordination of services, with attention to creating comprehensive coverage for all types of needs to overcome the potential for fragmentation of services and separation of care providers.

For children and adolescents typically receiving medical care in pediatric and family medicine clinics, integrated care is often delivered in primary care settings. These settings, often community-based practices, are places where many children are seen and where behavioral health issues initially present (Stancin, 2005; Wildman & Stancin, 2004). The primary care provider for children, whether a pediatrician or a family medicine physician, plays a significant role in identifying, treating, and referring children with psychosocial problems; the psychologist working in these primary care settings has a similar responsibility. About half of all pediatric visits have been found to involve behavioral, psychosocial, and educational concerns (Cassidy & Jellinek, 1998). However, primary care providers for children and adolescents underidentify children with developmental and behavioral problems (e.g., Costello et al., 1988; Lavigne et al., 1993). Investigations estimated that four out of five children with diagnosable behavioral and emotional problems are not identified by their primary care physicians and that even fewer receive behavioral or mental health services.

Primary care might most easily be differentiated from tertiary care, which takes place in children's hospitals, for example. (Integrated care does occur in tertiary-care inpatient units, but potentially with less frequency given that fewer numbers of children will be severely injured or ill enough to be hospitalized compared with the majority of children seen in primary care). The concepts of both integrated care and primary care have been present in the field since its inception in the late 1970s (Wright, 1979; Wright & Burns, 1986). Around the same time, Carolyn Schroeder, through her collaborative psychology practice for children and adolescents colocated in a private pediatrics clinic, demonstrated these early concepts in action (Schroeder, 1979; Schroeder, Goolsby, & Stangler, 1975).

Integrated care in pediatrics will also enhance interdisciplinary and interprofessional interactions that have been inherent in pediatric psychology. Gerry (2002) conceptualized integration of services as "personalized and caring. Where co-occurring needs are evident, service providers coordinate their efforts, and they treat individuals and families in need as partners. Working together, service providers tailor their services to fit what children, parents, and families want and need" (pp. 66–67). This type of integrated approach is inherently important because psychological–behavioral concerns present themselves in what is typically thought of as physical health arenas. These ideas coalesced in what has been labeled in recent health care reform (and much earlier in pediatrics) as the patient-centered medical home.

Medical Home

As noted by Roberts, Aylward, and Wu (Chapter 1, this volume) the American Academy of Pediatrics (1992) set out the concepts of a medical home (now adopted and updated by other groups and used in recent health care reform efforts), encompassing medical and health care services for children and adolescents, which should be accessible, continuous, comprehensive, family-centered, coordinated, compassionate, and culturally effective (Kleinsorge, Roberts, Roy, & Rapoff, 2010; Long et al., 2012). A medical home includes integrated care with availability of multiple services and mechanisms for easy referral and follow-through care, such as with the primary care psychologists. Of course, integrated care will not just be applied in primary care settings; children's hospitals will, for example, also utilize a collaborative team approach often in dealing with the more serious end of the continuum of children's problems. As the health care environment changes over the next years, integrated care concepts will be invoked as cost-effective approaches to improving children's health.

CONCLUSION

As seen in this chapter, the practice of pediatric psychology continues to evolve and expand in novel and exciting ways. This evolution and expansion is evident not only in the breadth of interventions that continue to be developed and the settings within which they are applied but also in the integration of pediatric psychology in broader medical systems. Indeed, the collaboration between pediatric psychologist and health care provider is at the heart of the field of pediatric psychology and appears poised only to increase in the coming years. To truly utilize the field's expertise and training, we need to continue to identify opportunities for meaningful collaboration with other health care providers, develop effective interventions for children and families, and advocate for thoughtful inclusion of pediatric psychology services into systems of care.

REFERENCES

American Academy of Pediatrics Task Force on the Definition of the Medical Home. (1992). The medical home. *Pediatrics, 90,* 774.

Carter, B. D., Kronenberger, W. G., Baker, J., Grimes, L. M., Crabtree, V. M., Smith, C., et al. (2003). Inpatient pediatric consultation-liaison: A case-controlled study. *Journal of Pediatric Psychology, 28*(6), 423–432.

Cassidy, L. J., & Jellinek, M. S. (1998). Approaches to recognition and management of childhood psychiatric disorders in pediatric primary care. *Pediatric Clinics of North America, 45,* 1037–1052.

Charlop, M. H., Parrish, J. M., Fenton, L. R., & Cataldo, M. F. (1987). Evaluation of hospital-based outpatient pediatric psychology services. *Journal of Pediatric Psychology, 12*(4), 485–503.

Costello, E. J., Edelbrook, C., Costello, A. J., Dullcan, M. K., Burns, B. J., & Brent, D. (1988). Psychopathology in pediatric primary care: The new hidden morbidity. *Pediatrics, 82,* 415–424.

Drotar, D. (1977). Clinical psychological practice in a pediatric hospital. *Professional Psychology, 8*(1), 72–80.

Drotar, D. (1995). *Consulting with pediatricians.* New York: Plenum.

Finney, J. W., Riley, A. W., & Cataldo, M. F. (1991). Psychology in primary health care: Effects of brief targeted therapy on children's medical care utilization. *Journal of Pediatric Psychology, 16*(4), 447–461.

Gelfand, K. C., Geffken, G., Lewin, A., Heidgerken, A., Grove, M. J., Malasanos, T., et al. (2004). An initial evaluation of the design of pediatric psychology consultation service with children with diabetes. *Journal of Child Health Care, 8*(2), 113–123.

Gerry, M. (2002). Service integration and achieving the goals of school reform. In W. Sailor (Ed.), *Whole-school success and inclusive education: Building partnerships for learning, achievement, and accountability* (pp. 63–76). New York: Teachers College Press.

Gröne, O., & Garcia-Barbero, M. (2001). A position paper of the WHO European office for integrated health care services. *International Journal of Integrated Care, 1*, e21.

Hickson, G. B., Altemeier, W. A., & O'Connor, S. (1983). Concerns of mothers seeking care in private pediatric offices: Opportunities for expanding services. *Pediatrics, 72,* 619–624.

Kleinsorge, C. A., Roberts, M. C., Roy, K. M., & Rapoff, M. A. (2010). The program evaluation of services in a primary care clinic: Attaining a medical home. *Clinical Pediatrics, 49*(6), 548–559.

Krahn, G. L., Eisert, D., & Fifield, B. (1990). Obtaining parental perceptions of the quality of services for children with special health needs. *Journal of Pediatric Psychology, 15*(6), 761–774.

Lavigne, J. V., Binns, H. J., Christoffel, K. K., Rosenbaum, D., Arend, R., Smith, K., et al. (1993). Behavioral and emotional problems among preschool children in pediatric primary care: Prevalence and pediatricians' recognition. *Pediatrics, 91,* 649–655.

Long, W. E., Bauchner, H., Sege, R. D., Cabral, H. J., & Garg, A. (2012). The value of the medical home for children without special health care needs. *Pediatrics, 129,* 87–98.

Magrab, P. R., & Davitt, M. K. (1975). The pediatric psychologist and the developmental follow-up of intensive care nursery infants. *Journal of Clinical Child Psychology, 4*(3), 16–18.

Olson, R. A., Holden, E. W., Friedman, A., & Faust, J. (1988). Psychological consultation in a children's hospital: An evaluation of services. *Journal of Pediatric Psychology, 13*(4), 479–492.

O'Malley, J. E., & Koocher, G. P. (1977). Psychological consultation to a pediatric oncology unit: Obstacles to effective intervention. *Journal of Pediatric Psychology, 2*(2), 54–57.

Opipari-Arrigan, L., Stark, L., & Drotar, D. (2006). Benchmarks for work performance of pediatric psychologists. *Journal of Pediatric Psychology, 31*(6), 630–642.

Roberts, M. C. (1986). *Pediatric psychology: Psychological interventions and strategies for pediatric problems.* New York: Pergamon Press.

Roberts, M. C., Canter, K. S., & Odar, C. C. (2012). Commentary: A call to action to secure the future of pediatric psychology: Resonating to the points of Rozensky and Janicke (2012). *Journal of Pediatric Psychology, 37*(4), 369–375.

Rodrigue, J. R., Hoffmann, R. G., Rayfield, A., & Lescano, C. (1995). Evaluating pediatric psychology consultation services in a medical setting: An example. *Journal of Clinical Psychology in Medical Settings, 2*(1), 89–107.

Rozensky, R. H., & Janicke, D. M. (2012). Commentary: Healthcare reform and psychology's workforce: Preparing for the future of pediatric psychology. *Journal of Pediatric Psychology, 37*(4), 359–368.

Schroeder, C. S. (1979). Psychologists in a private pediatric practice. *Journal of Pediatric Psychology, 4*(1), 5–18.

Schroeder, C. S. (2004). A collaborative practice in primary care. In B. G. Wildman & T. Stancin (Eds.), *Treating children's psychosocial problems in primary care* (pp. 1–34). Charlotte, NC: Information Age.

Schroeder, C., Goolsby, E., & Stangler, S. (1975). Preventive services in a private pediatric practice. *Journal of Clinical Child Psychology, 4*(3), 32–33.

Singer, L., & Drotar, D. (1989). Psychological practice in a pediatric rehabilitation hospital. *Journal of Pediatric Psychology, 14*(4), 479–489.

Sobel, A. B., Roberts, M. C., Rapoff, M. A., & Barnard, M. U. (2001). Problems and interventions of a pediatric psychology clinic in a medical setting: A retrospective analysis. *Cognitive and Behavioral Practice, 8*, 11–17.

Sobel, A. B., Roberts, M. C., Rayfield, A., Barnard, M. U., & Rapoff, M. A. (2001). Evaluating outpatient pediatric psychology services in a primary care setting. *Journal of Pediatric Psychology, 26*, 395–405.

Stancin, T. (2005). Mental health services for children in pediatric primary care settings. In R. G. Steele & M. C. Roberts (Eds.), *Handbook of mental health services for children, adolescents, and families* (pp. 85–101). New York: Kluwer Academic/Plenum.

Stancin, T., Perrin, E. C., & Ramirez, L. (2009). Pediatric psychology and primary care. In M. C. Roberts & R. G. Steele (Eds.), *Handbook of pediatric psychology* (4th ed., pp. 630–648). New York: Guilford Press.

Wildman, B. G., & Stancin, T. (2004). *Treating children's psychosocial problems in primary care*. Greenwich, CT: Information Age.

Wright, L. (1967). The pediatric psychologist: A role model. *American Psychologist, 22*(4), 323–325.

Wright, L. (1979). Health care psychology: Prospects for the well-being of children. *American Psychologist, 34*(10), 1001–1006.

Wright, L., & Burns, B. J. (1986). Primary mental health care: A "find" for psychology? *Professional Psychology: Research and Practice, 17*(6), 560–564.

CHAPTER 3

Cross-Cutting Issues in Pediatric Psychology

YELENA P. WU
BRANDON S. AYLWARD
MICHAEL C. ROBERTS

In the last four decades, the field of pediatric psychology has expanded to encompass clinical practice with numerous medical populations across a variety of clinical settings, addressing a diversity of presenting problems and health promotion needs (see Roberts, Aylward, & Wu, Chapter 1, and Lassen, Wu, & Roberts, Chapter 2, this volume). Pediatric psychologists often specialize in treating certain pediatric populations (e.g., children with gastrointestinal disorders) or may provide services to multiple populations (e.g., as part of consultation–liaison services). Besides the variability in the medical populations and presenting problems that pediatric psychologists treat, there are also numerous cross-cutting issues that arise in clinical practice. Other chapters in this book (Chapters 11–26) provide in-depth accounts of how these issues can play out in individual cases; the goal of the current chapter is to provide an introduction to common theoretical frameworks that guide clinical practice and to cross-cutting presenting problems seen in practice. However, this chapter cannot be an exhaustive review of cross-cutting issues in pediatric psychology clinical practice.

THEORETICAL FRAMEWORKS
AND TREATMENT STRATEGIES

In clinical practice, pediatric psychologists draw on a variety of pediatric-specific theoretical frameworks that guide their assessment strategies and tools, conceptualization of the presenting problems (e.g., factors contributing to the problems), choice of intervention, and outcome monitoring. From an assessment standpoint, the use of a developmentally based, systems-oriented framework (e.g., Bronfenbrenner's social ecological model; Bronfenbrenner, 1979) can provide a context for understanding interactions between different domains of functioning and outcome (e.g., academic, social, emotional) and thereby provide a more complete account of the factors that influence the development, course, and consequences associated with a particular chronic illness (Steele & Aylward, 2009). Employing such a model can improve the assessment of functioning in children and adolescents with a chronic illness and help clinicians create comprehensive interventions that target multidimensional areas affected by health. The stress and coping (Wallander & Varni, 1992) and transactional stress and coping (Thompson, 1985) models describe medical characteristics, child functioning, socioecological factors (e.g., family adjustment), stress, and reactions to stress that affect adjustment to the medical condition and its associated challenges. The family systems model as applied to pediatric clinical practice includes addressing family interactions and promoting family competence in coping with a child's medical condition (Kazak, Simms, & Rourke, 2002). Family systems models connect with broader socioecological approaches for understanding and addressing the relationships between systemic factors (e.g., a health care team) and the family system (Kazak et al., 2002). Pediatric psychologists also assess child and family strengths and protective factors, which are important resources for families and can be built upon in treatment (Barakat, Pulgaron, & Daniel, 2009). Together, these and other pediatric frameworks recognize the multiple factors that may affect child and family coping and adjustment to medical problems and medical and psychosocial outcomes and that may require intervention.

In addition to theoretical frameworks specific to practice with medical populations, pediatric psychologists draw on various psychological therapy theories and practices for children, adolescents, and their families. For example, pediatric psychologists may draw on behavioral, cognitive-behavioral, family systems, stages of change, and psychodynamic theories. These foundational therapy techniques and theoretical backgrounds affect the content and process of interventions that pediatric psychologists implement. However, the techniques pediatric psychologists use to implement these interventions differ between psychologists, settings, and referral problems (see Lassen et al., Chapter 2, this volume). In the following sections, we describe several cross-cutting issues in the clinical practice of pediatric psychology.

TRAUMATIC MEDICAL STRESS

Pediatric medical traumatic stress (PMTS) has received increased recognition concomitant to a general increase in attention to traumatic stress in psychology and psychiatry. Pediatric medical traumatic stress has been defined as

> a set of psychological and physiological responses of children and their families to pain, injury, serious illness, medical procedures, and invasive or frightening treatment experiences. These responses may include symptoms of arousal, re-experiencing, and/or avoidance. They may vary in intensity, are related to the subjective experience of the event, and can become disruptive to functioning. (National Child Traumatic Stress Network, *www.nctsnet.org/trauma-types/medical-trauma*).

Kazak, Schneider, and Kassam-Adams (2009) extended this psychological phenomenon to include not only diagnosable disorders (e.g., posttraumatic stress disorder) but also a range of stress symptoms resulting from potentially traumatic events often inherent in pediatric conditions and medical care.

A growing literature is developing evidence for preventive and therapeutic interventions to address PMTS (Kazak et al., 2004; Stuber, Schneider, Kassam-Adams, Kazak, & Saxe, 2006). Psychological expertise can identify events that might lead to PMTS and intervene before, during, and after events to ameliorate PMTS-related problems. Because PMTS can manifest with any medically related event, pediatric psychology practitioners and clinical researchers will need to assess and intervene in a wide variety of situations.

REINTEGRATION TO SCHOOL AND HOME

The survival rate for children who have been injured or become critically ill has dramatically improved over a number of decades. Children who survive illness and treatment now return to home life, engage in community activities, and reintegrate into schools, often with the expectation that "things" will get back to normal. Over time, it has become increasingly understood that the child's and family's life will resume within a new "normal" (e.g., DuPaul, Power, & Shapiro, 2009; Madan-Swain, Katz, & La Gory, 2004).

The tasks of this reintegration process include reestablishing regular school attendance, catching up and maintaining academic performance, and coping with effects of medical treatments or illness on academic and cognitive functioning (DuPaul et al., 2009; also see Alderfer & Rourke, Chapter 8, this volume). During this reintegration process, children and their families may face psychosocial adjustment difficulties, including fostering the child's independence and autonomy.

Pediatric psychologists and other staff associated with children's hospitals, often partnering with school psychologists and school personnel, have developed interventions to ease the transition to the new normal of family life and reentry into schools (see Alderfer & Rourke, Chapter 8, this volume). Multifaceted programs have been implemented in a variety of modalities for different chronic conditions (Harris, 2009; McCarthy, Williams, & Plumer, 1998; Power, DuPaul, Shapiro, & Kazak, 2003; Prevatt, Heffer, & Lowe, 2000). Programs often include education through providing information about the illness to teachers and peers, strategies for managing a child's behavioral change, and medication monitoring. More comprehensive interventions may include skill building for the ill child (e.g., social skills) and teachers, vignettes and role plays on handling challenging behaviors, and ongoing professional consultation about pertinent issues. Canter and Roberts (2012) found, in a meta-analysis of school reentry program outcomes, that the programs were generally effective in increasing teacher and peer knowledge about a child's specific disease and in improving attitudes relating to ill children as they reintegrate into school and social activities. More work is needed in this area to build the evidence base for pediatric psychology services to competently enhance children's functioning after diagnosis and treatment, as well as during ongoing treatments.

TREATMENT REGIMEN ADHERENCE

Children with health conditions and their families are often asked to adhere to a treatment regimen that can include medication, other health practices (e.g., respiratory therapy, blood glucose monitoring), and lifestyle changes. However, children and families may not adhere to part of or all of the medical regimen. For example, children and their families may not implement all parts of the recommended treatment regimen, take medication as prescribed, attend health care appointments, or obtain medication or other supplies for the treatment regimen. Adherence to the treatment regimen can affect a child's symptoms, long-term health, and provider management of the child's health condition (e.g., dose increases; Rapoff, 2010).

Children and their families may be identified as "nonadherent" and may be seen by a pediatric psychologist in a number of scenarios. Health care providers may obtain information indicating that a patient is non-adherent, such as blood assay results indicating low medication levels in a child's system. Alternatively, a decline in a child's health outcomes may raise provider's suspicions that nonadherence to the medical regimen may be a contributing factor. Nonadherence may also surface in the course of a health care provider's conversations with children and families about factors that could influence adherence (e.g., parent mental health, child behavior problems).

Numerous factors can contribute to nonadherence. Factors related to the child and family include the child's age or developmental level, cognitive abilities, child behavior problems, adjustment and coping, values or attitudes toward the medical regimen, understanding of the rationale for and implementation of the regimen, organizational abilities, and family resources. The health condition and the regimen itself may also present challenges, such as fluctuating illness course, presence of side effects, and regimen complexity. Moreover, the relationship between patients, their families, and health care providers can influence adherence (Rapoff, 2010; Seid, Sobo, Gelhard, & Varni, 2004).

A number of adherence assessments and interventions to promote adherence behaviors have been developed and tested (Graves, Roberts, Rapoff, & Boyer, 2010; Kahana, Drotar, & Frazier, 2008; Quittner, Modi, Lemanek, Ievers-Landis, & Rapoff, 2008; Wu & Roberts, 2008). In clinical practice, interventions such as problem-solving approaches are typically tailored to the specific barriers or factors contributing to the regimen non-adherence. Common adherence interventions include adherence prompts (e.g., cell phone texts, verbal reminders) that prevent forgetting and planning ahead for potential adherence problems. Educational interventions can be used to address knowledge or skills deficits but are not typically effective in increasing adherence by themselves. Behavioral interventions include self- or caregiver monitoring of adherence and use of incentives or other behavior management strategies to promote adherence (Rapoff, 2010). For adolescents and caregivers, techniques such as motivational interviewing can be used to initiate open discussions about an individual's reasons for adhering or not adhering to the prescribed regimen.

PATIENT AND FAMILY DIVERSITY

Pediatric psychologists work with patients and families from diverse backgrounds who are diverse in numerous ways (e.g., cultural, ethnic, socioeconomic, geographic, sexual orientation). Pediatric psychologists incorporate their understanding of a child's or family's unique diverse characteristics into their case conceptualization and into their choice of interventions that will best fit a family's needs and preferences. A child's or family's background and culture can affect beliefs about the causes and maintaining factors contributing to illness, methods of coping with or managing illness, manifestations of symptoms, family communication about the illness or symptoms, the extent to which medical treatments are acceptable to the family, and stigma associated with a medical condition and recommended treatments. A growing literature focuses on how aspects of diversity and a provider's own competence in working with diverse populations affect clinical care (Bernal, 2006).

Although many pediatric psychologists use empirically supported assessments and treatments in clinical practice, fewer clinical strategies are validated for use with diverse populations (Clay, Mordhorst, & Lehn, 2002; La Roche & Christopher, 2008). Consequently, general models for incorporating issues of diversity into clinical practice have been proposed (Clay, 2007; Liu & Clay, 2002). One model consists of understanding the impact diversity may have on the child, family, and presenting issues; assessing need for collaborating with or referring to others with expertise in the salient diversity issues; deciding the extent to which diversity issues are incorporated in treatment; reviewing existing evidence-based practices and considering whether modifications may better meet the needs of diverse families; and implementing interventions with a focus on the families' strengths (Clay, 2007). Specific models for incorporating aspects of diversity into case conceptualization for certain pediatric populations have been proposed (e.g., transplantation; Maloney, Clay, & Robinson, 2005).

In pediatric psychology, a growing number of psychologists have documented culturally specific interventions provided to certain pediatric populations (Kaslow et al., 1997; Schwartz, Radcliffe, & Barakat, 2007). For example, Schwartz and colleagues (2007) described ways in which a pain management intervention for African American adolescents with sickle cell disease was modified to promote patient engagement. In addition to modifying hospital or clinic-based interventions, pediatric psychologists can also strive to better meet the needs of diverse patients and families by collaborating with individuals and organizations within diverse communities (e.g., religious organizations, community centers) and working with schools (Tucker, 2002).

ADJUSTMENT TO CHRONIC ILLNESS

The functional consequences of a particular chronic illness can be widespread and have a negative effect on many domains of daily life for the child and family. For instance, when a child is diagnosed with type 1 diabetes, his or her new medical regimen of testing blood glucose levels multiple times a day, administering insulin, and attending closely to diet could affect home and school life, as well as participation in other activities such as sports. In addition, routine medical visits may place additional burden on the family due to parental work absences.

Overall, the impact of the illness can be linked to the experience of the illness itself, to the developmental period of the child, and to psychosocial difficulties resulting from the interaction between the illness symptoms, the child, and the child's immediate environment (Miauton, Narring, & Michaud, 2003). These dynamic factors all must be considered when examining the child's and family's adjustment to the medical condition and its associated challenges. In addition, other factors, such as the duration of illness and "typical" course of adjustment, should be given consideration. Factors influencing adjustment to a chronic illness can be thought of as existing on a continuum, with some serving as protective factors (e.g., family support, adaptive coping styles) and others potentially negatively affecting the medical situation (e.g., ignoring medical care as a way of coping with "bad" news). In addition, certain patterns of adjustment are more or less expected at different times. For example, a tearful reaction to news from the medical team that their child has just been diagnosed with cancer would likely be expected, whereas a caregiver who expresses hopelessness, frequent tearfulness, and avoidance behaviors concerning medical care 6 months following a diagnosis may suggest more serious problems, such as depressive symptoms.

Adjustment to a chronic illness may not involve just the child and his or her caregivers. For example, a sibling of the child may display increased argumentative and noncompliant behaviors in response to the change in the family's routine and decreased parental positive attention. Ultimately, negative adjustment on the part of any member of a child's family or larger social context could affect a child's medical course or adjustment. Thus the pediatric psychologist often considers a myriad of factors and "key players" in a child's life when assessing the impact an illness has on a child and family, all with different intervention implications.

OUTCOME MEASUREMENT

From the outset, the field of pediatric psychology was defined by improving patient outcomes through the application of interventions for children and adolescents with chronic illness. Given increasing health care costs and global aims for improving health care (Institute of Medicine, 2001;

Kohn, Corrigan, & Donaldson, 1999), there is an increased emphasis on demonstrating the effectiveness of clinical services on objective measures such as reduced health care costs and improved functioning in children and adolescents with chronic illness. This underscores the need for integrating evidence-based interventions into clinical care, a call that has been further emphasized within the field of pediatric psychology, to bridge the gap between clinical practice and research (Drotar, 2010; Drotar & Lemanek, 2001).

Outcome measurement can be based on measures for an individual patient (Drotar, 2011), as well as for the population of patients with a similar condition (e.g., patients with chronic pain). These outcomes include measures of social and emotional functioning, cognitive development, adherence and self-management, and family functioning, to name a few. From an analytical standpoint, assessment of outcomes can be accomplished using traditional statistics (e.g., group comparisons, descriptive analysis), small-n designs (e.g., time-series analyses), and quality improvement science methods.

Quality improvement science aims to (1) examine outcomes over time, (2) improve delivery of evidence-based therapies by reducing variation, (3) provide feedback at the point of care and mitigate any significant changes in treatment progress, and (4) use scale-up methods to more readily disseminate clinical improvements to other patients or settings (Kotagal & Nolan, 2010). As part of quality improvement science, clinical data (e.g., symptom frequency) are presented in a statistical control chart so that providers can view the effectiveness of patients' treatment plans over time and evaluate outcomes using statistically derived decision rules. Ultimately, use of these methods can allow understanding of data at the point of care, as well as providing a way to systematically make adaptations to treatment interventions to improve outcomes (Stark, 2010).

EVIDENCE-BASED PRACTICE

A Delphic poll on the future of pediatric psychology revealed a high priority given to demonstrating "viability through empirical support for treatment interventions" with attention to improved health outcomes, medical cost offset, and effectiveness of services (Brown & Roberts, 2000). Over the years of its development, pediatric psychology has moved from an intuitive approach to more of an empirical one in terms of its improved understanding of children and families in medical situations, assessment techniques, and clinical intervention approaches. In the movement to establish empirically supported treatments (ESTs) for clinical psychology, pediatric and clinical child psychology advanced the need for scientifically supported treatments of psychosocial and pediatric problems (Chambless & Ollendick, 2001; Lonigan, Elbert, & Johnson, 1998; Roberts & James, 2008; Spirito, 1999). A series of articles published in the *Journal of Pediatric Psychology* covered treatments for such conditions as recurrent abdominal pain (Janicke & Finney, 1999), procedure-related pain (Powers, 1999), disease-related pain (Walco, Sterling, Conte, & Engel, 1999), severe feeding problems (Kerwin, 1999), constipation and encopresis (McGrath, Mellon, & Murphy, 2000), and nocturnal enuresis (Mellon & McGrath, 2000). A related resource presented evaluations of evidence-based assessment pediatric concerns (Cohen, La Greca, Blount, Kazak, Holmbeck, & Lemanek, 2008).

Evidence-based practice (EBP) includes the scientific evidence base comprising ESTs but also incorporates two other key elements. In professional psychology, EBP "is the integration of best available research with clinical expertise in the context of patient characteristics, culture and preferences" (American Psychological Association [APA] Task Force on Evidence-Based Practice, 2006, p. 273). A later report provided a more directly relevant application of EBP for child and adolescent practice, including pediatric psychology (Kazak et al., 2010). EBP in psychology gives equal weight to the three components of the research base, patient characteristics, and clinical judgment. Within pediatric psychology, the research base for assessment and treatment strategies is present for many clinical applications and continues to build. However, there has been considerably less empirical investigation of the two other elements of patient characteristics and values and clinician expertise and judgment. The *Handbook of Pediatric Psychology* (Roberts & Steele, 2009) and the chapters in the present volume portray, to the extent possible, application of the three components of EBP in pediatric psychology. The chapters in this book demonstrate the range of EBP through discussions of the empirical literature as applied to real-world clinical practice with considerations of the patient's characteristics that may modify a treatment protocol or manualized approach.

COLLABORATION AND CONSULTATION

Pediatric psychologists have always engaged in consultation with other professionals, most often pediatricians and other physicians, nurses, social workers, and teachers. These interactions, frequently over an identified patient and particular needs for assessment and intervention, invoke collaboration and coordination of clinical or other activities to improve children's psychosocial functioning and health (Brown, 2004; Drotar, 1995; Carter, Kronenberger, Scott, & Ernst, 2009). A number of conceptual models have categorized collaboration and consultation (Drotar, 1995; Roberts & Wright, 1982; Roberts, 1986; Mullins, Gillman, & Harbeck, 1992): (1) the *independent functions model*, in which the psychologist provides assessment and treatment to a patient or family without extensive interaction with a referring pediatrician; in which exchanges of information occur before and after contact with the patient; and which may involve "curbside consultation" or written reports; (2) the *indirect consultation model*, in which the psychologist provides information to the pediatrician or staff about how to handle a particular case or situation but does not interact directly with the patient; (3) the *collaborative team model*, in which multiple disciplines work together on a shared health care protocol, with joint responsibility for patients and decision making and highly interactive collaboration; and (4) the *systems-based consultation*, in which the psychologist partners to make systemic changes on medical units to be more responsive to child and family needs and consults on procedural as well as structural changes in the health care environment. The pediatric psychologist often combines these functions in clinical practice, depending on the situation.

During consultation and collaboration, obstacles may occur, including administrative issues, a physical space with limited proximity to other providers, differing perceptions of professional roles and boundaries, and differences in professional cultures (e.g., approaches to case conceptualization, jargon used). These obstacles can be overcome with a commitment to interprofessional/interdisciplinary cooperation and respect for others' contributions and competence (Drotar, 1995).

As the health care environment changes, the field anticipates a greater emphasis on integrated health care arrangements and team collaborative models to patient care with enhanced communication and agreement in efficient and effective care (Rozensky & Janicke, 2012; Roberts, Canter, & Odar, 2012). Interprofessional approaches will require systematic coordination of health care through mutual decision making, joint interactions, and collaborative functions by different professionals to deliver services.

SUMMARY

As is evident from the current chapter and others in this volume, pediatric psychologists encounter a variety of presenting problems in clinical practice. Some of these presenting problems and the strategies used to address these problems extend across illness populations. In their work with individual children and families, pediatric psychologists provide clinical care by integrating relevant theoretical frameworks and therapies and through their knowledge of the unique aspects of the child's health condition, the empirical literature on the child's and family's presenting problems, and their conceptualizations of factors influencing health in the child and family.

REFERENCES

American Psychological Association Task Force on Evidence-Based Practice. (2006). Evidence-based practice in psychology. *American Psychologist, 61,* 271–285.

Barakat, L. P., Pulgaron, E. R., & Daniel, L. C. (2009). Positive psychology in pediatric psychology. In M. C. Roberts & R. G. Steele (Eds.), *Handbook of pediatric psychology* (4th ed., pp. 763–773). New York: Guilford Press.

Bernal, G. (2006). Intervention development and cultural adaptation research with diverse families. *Family Process, 45,* 143–151.

Bronfenbrenner, U. (1979). *The ecology of human development.* Cambridge, MA: Harvard University Press.

Brown, K. J., & Roberts, M. C. (2000). Future issues in pediatric psychology: Delphic survey. *Journal of Clinical Psychology in Medical Settings, 7*(1), 5–15.

Brown, R. T. (Ed.). (2004). *Handbook of pediatric psychology in school settings.* Mahwah, NJ: Erlbaum.

Canter, K. S., & Roberts, M. C. (2012). A systematic and quantitative review of interventions to facilitate school reentry for children with chronic health conditions. *Journal of Pediatric Psychology, 37*(10), 1065–1075.

Carter, B. D., Kronenberger, W. G., Scott, E., & Ernst, M. M. (2009). Inpatient pediatric consultation–liaison. In M. C. Roberts & R. G. Steele (Eds.), *Handbook of pediatric psychology* (pp. 114–129). New York: Guilford Press.

Chambless, D. L., & Ollendick, T. H. (2001). Empirically supported psychological interventions: Controversies and evidence. *Annual Review of Psychology, 52,* 685–716.

Clay, D. L. (2007). Culturally competent interventions in schools for children with physical health problems. *Psychology in the Schools, 44,* 389–396.

Clay, D. L., Mordhorst, M. J., & Lehn, L. (2002). Empirically supported treatments in pediatric psychology: Where is the diversity? *Journal of Pediatric Psychology, 27,* 325–337.

Cohen, L. L., La Greca, A. M., Blount, R. L., Kazak, A. E., Holmbeck, G. N., & Lemanek, K. L. (2008). Introduction to special issue: Evidence-based assessment in pediatric psychology. *Journal of Pediatric Psychology, 33*(9), 911–915.

Drotar, D. (1995). *Consulting with pediatricians.* New York: Plenum.

Drotar, D. (2010).Integrating research and practice: The role of the *Journal of Pediatric Psychology* [Editorial]. *Journal of Pediatric Psychology, 35,* 111–113.

Drotar, D. (2011). Guidance for submitting and reviewing case reports and series in the *Journal of Pediatric Psychology* [Editorial]. *Journal of Pediatric Psychology, 36,* 951–958.

Drotar, D., & Lemanek, K. (2001). Steps toward a clinically relevant science of interventions in pediatric psychology: Introduction to the special issue. *Journal of Pediatric Psychology, 26,* 385–394.

DuPaul, G. J., Power, T. J., & Shapiro, E. S. (2009). Schools and integration/reintegration into schools. In M. C. Roberts & R. G. Steele (Eds.), *Handbook of pediatric psychology* (pp. 689–702). New York: Guilford Press.

Graves, M. M., Roberts, M. C., Rapoff, M., & Boyer, A. (2010). The efficacy of adherence interventions for chronically ill children: A meta-analytic review. *Journal of Pediatric Psychology, 35,* 368–382.

Harris, M. S. (2009). School reintegration and adolescents with cancer: The role of school psychologists. *Psychology in the Schools, 46*(7), 579–592.

Institute of Medicine. (2001). *Crossing the quality chasm: A new health system for the 21st century.* Washington, DC: National Academies Press.

Janicke, D. M., & Finney, J. W. (1999). Empirically supported treatments in pediatric psychology: Recurrent abdominal pain. *Journal of Pediatric Psychology, 24,* 115–128.

Kahana, S., Drotar, D., & Frazier, T. (2008). Meta-analysis of psychological interventions to promote adherence to treatment in pediatric chronic health conditions. *Journal of Pediatric Psychology, 33,* 590–611.

Kaslow, N. J., Collins, M. H., Loundy, M. R., Brown, F., Hollins, L. D., & Eckman, J. (1997). Empirically validated family interventions for pediatric psychology: Sickle cell disease as an exemplar. *Journal of Pediatric Psychology, 22,* 213–227.

Kazak, A., Alderfer, M., Streisand, R., Simms, S., Rourke, M., Barakat, L., et al. (2004). Treatments of posttraumatic stress symptoms in adolescent survivors of childhood cancer and their families: A randomized clinical trial. *Journal of Family Psychology, 18,* 493–504.

Kazak, A. E., Hoagwood, K., Weisz, J. R., Hood, K., Kratochwill, T. R., Vargas, L. A., et al. (2010). A meta-systems approach to evidence-based practice for children and adolescents. *American Psychologist, 64,* 85–97.

Kazak, A. E., Schneider, S., & Kassam-Adams, N. (2009). Pediatric medical traumatic stress. In M. C. Roberts & R. G. Steele (Eds.), *Handbook of pediatric psychology* (pp. 205–215). New York: Guilford Press.

Kazak, A. E., Simms, S., & Rourke, M. T. (2002). Family systems practice in pediatric psychology. *Journal of Pediatric Psychology, 27,* 133–143.

Kerwin, M. E. (1999). Empirically supported treatments in pediatric psychology: Severe feeding problems. *Journal of Pediatric Psychology, 24,* 193–214.

Kohn, L. T., Corrigan, J. M., & Donaldson, M. S. (Eds.). (1999). *To err is human: Building a safer health system.* Washington, DC: National Academy Press.

Kotagal, U., & Nolan, T. (2010). Commentary: The application of quality improvement in pediatric psychology: Observations and applications. *Journal of Pediatric Psychology, 35,* 42–44.

La Roche, M., & Christopher, M. S. (2008). Culture and empirically supported treatments: On the road to a collision? *Culture and Psychology, 14,* 333–356.

Liu, W. M., & Clay, D. L. (2002). Multicultural counseling competencies: Guidelines in working with children and adolescents. *Journal of Mental Health Counseling, 24,* 177–187.

Lonigan, C. J., Elbert, J. C., & Johnson, S. B. (1998). Empirically supported psychosocial interventions for children: An overview. *Journal of Clinical Child Psychology, 27,* 138–145.

Madan-Swain, A., Katz, E. R., & La Gory, J. (2004). School and social reintegration after a serious illness or injury. In R. T. Brown (Ed.), *Handbook of pediatric psychology in school settings* (pp. 637–655). Mahwah, NJ: Erlbaum.

Maloney, R., Clay, D. L., & Robinson, J. (2005). Sociocultural issues in pediatric transplantation: A conceptual model. *Journal of Pediatric Psychology, 30,* 235–246.

McCarthy, A. M., Williams, J., & Plumer, C. (1998). Evaluation of a school reentry nursing intervention for children with cancer. *Journal of Pediatric Oncology Nursing, 15*(3), 143–152.

McGrath, M. L., Mellon, M. W., & Murphy, L. (2000). Empirically supported treatments in pediatric psychology: Constipation and encopresis. *Journal of Pediatric Psychology, 25,* 225–254.

Mellon, M. W., & McGrath, M. L. (2000). Empirically supported treatments in pediatric psychology: Nocturnal enuresis. *Journal of Pediatric Psychology, 25,* 193–214.

Miauton, L., Narring, F., & Michaud, P. A. (2003). Chronic illness, lifestyle and emotional health in adolescence: Results of a cross-sectional survey on the health of 15–20-year-olds in Switzerland. *European Journal of Pediatrics, 162,* 682–689.

Mullins, L. D., Gillman, J., & Harbeck, C. (1992). Multiple-level interventions in pediatric psychology settings: A behavioral systems perspective. In A. M. La Greca, L. J. Siegel, J. L. Wallander, & C. E. Walker (Eds.), *Stress and coping in child health* (pp. 371–399). New York: Guilford Press.

National Child Traumatic Stress Network. (n.d.). *Pediatric medical traumatic stress.* Retrieved from *www.nctsnet.org/trauma-types/medical-trauma.*

Power, T. J., DuPaul, G. J., Shapiro, E. S., & Kazak, A. E. (2003). *Promoting children's health: Integrating school, family, and community.* New York: Guilford Press.

Powers, S. W. (1999). Empirically supported treatments in pediatric psychology: Procedure-related pain. *Journal of Pediatric Psychology, 24,* 131–146.

Prevatt, F. F., Heffer, R. W., & Lowe, P. A. (2000). A review of school reintegration programs for children with cancer. *Journal of School Psychology, 38*(5), 447–467.

Quittner, A. L., Modi, A. C., Lemanek, K. L., Ievers-Landis, C. E., & Rapoff, M. A. (2008). Evidence-based assessment of adherence to medical treatments in pediatric psychology. *Journal of Pediatric Psychology, 33,* 916–936.

Rapoff, M. A. (2010). *Adherence to pediatric medical regimens* (2nd ed.). New York: Springer.

Roberts, M. C. (1986). *Pediatric psychology: Psychological interventions and strategies for pediatric problems.* New York: Pergamon Press.

Roberts, M. C., Canter, K.S., & Odar, C.C. (2012). Commentary: A call to action to secure the future of pediatric psychology: Resonating to the points of Rozensky and Janicke (2012). *Journal of Pediatric Psychology, 37*(4), 369–375.

Roberts, M. C., & James, R. L. (2008). Empirically supported treatments and evidence-based practice for children and adolescents. In R. G. Steele, D. Elkin, & M. C. Roberts (Eds.), *Handbook of evidence-based therapies for children and adolescents* (pp. 9–24). New York: Springer.

Roberts, M. C., & Steele, R. C. (Eds.). (2009). *Handbook of pediatric psychology* (4th ed.). New York: Guilford Press.

Roberts, M. C., & Wright, L. (1982). Role of the pediatric psychologist as consultant to pediatricians. In J. Tuma (Ed.), *Handbook for the practice of pediatric psychology* (pp. 251–289). New York: Wiley-Interscience.

Rozensky, R. H., & Janicke, D. M. (2012). Commentary: Healthcare reform and psychology's workforce: Preparing for the future of pediatric psychology. *Journal of Pediatric Psychology, 37*(4), 359–368.

Schwartz, L. A., Radcliffe, J., & Barakat, L. P. (2007). The development of a culturally sensitive pediatric pain management intervention for African American adolescents with sickle cell disease. *Children's Health Care, 36,* 267–283.

Seid, M., Sobo, E. J., Gelhard, L. R, & Varni, J. W. (2004). Parents' reports of barriers to care for children with special health needs: Development and validation of the Barriers to Care Questionnaire. *Ambulatory Pediatrics, 4,* 323–331.

Spirito, A. (1999). Introduction: Special series on empirically supported treatments in pediatric psychology. *Journal of Pediatric Psychology, 24,* 87–90.

Stark, L. J. (2010). Introduction to the special issue: Quality improvement in pediatric psychology. *Journal of Pediatric Psychology, 35,* 1–5.

Steele, R. G., & Aylward, B. S. (2009). An overview of systems in pediatric psychology research and practice. In M. C. Roberts & R. G. Steele (Eds.), *Handbook of pediatric psychology* (4th ed., pp. 649–655). New York: Guilford Press.

Stuber, M. L., Schneider, S., Kassam-Adams, N., Kazak, A. E., & Saxe, G. (2006). The Medical Traumatic Stress Toolkit. *CNS Spectrums, 11,* 137–142.

Thompson, R. J. (1985). Coping with the stress of chronic childhood illness. In A. N. O'Quinn (Ed.), *Management of chronic disorders of childhood* (pp. 11–41). Boston: Hall.

Tucker, C. M. (2002). Expanding pediatric psychology beyond hospital walls to meet the health care needs of ethnic minority children. *Journal of Pediatric Psychology, 27,* 315–323.

Walco, G. A., Sterling, C. N., Conte, P. M., & Engel, R. G. (1999). Empirically supported treatments in pediatric psychology: Disease-related pain. *Journal of Pediatric Psychology, 24,* 155–167.

Wallander, J. L., & Varni, J. W. (1992). Adjustment in children with chronic physical disorders: Programmatic research on a disability-stress-coping model. In A. M. La Greca, L. Siegal, J. L. Wallander, & C. E. Walker (Eds.), *Stress and coping with pediatric conditions* (pp. 279–298). New York: Guilford Press.

Wu, Y. P., & Roberts, M. C. (2008). A meta-analysis of interventions to increase adherence to medication regimens for pediatric otitis media and streptococcal pharyngitis. *Journal of Pediatric Psychology, 33,* 789–796.

CHAPTER 4

Financial and Organizational Issues of Pediatric Psychology Practice

CHRISTINA L. DUNCAN
ALLISON G. DEMPSEY

The purpose of this chapter is to provide an overview of service delivery in pediatric psychology, as well as associated administrative/organizational and financial tasks that are critical to developing and maintaining a success-ful (and profitable) clinical service position. Although the information con-tained within this chapter is current as of 2013, it may be less accurate over time, particularly because financial policies and practices evolve.

MODELS OF SERVICE DELIVERY

To establish an effective practice, pediatric psychologists need to forge col-laborative relationships and share psychological information (e.g., princi-ples, assessment findings, intervention plans) clearly with other health care professionals, as well as take the initiative to develop and sustain a record of productivity (Carpenter, 1989). Pediatric psychologists are equipped with the expertise necessary to function in a variety of roles (e.g., consultant, collaborator, direct clinician) across a wide range of settings, such as private practice, ambulatory primary care clinics, subspecialty medical clinics, hospitals, rehabilitation facilities, school-based clinics, and summer camps. Indeed, since the inception of the field of pediatric psychology, the scope and breadth of our services has expanded greatly. Common models of service delivery are described in some detail in the following. For a more comprehensive overview of service delivery settings, see Lassen, Wu, and Roberts (Chapter 2); Carter, Thompson, and Thompson (Chapter 5); Stancin, Sturm, and Ramirez (Chapter 6); and Alderfer and Rourke (Chapter 8) in this volume.

In-Clinic Consultation

Behavioral health issues are common to primary care practice and significantly lengthen the time of pediatrician visits (Meadows, Valleley, Haack, Thorson, & Evans, 2011). Yet reimbursement to pediatricians is significantly lower for billing codes used during behavioral visits when compared with medical visits. This situation lends some support for having psychologists available "in-house" (in clinic) to address behavioral health issues in patients (Meadows et al., 2011). Family follow-through with behavioral health services also tends to be greater with this model of service delivery, as patients are seen in an environment that is comfortable to them and are not required to contact an outside practice to arrange plans for subsequent appointments. Whether in a primary care or medical subspecialty clinic, inside or outside of a hospital, this consultation can take various forms: seeing every patient as part of a multidisciplinary care approach (as in subspecialty pediatric services); providing direct clinical services (e.g., screening, brief intervention) to patients with psychosocial needs; and providing consultation and guidance to health care staff on identifying and managing behavioral health issues. Appointments typically fit within a fast-paced clinic schedule and its routine for patient follow-up. Thus psychologists usually conduct a screening, as opposed to a comprehensive diagnostic evaluation, and utilize brief interventions. When a patient requires more extensive services, the family is provided with a referral for services outside of the pediatric clinic.

Outpatient Referral Service

At times, it is not possible for a pediatric psychologist to be physically present in pediatric clinics, especially on a routine basis. Therefore, an alternative practice arrangement is one in which the pediatric psychologist forms partnerships with pediatric practices, accepting referrals for patients and families with behavioral health concerns. It is important to recognize that psychologists usually are the ones who initiate these partnerships, and specific professional behaviors help to sustain it. For example, the psychologist should make every effort to provide timely appointments based on the need of the case (e.g., urgent vs. routine) and to establish agreed-upon standards for consistent communication (e.g., therapy progress updates via brief letter to referring pediatrician; regular joint meetings). Certainly, communication among the psychologist, pediatric staff, and family is key to the success of this practice arrangement. The psychologist also should inform the pediatric practice staff of any limitations in referrals, such as insurance coverage. Although patients may have medical insurance, mental health benefits may not be covered by their particular plan, or such benefits may be carved out to a different insurance company for whom the provider is not listed as "in-network." Session length and schedule would be similar to that in any psychology private practice. Suggestions for promoting a psychology private practice would apply to this model of service delivery, including a focus on marketing, ease of appointment scheduling, and other approaches that facilitate maintaining a patient base.

Consultation–Liaison Service

Similar to working within a pediatric subspecialty clinic, psychologists who are part of a multidisciplinary team often serve specific populations during hospitalizations (Brosig & Zahrt, 2006). In this setting, psychologists deliver a variety of services, such as conducting psychological evaluations and testing, assisting with disease management, providing skills training in coping and pain management, establishing behavior modification plans (e.g., to promote patient cooperation, adherence to regimen), and providing patient and family support (Brosig & Zahrt, 2006; see Carter et al., Chapter 5, this volume, for more details). Although it varies as a function of the particular hospital, consults come from general pediatrics, as well as various specialty areas (e.g., trauma, hematology/oncology, transplant, feeding). Session length and schedule vary with the presenting concern and intervention needs. Oftentimes, inpatient hospitalization affords the opportunity to engage in more intensive psychotherapy on a more frequent basis (e.g., daily). Yet psychologists need to be aware that the patient's schedule fluctuates during a hospital stay and that there will be times when the patient will not be available.

Getting Patient Referrals across Service Delivery

Whether a psychologist is working in a hospital, an ambulatory clinic, or private practice, the first step in a pediatric psychology practice is to establish a referral base. A psychologist can garner patient referrals by taking the initiative to meet with physicians and pediatric practices in person, sharing concise information regarding areas of psychological expertise and potential collaboration, and providing them with contact information (e.g., business card, practice flyer) that can be shared with others. Once a pediatric psychologist establishes an effective referral base and referring providers experience positive outcomes when collaborating with the psychologist (e.g., seeing improvement in patients), additional referrals from those providers will likely continue. Psychologists also experience an increase in patient referrals as a result of delivering presentations on topics of expertise during grand rounds, in continuing medical education (CME) sessions, in community-based seminars, and on patient education days. When patient referrals involve families seeking behavioral health services outside of their pediatric clinic, it also is helpful to have a professional website for them to access so that they can better "connect" with the practitioner and thus feel more comfortable scheduling an appointment.

FINANCIAL ISSUES IN PEDIATRIC PSYCHOLOGY

Billing for Clinical Services

Pediatric psychologists typically are reimbursed for their services through fee-for-service arrangements or out-of-pocket pay from families, as well as through insurance payments. Reimbursement from insurers for services is critical to the practice of pediatric psychology. Most often, this reimbursement is obtained via two different sets of billing codes. First, pediatric psychologists can bill traditional current procedural terminology (CPT) codes for services that target issues related to a patient meeting criteria for a mental health diagnosis. Second, as of 2002, pediatric psychologists can bill with health and behavior (H&B) codes, which are designed to be used when a patient does not meet criteria for a mental health diagnosis but when clinical services are rendered to address a health-related concern. (Table 4.1 provides a brief description of the codes and example situations for their use; refer to Noll & Fischer, 2004, for a more detailed description of H&B codes and their applications.) Indeed, the diagnosis submitted with the H&B code is a medical condition (e.g., cystic fibrosis), rather than a mental health diagnosis. The approval of H&B codes filled a critical gap for the practice of pediatric psychologists, as the scope of our clinical work often addresses the adjustment to and management of acute and chronic health conditions or the promotion of healthy behaviors and health-related quality of life (Drotar, 2012). Prior to the approval of the H&B codes, pediatric psychologists felt pressured to provide a mental health diagnosis for their clinical services, even when the primary referral was directly related to the youth's medical diagnosis.

TABLE 4.1. H&B Codes

Code	Description	Example	Unit
96150	Initial assessment that focuses on biological, psychological, and social factors that may affect health and intervention	Evaluation of patient who is newly diagnosed with leukemia	15 minutes
96151	Reassessment and need for further treatment	Reevaluation of patient adjustment to amputation	15 minutes
96152	Individual intervention focusing on behavioral, cognitive, or social factors that affect a patient's health	Individual psychotherapy to teach pain management strategies to a patient with Crohn's disease	15 minutes
96153	Group intervention that provides educational information, cognitive-behavioral intervention, or social support	Group therapy to promote adherence in adolescents with type 1 diabetes	15 minutes
96154	Family-based intervention with patient present	Family therapy to encourage patient cooperation with dressing changes at home for a burn injury	15 minutes
96155	Family-based intervention without patient present	Family therapy to address grief reaction in response to a comatose patient with a brain injury	15 minutes

Practical Issues in Using H&B Codes

There are several practical issues to consider when using H&B codes. First, H&B codes are used to bill in 15-minute increments for face-to-face time. Consequently, although some traditional CPT codes allow the clinician to include time spent scoring and interpreting test results as well as reviewing records and writing reports, the H&B codes do not cover such activities. Also, time spent in collaborative care, consultation, and multidisciplinary case management is not reimbursable via H&B codes. Second, unlike traditional CPT codes, funding for H&B code reimbursement should be taken from the medical portion of the individual's insurance plan (which often has more extensive funds than mental health coverage). However, this funding approach has not been adopted within some states and by some insurance carriers (e.g., Woods & Gillaspy, 2012). Although preauthorization should not be required when using the patient's medical benefits, many insurers require preauthorization before submitting bills for H&B codes (Brosig, 2012). Third, some insurance companies have restrictions against same-day billing of services for both physical health and behavioral health services. This restriction is particularly problematic when pediatric psychologists provide their services within an outpatient multidisciplinary clinic or through inpatient pediatric consultation. Fourth, psychologists also cannot bill for traditional CPT codes (with a psychiatric diagnosis) and H&B codes (with a medical diagnosis) on the same day. When a patient qualifies for a mental health diagnosis in addition to his or her medical diagnosis, the pediatric psychologist should use the CPT code that best reflects the referral needs of the patient and the principal service delivered. Fifth, when a patient has more than one medical diagnosis, the psychologist should report the one that is most relevant to the focus of the clinical service provided. It also is important that physician documentation exist in the patient's record to support any medical diagnosis listed with an H&B code. Finally, the role of trainees in providing and receiving reimbursement for services under the supervision of licensed psychologists also has varied across states and insurers. Taking a proactive approach to obtaining approval for trainee reimbursement from Medicaid and commercial insurers has met with some success (e.g., Woods & Gillaspy, 2012).

Reimbursement Concerns with H&B Codes

Though approval of the H&B codes opened new avenues for reimbursement for pediatric psychology services, this means of reimbursement has not been without significant challenges. Indeed, success with and rate of reimbursement through H&B codes has varied within and across institutions since the inception of these codes. A special issue of the *Journal of Pediatric Psychology* (Vol. 37, No. 5) reported on the detailed experiences of practitioners using H&B codes within different programs across the United States (Drotar, 2012). This issue serves as an excellent resource for clinicians seeking to use and obtain reimbursement for the H&B codes.

Pediatric psychologists must take an active effort in monitoring and advocating for reimbursement of H&B codes, particularly because both commercial and Medicaid insurance policies vary state to state. Given this variation, it has been recommended that a collaborative approach should be taken by the Society of Pediatric Psychology, state psychological associations, and the American Psychological Association (APA) to facilitate reimbursement in a judicious manner (Drotar, 2012). Indeed, with future changes in the health care system (e.g., the Patient Protection and Affordable Care Act, or ACA, slated to begin implementation in 2014), pediatric psychologists will need to work together to ensure not only that children and families receive important behavioral health services but also that pediatric psychologists are compensated adequately and consistently for providing them (Drotar, 2012).

At the local and state levels, several strategies have been recommended to optimize reimbursement (e.g., Brosig, 2012; Duke, Guion, Freeman, Wilson, & Harris, 2012). Suggestions have included: (1) explaining to insurers the need for and unique impact of specific pediatric psychology services; (2) clarifying that these services, as well as a psychologist's collaborative efforts within a multidisciplinary care approach, often are not available from local in-network providers (e.g., community mental health centers); (3) communicating directly with insurers prior to submitting claims to educate them about appropriate use of the codes; (4) monitoring and responding to denied claims; (5) keeping a record of successful reimbursement (as evidence to use when advocating for approval from new insurers); and (6) having parents, physicians, and physician state organizations join psychologists in advocacy efforts. State Medicaid programs should be targeted specifically for approved reimbursement, as private insurance companies tend to follow the standard set by Medicaid. Serving as an excellent example, Woods and Gillaspy (2012) provide a detailed account of the steps they took to secure Medicaid support in Oklahoma.

Though these recommendations for facilitating reimbursement of H&B codes seem rather straightforward, some practitioners may lack the support necessary to dedicate significant time and staff to such efforts. For example, H&B codes were designed to be used by health psychologists, who often work in fast-paced clinic and hospital settings, yet these codes often require preauthorization (Duke et al., 2012). It has been suggested that reimbursement rates will improve and that clinician billable time will be more readily available when programs hire billing staff or an insurance verification specialist whose role is to educate and communicate with insurance companies and maintain consistent tracking of denials and appeals (Brosig & Zahrt, 2006). Drotar (2012) also suggested that when institutions are positioned such that they provide the lion's share of health care to children and families in the geographic region, these institutions may be in a position of power that affords them the opportunity to negotiate at a higher level and to place pressure on insurance companies to compensate behavioral health services if these companies are to maintain other large health care contracts with the institution. Drotar further noted that to enhance our advocacy efforts for funding it will be important for pediatric psychology to conduct a large-scale evaluation of the cost-effectiveness and financial value of the services we provide, particularly with the H&B codes. Ideally, a partnership between pediatric psychologists and insurance companies can be developed such that they both "win" when evidence-based psychological services are funded within pediatric health care and these

behavioral health care services offset later costs to the insurance companies by reducing patients' health care utilization and health complications
(e.g., avoiding costly hospitalization for diabetic ketoacidosis by promoting
adherence; e.g., Duke et al., 2012).

Other Financial Models for Pediatric Psychology

Because of limited acceptance of insurance claims and overall percentage
of financial return for both traditional CPT and H&B codes, pediatric
psychologists often must identify alternative funding streams within their
institutions. It is most common that a mix of funding sources support clinical pediatric psychology programs. For example, psychologists' salaries
can be covered by hospital or clinic service fees as an overhead expense
(Rae, 2004), recognizing that pediatric psychology services are valuable
despite their limited funding. Similarly, psychologists can devise an agreement with hospital-based subspecialty clinics or community-based primary
care clinics to pay their salaries to provide clinical and research consultation, regardless of billing (Rae, 2004). In this scenario, pediatric psychology services may be "bundled" so that the psychologist's fee is included as
part of the overall clinic visit or hospitalization fee (Rae, 2004). Families
can then access psychology services in settings where they typically are seen
(i.e., medical clinics). Lastly, a psychologist can establish a private practice
within an outpatient pediatric clinic, accepting referrals from the physicians, and choosing from a few different funding mechanisms, including
working as a partner in the practice, being employed by the practice with
a fixed salary or a salary based upon monies billed or collected, or establishing an independent practice that pays overhead (e.g., for administrative
support) to the practice (Schroeder, 1996). In each of these scenarios, it is
important to consider the potential impact that these arrangements have on
the fiscal viability of the departments and programs involved, as well as the
individual psychologist (Brosig & Zahrt, 2006).

ADMINISTRATIVE TASKS

Credentialing

Before starting clinical services at a hospital or other health care organization, the institution will need to verify the psychologist's credentials. The
purpose of credentialing is to formally recognize a practitioner's qualifi-
cations and competence to ensure patient safety (Robiner, Dixon, Miner,
& Hong, 2010). Each institution or organization is responsible for establishing its own credentialing procedures (for a review of this process, see
Rauch, 2012). Generally, it can be extremely time-consuming and may

be arduous in the amount of paperwork and supporting documentation required. However, credentials banking programs (e.g., Association of State and Provincial Psychology Boards [ASPPB], National Health Register) are tools that trainees and psychologists can use to facilitate the credentialing process, as these programs serve as repositories of licensure-related information (e.g., licensure exam scores, transcripts, letters of recommendation). Additionally, the American Board of Professional Psychology (ABPP; *www.abpp.org*) has an early-entry program for graduate students and interns to start the board certification process before yet being licensed. Overall, a psychologist likely will need to provide evidence of degree, current and previous state licensures and certifications, previous employment and malpractice history, criminal background check, vaccination record and current tuberculosis test, and professional references. To expedite the process, the psychologist should be as thorough as possible in gaining supporting documentation of professional history and explaining anything unusual (e.g., gaps in employment history). It is also important to check all documentation, as errors or omitted information can delay the process further. Moreover, obtaining board certification in a specialty of psychology pertaining to health care (e.g., from the American Board of Clinical Child and Adolescent Psychology) is one possible indicator of competence and can facilitate the credentialing process. Indeed, in the practice of pediatric psychology, increasingly more hospitals are either requiring new practitioners to become board certified or giving them incentives to do so.

A second step in the credentialing process, after verifying subjective and objective indicators of qualification and competency, is the delineation of clinical privileges for the practitioner. In this step, appointed individuals involved in the credentialing process specify the types of patient care services that the psychologist is approved to deliver in the hospital, such as assessment, intervention, and administrative services. As an additional complicating factor, some institutions, such as medical schools, may be affiliated with an independent hospital or clinic. If the psychologist is expecting to provide services in both agencies, such as an outpatient clinic in the medical school and consultation–liaison services at the affiliated hospital, then credentialing will likely need to occur separately for each agency.

In some organizations, an employment contract cannot be executed until the credentialing and privileges process is complete. Approval is for a time-limited period, and reappointment is required at a minimum of every 2 years. During the reappointment process, information such as professional performance may be reviewed. Additionally, the institution likely will request updated information and documentation, such as licensure and continuing education credits, any personal or malpractice litigation, and current liability insurance (Rauch, 2012).

Insurance Paneling

Credentialing is the first step in the process to begin providing psychological services. For those psychologists who bill patients individually and not through third-party payers, credentialing is sufficient to begin service delivery. However, if the psychologist is involved with a hospital or clinic that accepts insurance (as most do), then the health care organization will need to add the practitioner to insurance panels so he or she may bill for provided services as an in-network provider. Each insurance company may differ in its application requirements; thus evidence of training, licensure, and malpractice insurance may be requested by each individual insurance company. It takes approximately 3 months to be approved and added to an insurance panel. The majority of insurance plans will not reimburse for charges until the psychologist is listed as in-network. However, some will allow bills to be submitted retroactively from the time the application was submitted. For this reason, it is important to be knowledgeable regarding the rules and procedures for specific insurance companies and plans.

MEASURING PRODUCTIVITY

Establishing a Business Plan

When opening a position for a new psychologist, the institution usually develops a business plan to determine how the psychologist's salary, benefits, and operating costs (e.g., travel, software, instruments/measures) will be covered. In institutions in which psychology has a large presence, the new psychologist may not need to be involved in this process, as it has likely been completed with previous hires. However, when psychology is not well represented in the health care agency, the psychologist may need to work with administrators to develop a business plan. Having a psychologist involved in this process is critical, as administrators in a health care agency tend to be much more knowledgeable about medical than about behavioral health, costs, and reimbursement rates.

When developing a business plan, the psychologist's salary and benefits will be compared with the expected generated income from the position. This income may consist of time purchased by clinics or grants and/or by billing per service delivered. The psychologist will need to estimate the patient flow, types of services to be provided, and corresponding billing codes. That is, the psychologist will need to project the number of annual units billed for each code. Whether taking part in developing the business plan or not, the psychologist should be aware of billing and reimbursement rates to protect him- or herself when committing to particular earnings as part of the position. Billing staff at the institution will be able to provide this information to the psychologist. Alternatively, the psychologist can contact the insurance companies directly to determine rates of reimbursement for each billing code that will be used. Also of critical importance in agreeing to a specific billing load, the psychologist should determine whether the institution is basing the employment contract on services billed or actual monies collected. Unfortunately, reimbursement rates for psychological services tend to be low. Although reasonable fees may be set for services, actual reimbursement rates from managed-care insurance companies may be much lower. Finally, some services may not be reimbursed at all by some insurance companies. For example, some insurance plans will reimburse for only individual therapy and will deny claims for family therapy.

Finally, the value of the psychologist in the health care setting may be to prevent increased medical costs associated with nonadherence and psychological factors that affect the presentation of a medical disorder, rather than merely to generate income through billing for service delivery. Therefore, the psychologist may need to work with administration to develop a method for quantifying the value of the preventative services, such as reduced visits to the emergency department and decreased rates of surgical complications. The American Psychological Association Practice Directorate (*www.apapracticecentral.org/*) has many online resources to help in developing a business plan for independent practitioners. The psychologist in the health care agency may find this information useful in establishing a business plan for services delivered.

Relative Value Units

In addition to services billed, many institutions measure productivity of staff in relative value units (RVU). Health care service delivery has been undergoing a reform in service reimbursement over the past two decades. As part of this reform, the Resource-Based Relative Value Scale (RBRVS) emerged as a way to quantify service delivery to inform uniform Medicare reimbursement rates (for a comprehensive description of the development of the RBRVS system, see Hsiao, Braun, Dunn, & Becker, 1988). The scale has since been expanded to include pediatric services. The RVU assigned to various services was determined by a panel of health care professionals for specific CPT billing codes. The RVU considers the time spent to prepare for a patient (preservice work), to deliver services (intraservice work), and to conduct postvisit activities (postservice work), such as charting. Fee schedules for provider compensation are then calculated from these RVUs. Many agencies are now basing contracts and productivity assessments on generated RVUs rather than on billing or reimbursement rates. In such cases, psychologists may need to negotiate the amount of RVUs required for their positions when developing a business plan and/or at the time of hire, as well as during annual reviews of provider productivity. To be prepared for such negotiations, the psychologist should be aware of the standard RVUs of the services he or she expects to deliver. There are RVUs attached to both CPT and H&B billing codes. The psychologist should contact his or her state Medicaid agency to learn about the most updated RVUs attached to these codes. The psychologist should also be aware of the limitations of applying RVUs to pediatric psychology practice, as various services (e.g., school consultation) are not recognized in the RVU system (for a review, see Opipari-Arrigan, Stark, & Drotar, 2006).

CONSENT AND RECORD KEEPING

Other critical issues that the pediatric psychologist must consider when working in a health care agency relate to consent, record keeping, and confidentiality. Of course, the same principles, ethics, and guidelines outlined by the APA and state licensing boards apply to work completed in pediatric psychology settings. However, the multidisciplinary setting involved in pediatric psychology practice presents special considerations.

Consent

First, pediatric psychologists must consider the best method for obtaining informed consent from caregivers. Professionals in health care settings are generally required to obtain informed consent from patients to administer health care services. Additionally, health care professionals are required by law to inform the patient of their privacy practices, which detail what types of information may be shared and with whom (e.g., third-party payers). Although services provided by the psychologist certainly fall under this consent, the language contained in the general medical consent may not be sufficient to meet consent criteria for mental health services advised by APA and regulated by state boards of psychology. Therefore, a separate consent may be needed for psychology services detailing the following items: services that may be provided, how testing information may be used, presence of trainees, use of audio or video recording, confidentiality and its limits, and billing and payment issues. Many state boards of psychology and liability insurance companies have legal experts available to provide consultation to psychologists. It is recommended that the pediatric psychologist have the consent form reviewed by professionals knowledgeable about legal issues related to psychology practice to make sure that the consent form adequately addresses pertinent and unique issues.

MEDICAL AND MENTAL HEALTH RECORDS

An additional challenge facing pediatric psychology practice relates to record keeping. Many health care agencies, particularly large agencies, have adopted electronic medical record (EMR) systems. Although such systems certainly have benefits for patient care, such as ease of coordination of care across providers and reductions in medical errors, increased threats to security of records and patient confidentiality exist (for a review, see Richards, 2009). In contrast to traditional paper-based notes, EMRs are accessible to many providers within a hospital setting. Although EMRs are a helpful tool in multidisciplinary care and allow psychologists to communicate with other members of a medical team with ease, they also a pose a unique challenge, as the psychologist must consider how to balance professional communication with patient confidentiality. That is, information contained in mental health records progress notes may not be appropriate for other providers to access. Even if providers do not open patient notes, they will likely be able to see the number and type of mental health visits, as well as billing codes and diagnoses, in the EMR system.

The psychologist needs to take several steps to protect the confidentiality and privacy of the patient and family. First, the psychologist must consider how to find a balance between appropriately documenting services, promoting coordination of care, and also protecting the privacy of the individual patient. Additionally, if psychology notes are entered into EMR, the psychologist will need to work with individuals involved in medical records to determine the types of additional security that may be available for mental health records. This may include using a separate system for mental health records that cannot be accessed by other providers, "locking" notes so that only designated persons may see or access them, or allowing "glass" to be laid over the notes so that if other providers try to access them, they are required to verify that they have the right to access them and so that a clear record of people who have accessed the notes is available (i.e., "breaking the glass"). Some systems allow only parts of notes to be viewed by medical providers, such as the mental status, diagnoses, and treatment plans. Regardless of the system used, the psychologist should inform the patient and caregivers both verbally and in writing of the use of EMRs and how mental health records are protected within the system. For a comprehensive review and suggestions for maintaining EMRs, see Steinfeld and Keyes (2011).

When using an EMR system, the psychologist will need to work with medical records and information technology services to develop a template within the EMR system that will prompt the psychologist to provide necessary information for each visit (Steinfeld & Keyes, 2011). Additionally, although the psychologist may use an EMR system to document services, paper files may still need to be maintained to store test protocols, as scanning protocols into the system poses a threat to test security and may violate copyright laws. The psychologist will need to determine where and how these records will be securely maintained, stored, and accessed.

CONCLUSION

Pediatric psychology services are provided across a range of settings and involve a multitude of organizational, financial, and pragmatic factors to consider. Roberts, Brown, and Puddy (2002) argue that more programmatic research in pediatric psychology service systems and practice should be conducted to advance our field and demonstrate our worth as a profession. Based on the relevant studies they reviewed, Roberts and colleagues concluded the following: (1) Pediatric psychology services are used when they are made available to families; (2) pediatric psychologists receive relevant referrals for clinical service; (3) pediatric psychologists are effective in modifying behavior; and (4) consumers (e.g., patients, families) generally are satisfied with the pediatric psychology services received. Yet, just as pediatric psychology has evolved and adapted in the past, our profession should anticipate and prepare for "challenges and opportunities" associated with impending, significant reform in our health care system (Rozensky & Janicke, 2012, p. 366). To remain viable and respected as a profession, we need to take a proactive approach to establish a solid basis of evidence and value for the work that we do, to advocate for appropriate funding and reimbursement for the services we provide and the roles we fill within children's health care, and to prepare ourselves for the changing times ahead.

REFERENCES

Brosig, C. L. (2012). Commentary: The use of health and behavioral codes in a pediatric cardiology setting. *Journal of Pediatric Psychology*, *37*, 514–518.

Brosig, C. L., & Zahrt, D. M. (2006). Evolution of an inpatient pediatric psychology consultation service: Issues related to reimbursement and use of health and behavior codes. *Journal of Clinical Psychology in Medical Settings*, *13*, 425–429.

Carpenter, P. J. (1989). Establishing the role of the pediatric psychologist in a university medical center-based oncology service. *Training and Practice in Professional Psychology*, *3*, 21–28.

Drotar, D. (2012). Introduction to the special issue: Pediatric psychologists' experiences in obtaining reimbursement for the use of health and behavior codes. *Journal of Pediatric Psychology*, *37*, 479–485.

Duke, D., Guion, K., Freeman, K. A., Wilson, A. C., & Harris, M. A. (2012).

Commentary: Health & behavior codes: Great idea, questionable outcome. *Journal of Pediatric Psychology, 37,* 491–495.

Hsiao, W. C., Braun, P., Dunn, D., & Becker, E. R. (1988). Resource-based relative values: An overview. *Journal of the American Medical Association, 260*(16), 2347–2353.

Meadows, T., Valleley, R., Haack, M. K., Thorson, R., & Evans, J. (2011). Physician "costs" in providing behavioral health in primary care. *Clinical Pediatrics, 50,* 447–455.

Noll, R. B., & Fischer, S. (2004). Commentary: Health and behavior CPT codes: An opportunity to revolutionize reimbursement in pediatric psychology. *Journal of Pediatric Psychology, 29,* 571–578.

Opipari-Arrigan, L., Stark, L., & Drotar, D. (2006). Benchmarks for work performance of pediatric psychologists. *Journal of Pediatric Psychology, 31,* 630–642.

Rae, W. A. (2004). Financing pediatric psychology services: Buddy, can you spare a dime? *Journal of Pediatric Psychology, 29,* 47–52.

Rauch, D. A. (2012). Clinical report: Medical staff appointment and delineation of pediatric privileges in hospitals. *Pediatrics, 129*(4), 782–783.

Richards, M. M. (2009). Electronic medical records: Confidentiality issues in the time of HIPAA. *Professional Psychology: Research and Practice, 40,* 550–556.

Roberts, M. C., Brown, K. J., & Puddy, R. W. (2002). Service delivery issues and program evaluation in pediatric psychology. *Journal of Clinical Psychology in Medical Settings, 9,* 3–13.

Robiner, W. N., Dixon, K. E., Miner, J. L., & Hong, B. A. (2010). Hospital privileges for psychologists in the era of competencies and increased accountability. *Journal of Clinical Psychology in Medical Settings, 17,* 301–314.

Rozensky, R. H., & Janicke, D. M. (2012). Commentary: Healthcare reform and psychology's workforce: Preparing for the future of pediatric psychology. *Journal of Pediatric Psychology, 37,* 359–368.

Schroeder, C. (1996). Psychologists and pediatricians in collaborative practice. In R. J. Resnick & R. H. Rozensky (Eds.), *Health psychology through the life span: Practice and research opportunities* (pp. 109–131). Washington, DC: American Psychological Association.

Steinfeld, B. I., & Keyes, J. A. (2011). Electronic medical records in a multidisciplinary health care setting: A clinical perspective. *Professional Psychology: Research and Practice, 42,* 426–432.

Woods, K., & Gillaspy, S. (2012). Medical reimbursement and utilization of health and behavior codes. *Journal of Pediatric Psychology, 37,* 503–508.

PART II

CLINICAL ROLES IN PEDIATRIC PSYCHOLOGY

CHAPTER 5

Pediatric Consultation–Liaison

The Psychological Hospitalist

BRYAN D. CARTER
SUZANNE M. THOMPSON
AIMEE N. THOMPSON

Many pediatric psychologists perform consultation–liaison (C-L) services in inpatient pediatric hospital settings as their primary clinical responsibility. Fortunately, there is an expanding clinical and evidence-based literature to support C-L activities, including those that provide an overview of psychologist roles and functions (e.g., Drotar, 1995; Carter & von Weiss, 2005; Carter, Kronenberger, Scott, & Ernst, 2009) and those that are somewhat encyclopedic in scope (Ernst et al., in press; Fritz, Mattison, Nurcombe, & Spirito, 1993), as well as articles that address specific systems-level roles and interventions (Kazak, Sims, & Rourke, 2002). The current chapter employs a case-based approach to illustrate evidence-based and clinical applications relevant to pediatric psychologist roles and functions in providing C-L services.

PSYCHOLOGIST AS HOSPITALIST

The Society of Hospital Medicine defines a hospital medicine practitioner as a physician or nonphysician provider whose primary focus is the clinical care of hospitalized patients and whose responsibilities also include teaching, research, and leadership related to hospital care (Society of Hospital Medicine, 2009). In many ways the pediatric psychologist providing C-L services in the academic children's hospital setting can be seen as functioning as a "pediatric psychological hospitalist" in that the psychologist is responsible for the myriad of psychosocial issues and factors affecting medically hospitalized children. These roles and responsibilities often include the following:

- Providing prompt and evidence-based attention to psychosocial care needs that may have an impact on patient and family coping and adherence.
- Providing a differential diagnosis of psychosocial conditions that may produce symptoms suggesting an underlying organic disease.
- Providing behavioral health interventions that enhance coping/ adjustment and facilitate the performance of medical procedures and care.
- Developing and employing quality and process improvement techniques that enhance patient/family understanding of medical conditions and maximize treatment adherence.
- Collaborating, communicating, and coordinating with all health care providers and specialty teams caring for hospitalized patients.
- Safe and smooth transitioning of patient psychosocial care within the hospital and from the hospital to the community and regional resources.
- Providing local and national leadership in integrating teaching and research on psychosocial aspects of pediatric hospital care.

In-hospital C-L psychologists are increasingly actively involved in attending to the multiple patient-, family-, and systems-level aspects of inpatient care. In parallel to the growing use of pediatricians as full-time hospitalists in the children's hospital setting, it may be time to more clearly delineate a "psychological hospitalist" role to ensure addressing the many psychosocial factors that affect patient and family welfare, treatment adherence, health care utilization, and long-term functioning beyond the hospital.

PEDIATRIC C-L MODELS AND ROLES

C-L services can be characterized on a variety of dimensions, including team disciplinary makeup, range of services provided, scope of targeted populations and issues, team member functions, and theoretical/conceptual model of the service (Carter et al., 2009). In the academic medical center setting, the C-L psychologist often has the added responsibility of providing "liaison" via didactics, lectures, and grand rounds, as well as service and specialty rounds. This provides a unique opportunity for the psychologist to educate his or her medical colleagues about the many biopsychosocial issues involved in providing inpatient pediatric care, as well as serve as a role model for the empathetic and sensitive communication skills that are important in guiding pediatric patients and their families through the often bewildering experience of diagnosis and treatment in the inpatient hospital environment.

CASE STUDIES IN INPATIENT PEDIATRIC C-L: PRACTICE ARENAS

The roles and responsibilities of the pediatric C-L psychologist have been previously organized according to practice arenas as the five C's of C-L: crisis, coping, compliance (adherence), communication, and collaboration (Carter et al., 2009). This chapter employs these practice arenas for conceptualizing case studies that will elucidate the different roles and evidence-based interventions applicable to the clinical practice of pediatric psychology in the inpatient pediatric hospital setting.

Crisis

When in "crisis" (e.g., new-onset illness, self-injurious behavior, changes in health, traumatic injury), patient and family are in a heightened emotional state of shock and disbelief, which affects coping and decision making (Drotar & Zagorski, 2001). Often the times of heightened risk come during the initial evaluation, the arrival at a diagnosis, a sudden significant decline in the patient's condition, and the determination of a medical treatment approach (Barlow & Ellard, 2006). Failure to address these crises may place the patient and family at higher risk for future adjustment difficulties (Koocher, Curtiss, Pollin, & Patton, 2001).

Case Example 1: Amy

Amy, a 16-year-old female with no previous history of psychiatric or medical problems, presented with multiple injuries sustained in a motor vehicle accident in which she was the driver. Amy's 12-year-old brother, the sole passenger, died of injuries he sustained in the accident. Conflicting and erroneous information about the details of the accident fueled Amy's ruminations (e.g., "What if I hit the car first? What if I was distracted and it was my fault?"). No signs of traumatic brain injury were observed. Contact was initiated with Amy and her family after her transfer from the pediatric intensive care unit to the trauma unit and continued for the duration of her 2-week hospital stay.

An immediate concern of the trauma unit staff was the level of emotional distress on the part of Amy's parents and its impact on the patient. The mother expressed vague suicidal ideation (e.g., "There's no point in going on," "I have lost my son; if anything happens to my daughter I have no reason to live"), and a constant companion was provided. Amy was seen by the C-L psychologist every other day and gently encouraged to recount her traumatic experience and grieve the loss of her brother. The parents proved difficult to engage, often avoiding meaningful interaction by focusing on the usually large group of visitors in the room. Attending the memorial service on a hospital pass made the brother's death more "real" and allowed Amy to more actively work on her grief and feelings of guilt. Prior to discharge, the family was given information on warning signs of complicated grief and posttraumatic stress.

At a 4-month postdischarge follow-up, Amy appeared depressed, with symptoms of posttraumatic stress. Her personal bereavement was complicated by the parents' extreme grief, which fueled Amy's continued feelings of guilt and responsibility for her brother's death. She ruminated over what she could have done differently to prevent the collision and had intrusive images of reliving the accident. Amy benefited from time-limited follow-up by the C-L psychologist employing behavioral activation (Curry & Becker, 2008), relaxation training (Kendall, Furr, & Podell, 2010; Silverman & Pina, 2008), cognitive therapy for her guilt-inducing thoughts (Cohen, Mannarino, & Deblinger, 2006), verbally recounting the accident (Cohen et al., 2006), and supportive interventions around anniversary dates. Trauma-focused cognitive-behavioral therapy (TF-CBT; Cohen et al., 2006) proved particularly effective in decreasing posttraumatic stress disorder (PTSD) symptoms, improving school attendance and performance, and peer involvement. Family sessions improved family communication, clarified misunderstandings and associated intrusive negative thoughts, and facilitated the grief process. Amy continued to experience appropriate intermittent grief and sadness but was able to hold a part-time job and resume driving. Amy and her parents became more skilled at articulating and expressing feelings with one another and benefited from putting energies into planning a memorial project for her brother at his school. The patient's recovery from the psychological impact of her injuries and loss was gradual, with in-hospital psychological intervention helping with crisis management and, in this case, setting the stage for necessary posthospitalization intervention.

Coping

One of the roles that the pediatric C-L psychologist often fulfills is facilitating patient and family coping with the many stressors associated with acute and chronic childhood illness and injury (Harbeck-Weber, Fisher, & Dittner, 2003; Kazak, Schneider, & Kassam-Adams, 2009). Numerous aspects of hospitalization, diagnosis, and treatment can be stressful and traumatic, including the uncertainty of the outcome of a patient's condition, the intensity, duration, and type of treatments, the invasiveness of procedures (intubation, IVs, PICC lines, chest tubes, catheters, etc.), body image changes, among many other things. Certain chronic illnesses, such as childhood cancers, cystic fibrosis, diabetes, renal disease, sickle cell disease, and so forth, can produce long-term stressors for the patient and family via outpatient disease management demands, as well as frequent hospitalizations, high overall medical utilization, and complicated treatment regimens (Carter et al., 2009). Fortunately, there is evidence that early intervention in the course of a hospitalization can shorten the length of the child's hospital stay (Kishi, Meller, Kathol, & Swigart, 2004). Coping interventions may target such adaptations as facilitating patient and family acceptance, developing a coping style to match the stressor, establishing a routine, and identifying and maintaining personal control (Ernst et al., in press).

Case Example 2: Kristen

Kristen, a previously healthy and well-adjusted 13-year-old white female, was admitted to the intensive care unit after an ATV accident that occurred at her father's home. Her right femoral artery was crushed by the ATV handlebar when she accidently hit the accelerator instead of the brake, propelling the ATV into the wall of the garage. Due to significant blood loss and loss of consciousness, Kristen was transported by air to the hospital. The severity of the arterial damage necessitated a below-the-knee amputation of the right leg. As a highly competitive soccer player, the anticipated loss of her limb was overwhelming. Kristen and her parents asked to "talk to someone who could help us cope with all of this," and the attending surgeon put in a request for a psychological consultation.

Developmentally, Kristen's favored sport proved to be a major part of her identity and social linkage with her peers and community. She feared that the loss of her leg could present problems with peer acceptance and expressed concerns, bordering on phobia, of getting her prosthesis and the process of rehabilitation. Her hospital stay was complicated by a number of unanticipated surgeries and procedures, as well as difficulty matching the patient with an appropriate prosthetic, resulting in an extended stay of several weeks. However, her coping was facilitated by numerous protective factors, including strong parental, family, church, and community support and presence in the hospital, the family's openness and expressive communication skills, and her assertiveness and receptivity in requesting and processing information regarding her surgeries and rehabilitation.

Cognitive-behavioral therapy (CBT), which has been shown to be efficacious for a wide variety of pediatric mental and physical health-related concerns (Butler, Chapman, Forman, & Beck, 2006; Powers, Jones, & Jones, 2005), was employed to help Kristen identify, label, and monitor thoughts and feelings regarding her medical condition. The A-B-C (activating event–beliefs–consequences) model of CBT was introduced, and Kristen was taught to challenge negative thoughts using "evidence" available to dispute her distress-provoking cognitions (e.g., "I will never be able to play soccer again" vs. "It will take some rehabilitation, but there are amputee athletes who continue to play their sports and have meaningful lives"). Kristen responded well to an arranged meeting with a young adult who was competing in the regional paralympics games, asking numerous questions and expressing strong admiration for and taking encouragement from the athlete's dedication, determination, and accomplishments. In addition to CBT, negative thoughts about altered body image, identity, and hopelessness were addressed from an acceptance and commitment therapy (ACT) approach (Hayes, Luoma, Bond, Masuda, & Lillis, 2006; Greco & Hayes, 2008).

Kristen's disrupted sleep schedule, often seen in hospitalized children, necessitated establishing a consistent schedule and formal sleep hygiene intervention (Meltzer & Mindell, 2009). Although activity scheduling and behavioral activation (BA) have not been specifically tested in the hospital environment—which is the case for many interventions that the pediatric C-L psychologist may need to adapt for use with inpatients—they have been shown to be effective with a broad array of childhood conditions, particularly in addressing mood concerns (Dimidjian, et al., 2006; Jacobson, Martell, & Dimidjian, 2001). Kristen was also trained in the use of clinical biofeedback (galvanic skin response and heart rate variability) and Web-based diaphragmatic breathing practice (*www.copingclub.com*) to assist with general relaxation and stress management, as well as more realistic and empowering self-talk via CBT, all of which added to her development of a personal coping menu to employ at times of increased anxiety and challenge. Kristen made a successful transition from the children's hospital to inpatient rehabilitation and responded enthusiastically to getting her prosthetic leg fitted and returning home.

Compliance

Medical conditions seen in the children's hospital settings often call for patient and family compliance with complex treatments that necessitate long-term behavior change and lifestyle modifications. Failure to understand and comply with treatments is one of the major risk factors contributing to frequent hospitalization, excessive health care utilization, morbidity, and even mortality (Spirito & Kazak, 2006). When nonadherent behavior has a negative impact on patient progress and health outcomes, the C-L psychologist is frequently requested to intervene with such behaviors as refusal to cooperate with procedures and therapies, combative and aggressive behaviors, family dynamics that hamper effective collaboration, and even patients whose families may threaten to take the patient out of the hospital against medical advice (Carter et al., 2009; Ernst et al., in press). Poor patient/family compliance may be due to preexisting behavioral problems (Carter et al., 2003), skill deficits, fears or misunderstanding, efforts to exert control in the hospital setting due to overwhelming stress and feelings of lack of control, neurocognitive deficits, and even physiological factors such as sleep deprivation, pain, and adverse effects of medication. In such circumstances it is critical that the C-L psychologist base his or her interventions on an accurate assessment and understanding of the factors that are causing and maintaining poor treatment compliance.

Case Example 3: Brandon

Brandon was a 5-year-old male who was admitted to the hospital for evaluation of recurrent respiratory infections that had failed to respond to painful antibiotic injections by his primary care pediatrician. During his hospital stay he was diagnosed with cystic fibrosis (CF), family education was initiated, and medications and airway clearance treatments were begun. However, Brandon had become increasingly more uncooperative and even combative with the nurses and respiratory therapists who attempted to administer treatments, and on one occasion he bit a medical resident attempting to examine him. The hospital team was divided in their opinions as to the source of Brandon's oppositional and, at times, aggressive behavior. Some of the pediatric residents were convinced that the parents, who were in the midst of a divorce, were inconsistent in their discipline and failed to punish Brandon for his aggressive behaviors. At the residents' urging, a request was made by the attending pediatric pulmonologist for a psychological consultation, with the stated primary goal of assisting the parents in "more appropriate parenting, discipline, and limit setting" with the patient.

Upon the consultant's arrival on the unit, two of the residents approached the psychologist to voice their perspective that the parents needed to be firmer in employing consequences for the patient's difficult and uncooperative behaviors. However, the nurse assigned to Brandon observed the mother to be quite nurturing and appropriate in limit setting. Brandon was an only child, and his parents reported him to be a somewhat shy but happy child with no premorbid developmental, behavioral, or adjustment difficulties. They did note that he had never been comfortable going to his pediatrician and that the recent painful antibiotic injections had made him even more fearful of doctors. The parents admitted feeling overwhelmed at learning of their son's diagnosis with a chronic, genetic, potentially life-shortening illness with involved daily treatments.

Brandon's mother completed the Behavior Assessment System for Children (BASC-2; Reynolds & Kamphaus, 2012), and Brandon's nurse completed the 25-item Pediatric Inpatient Behavior Scale (PIBS; Kronenberger, Carter, & Thomas, 1997). The BASC-2 revealed no at-risk or clinically significant elevations except for a slight elevation on the Somatic Symptoms subscale, which is frequently seen in children with persistent medical concerns. The nurse's ratings on the PIBS indicated significant problems with noncompliance, anxiety, and distress.

The C-L psychologist conceptualized Brandon's noncompliance and combative behavior as a phobic response to his painful injections prior to admission and his sense of lack of control of the numerous aversive experiences in the hospital. In a further attempt to engage Brandon, he and his mother were shown a video on a digital tablet of another child, close to his age, engaging with the C-L psychologist in medical play with a toy medical kit and puppets. Brandon was quickly enthralled with the child's play in the video and, during the course of the day, had his mother replay the video several times. He then requested to "make my own movie" with the psychologist and was provided with a toy medical kit and several puppets and dolls. His initial medical play was somewhat aggressive, but with the psychologist's gentle guidance, his play gradually evolved into several playful scenarios (e.g., nebulizer treatments, chest physiotherapy [PT]) in which Brandon revealed a surprising level of knowledge and understanding about CF and treatments, despite his uncooperative behavior since admission with most attempted physical examinations and treatment interventions. In his play Brandon was able to demonstrate how chest PT helped "get the mucus out of the trees" (bronchi) in his lungs. Also, beliefs and misconceptions revealed in medical play (e.g., that the "patient" had to have a procedure because his behavior was "bad") were addressed and corrected in the play process.

Brandon was given a digital copy of the video of his own medical play, which was recorded on a multimedia "coping cart" (Novotney, 2010), and then viewed by him numerous times over the next day. He shared this with a child life worker who continued to work with Brandon in medical play. By the third day postreferral, Brandon's mood and demeanor had improved dramatically, and he was fully, even pleasantly, compliant with all examinations and treatment procedures. The concerned pediatric residents were particularly impressed with the rapid "overnight" change in the patient, which led to an excellent opportunity for the C-L psychologist to educate them as to how overwhelming fear and anxiety can often manifest as externalizing behaviors (Albano, Causey, & Carter, 2001). Brandon's improved adherence persisted on follow-up at the CF clinic, where the C-L psychologist attended twice a month (allowing for a *collaborative consultation* interaction between the patient and CF clinic team), including through his parents' divorce. Brandon was viewed by the CF team as a "model patient," due to his pleasant and accepting attitude and cooperation with his CF care.

Medical play has a long history in helping children cope with hospitalization and aversive medical experiences (Bratton, Ray, Rhine, & Jones, 2005). In cognitive-behavioral play therapy, the clinician models adaptive coping statements, skills, and strategies. The use of medical play provided Brandon a natural and enjoyable modality that facilitated rapport establishment and joining between the patient, the psychologist, his family, and the CF team (Kazak et al., 2002). This was necessary to help him to overcome the fear he had developed from his aversive medical experiences, to employ cognitive-behavioral strategies to correct his misperceptions and erroneous beliefs, and to engage in mastery of skills needed to comply with his CF treatment requirements. The visibility of Brandon's improved compliance, mood, and behavior also served to provide the medical residents with a more in-depth awareness of psychosocial issues in pediatric illness and hospitalization.

Communication

In the busy, complex multidisciplinary setting of the pediatric hospital, there are numerous opportunities for misunderstanding and miscommunication between patient and family and members of the medical team (Carter et al., 2009). As a member of the collaborative team, the C-L psychologist must demonstrate and model sensitivity to all concerned: patient, parents/family, and medical staff alike. Indeed, in addition to the "five C's of consultation" presented here and in previous writings (Carter et al., 2009; Carter & von Weiss, 2005), one could add what might be called the "three D's of consultation," that is, diplomacy, diplomacy, diplomacy! The C-L psychologist's involvement is often invaluable in diffusing patient and family defensiveness and conflict, sensitizing staff to relevant cultural traditions and values, and reframing behaviors on the part of patient and family and staff members to improve understanding and communication.

Case Example 4: Matt

Matt was a 6-year-old boy in the cardiac intensive care unit awaiting a heart transplant due to cardiomyopathy. The initial psychological consultation was requested because of nursing and staff concerns with the patient's uncharacteristic emotional withdrawal and uninterest in activities on the unit. In the course of his hospital stay, Matt's condition declined further, and he received a ventricular assist device (VAD). Due to his level of pain, he had been on high doses of narcotic medications. As his medical condition improved, Matt continued to complain of pain, which the medical team felt was mostly driven by anxiety and "emotional factors." Matt was noted to be significantly less distressed when staff engaged him in distraction and activities.

In contrast, Matt's mother was concerned that increased activity would likely exacerbate his pain and distress and was reluctant to have his pain medication doses reduced and have him "being pushed to do things." The mother said that, during Matt's most recent hospitalization, her reports of his pain levels to the team were met with praise and encouragement, and she saw the present response as insensitive and contradictory. "Lots of rest" and refraining from activities was what she felt was needed. The cardiology team's "rehabilitation approach," in which daily functioning expectations were set for the patient, was in direct contradiction to the most recent hospitalization experience.

After some discussion with the mother, it became apparent that the rationale for this change of approach by the cardiology team had not been clearly communicated to the mother, who, when anxious and unsure, often perceived medical information and procedures very concretely. The C-L psychologist's discussions with the cardiology team revealed their perception of the mother's objections to increased activity as indicative of an unhealthy parent–child enmeshment fostering a dependent "sick role," contributing to the patient's sullen mood and withdrawn behavior.

Who are the crucial staff members with whom to discuss the issues? What is the most effective communication style to use with each person? What is the most effective mode of dissemination of interpretations and suggested strategies to staff members who are caring for the patient? These are key questions that need to be addressed by the consultant and are illustrative of the not infrequent lengthy, indirect, and nonbillable professional time needed in performing complex hospital consultations (Bierenbaum et al., 2010).

Consistent with the *collaborative consultation* model (Drotar, 1995), a team "care conference" was held. After reviewing the history of the noted behavioral changes in Matt and a rationale for the recommended increased activities, the psychologist presented a formulation of the barriers to the mother's acceptance of the need for increased physical activity that included sensitizing the staff to the fact that the patient's behavior was not atypical for his age, for the multiple stressors experienced in the preceding weeks, and for the wearying lengthy hospitalization waiting for the transplant. Staff members were guided in specific strategies (e.g., listening to mother's concerns, reassurance that Matt's pain levels would be closely monitored and activities titrated accordingly) and in appropriate wording for communicating recommendations to the mother, along with brief role play to increase the accurate employment of these recommendations. This conference led to improvement in staff appreciation of the mother's perspective and concerns, improved sensitivity and trust in the relationship between the family and the team, and greater receptivity to team recommendations for increased behavioral activation (Dimidjian et al., 2006; Jacobson et al., 2001). This, in turn, resulted in Matt's increased engagement, improved mood, and reduced complaints of pain. In subsequent days team members on the unit were observed referring to mother and patient in more sensitive and supportive terms, rather than characterizing their interactions as pathological. With this basic perceptual and relational shift, the trust process between parent and team was strengthened, further supporting effective communication and care.

Collaboration

Interprofessional agreement regarding the goals of consultations has been shown to be associated with positive ratings by referring physicians on goal attainment, as well as on provider, patient, and parent/guardian satisfaction with C-L services (Carter et al., 2003). True collaboration can present a challenge in the busy children's hospital setting, where it may be difficult to meet and coordinate with everyone involved in the patient's care. However, without collaboration, turf issues may arise over professional role boundaries (Goldberg & Van Dyke, 2000). This can be particularly true for nonadmitting support services such as C-L psychology and psychiatry, child life, chaplaincy, social services, palliative care, and so forth. The development of competitive hostilities over these issues can be confusing and distressing for the patient and family and can have an adverse impact on the quality of patient care (Ernst et al., in press). However, with coordinated collaboration, the C-L psychologist can often avoid the trap of trying to be "all things to all people."

Case/Organizational Example

The C-L psychologist, who was in the process of establishing a pain management program within the hospital, was asked to see a 14-year-old male with Ewing sarcoma to assist him in coping with pain that had not fully abated with medical treatment. When the C-L psychologist went into the patient's room, a child life student was just leaving. The patient and parent expressed confusion when the C-L psychologist informed them that the oncologist had requested the consultation to help with pain management, as that was what the family understood the child life student to be doing in suggesting that the patient draw pictures to help him with developing relaxing imagery and in teaching him "breathing techniques." The psychologist discussed the situation with the referring oncologist, who was unaware of the child life involvement as child life could see any patient on the unit without a referral.

The child life service chief and C-L psychologist met and had a frank discussion about the overlapping and competing aspects of their services and agreed that there was more than enough work to go around for both services. There was also acknowledgement of similar conflicts with chaplaincy and palliative care, which had both recently added personnel to their teams. The hospital medical director was approached and agreed to establish a task force of the various support services to meet and address the concerns. The initial meeting was somewhat awkward, in that many in attendance seemed suspicious that the effort was intended to undermine their particular service. However, tensions decreased considerably when all agreed that there was more need than could be met by any one service and that patients and families would benefit if the services could more effectively communicate and delineate roles and areas of expertise.

The task force agreed to establish a hospital-based integrated support services group (ISSG) and met on a monthly basis. Initially, each service gave a presentation on its history, mission statement, personnel, and so forth. The most useful device was having each service give a case presentation and discuss how its team approached the process of referral, evaluation, and intervention. Although this led to identifying areas of service overlap, there was increased appreciation for how the differing professions possessed unique skills that could enhance effectiveness of services if coordinated and integrated through regular contact and improved communication. This understanding resulted in the establishment of a more formal organization of the ISSG, regular meetings with case- and systems-level rounds, and the development of an ISSG document that was integrated into the electronic medical records (EMR) system. This directory catalogued the services provided by each member of the ISSG, as well as contact information and referral procedures. This type of delineation and collaboration, representative of a *systems consultation* model, has been shown to significantly reduce the conflict and territorial disputes that can have a negative impact on patient care (Goldberg & Van Dyke, 2000).

THE FUTURE OF PEDIATRIC CONSULTATION-LIAISON

If pediatric C-L psychologists are going to further solidify our value as "pediatric psychological hospitalists" alongside our physician hospitalist colleagues, we need to establish more evidence-based assessments and interventions for use in the hospital setting. Difficulties with recruitment of patients who are physically impaired or distressed, diversity of illness types, multiple intrusions and unpredictability of patient availability, lack of well-developed measures relevant to in-hospital treatment goals, and so forth make C-L–related research most challenging (Carter et al., 2003; Carter et al., 2009). More integration and adaptation of child, adolescent, family, and systems-level assessment and intervention methodologies and protocols used in other clinical settings, along with clinical innovation in the hospital environment, is called for to ensure that C-L services remain an integral part of comprehensive patient care. Other C-L initiatives should include establishing systematic data collection procedures on such variables as referral patterns, clinical outcome ratings, service satisfaction data, qualitative methodology, and assessing the institutional impact of increased integration of pediatric behavioral medicine into policies and procedures.

REFERENCES

Albano, A. M., Causey, D., & Carter, B. D. (2001). Anxiety disorders in children. In C. E. Walker & M. C. Roberts (Eds.), *Handbook of clinical child psychology* (3rd ed., pp. 291–316). New York: Wiley.

Barlow, J. H., & Ellard, D. R. (2006). The psychosocial well-being of children with chronic disease, their parents and siblings: An overview of the research evidence base. *Child Care Health and Development, 32(1),* 19–31.

Bierenbaum, M., Carter, B. D., McCrary, K., Bowersox, S., Katsikas, S. & Furr, A. (2010, November). *Factors associated with increased non-reimbursable activity for an inpatient pediatric consultation–liaison service.* Poster presented at the annual convention of the Association for Behavioral and Cognitive Therapies, San Francisco, CA.

Bratton, S. C., Ray, D., Rhine, T., & Jones, L. (2005). The efficacy of play therapy with children: A meta-analytic review of treatment outcomes. *Professional Psychology: Research and Practice, 36(4),* 376–390.

Butler, A., Chapman, J., Forman, E., & Beck, A. (2006). The empirical status of cognitive- behavioral therapy: A review of meta-analyses. *Clinical Psychology Review, 26(1)*, 17–31.

Carter, B. D., Kronenberger, W. G., Baker, J., Grimes, L. M., Crabtree, V. M., Smith, C., et al. (2003). Inpatient pediatric consultation–liaison: A case-controlled study. *Journal of Pediatric Psychology, 28*, 425-432.

Carter, B. D., Kronenberger, W. G., Scott, E., & Ernst, M. M. (2009). Inpatient pediatric consultation–liaison. In M. C. Roberts & R. G. Steele (Eds.), *Handbook of pediatric psychology* (4th ed., pp. 114–129). New York: Guilford Press.

Carter, B. D., & Von Weiss, R. (2005). Pediatric consultation–liaison. In M. Roberts & R. Steele (Eds.), *Handbook of mental health services for children and adolescents* (pp. 63–82). New York: Kluwer.

Cohen, J. A., Mannarino, A. P., & Deblinger, E. (2006). *Treating trauma and traumatic grief in children and adolescents*. New York: Guilford Press.

Curry, J. F., & Becker, S. J. (2008). Empirically supported psychotherapies for adolescent depression and mood disorders. In R. G. Steele, T. D. Elkin, & M. C. Roberts (Eds.), *Handbook of evidence-based therapies for children and adolescents: Bridging science and practice* (pp. 161–176). New York: Springer.

Dimidjian, S., Hollon, S. D., Dobson, K. S ., Schmaling, K. B., Kohlenberg, R. J., Addis, M. E., et al. (2006). Randomized trial of behavioral activation, cognitive therapy, and antidepressant medication in the acute treatment of adults with major depression. *Journal of Consulting and Clinical Psychology, 74(4)*, 658–670.

Drotar, D. (1995). *Consulting with pediatricians: Psychological perspectives*. New York: Plenum.

Drotar, D., & Zagorski, L. (2001). Providing psychological services in pediatric settings in an era of managed care. In J. N. Hughes, A. M. La Greca, & J. C. Conoley (Eds.), *Handbook of psychological services for children and families* (pp. 89–104). New York: Oxford University Press.

Ernst, M. M., Piazza-Waggoner, C., Chabon, B., Murphy, M. K., Carey, J., & Roddenberry, A. (in press). The hospital-based consultation and liaison service. In C. M. Hunter, R. Kessler, & C. L. Hunter (Eds.), *Handbook of clinical psychology in medical settings: evidence-based assessment and intervention*. New York: Springer.

Fritz, G. K., Mattison, R. A., Nurcombe, H., & Spirito, A. (1993). *Child and adolescent mental health consultation in hospitals, schools, and courts*. Washington, DC: American Psychiatric Press.

Goldberg, R. J., & Van Dyke, C. (2000). Consultation psychiatry in the general hospital. In H. H. Goldman (Ed.), *Review of general psychiatry* (5th ed., pp. 522–529). Columbus, OH: McGraw-Hill.

Greco, L. A., & Hayes, S. C. (2008). *Acceptance and mindfulness treatments for children and adolescents: A practitioner's guide*. Oakland, CA: New Harbinger.

Harbeck-Weber, C., Fisher, J. L., & Dittner, C. A. (2003). Promoting coping and enhancing adaptation to illness. In M. C. Roberts (Ed.), *Handbook of pediatric psychology* (3rd ed., pp. 99–118). New York: Guilford Press.

Hayes, S. C., Luoma, J. B., Bond, F. W., Masuda, A., & Lillis, J. (2006). Acceptance and commitment therapy: Model, processes, and outcomes. *Behaviour Research and Therapy, 44(1),* 1–25.

Jacobson, N. S., Martell, C. R., & Dimidjian, S. (2001). Behavioral activation treatment for depression: Returning to contextual roots. *Clinical Psychology: Science and Practice, 8*(3), 255–270.

Kazak, A. E., Schneider, S., & Kassam-Adams, N. (2009). Pediatric medical traumatic stress. In M. C. Roberts & R. G. Steele (Eds.), *Handbook of pediatric psychology* (4th ed., pp. 205–215). New York: Guilford Press.

Kazak, A. E., Sims, S., & Rourke, T. (2002). Family systems practice in pediatric psychology. *Journal of Pediatric Psychology, 27,* 133–143.

Kendall, P. C., Furr, J. M, & Podell, J. L. (2010). Child-focused treatment of anxiety. In J. R. Weisz & A. E. Kazdin (Eds.), *Evidence-based psychotherapies for children and adolescents* (2nd ed., pp. 45–60). New York: Guilford Press.

Kishi, Y., Meller, W. H., Kathol, R. G., & Swigart, S. E. (2004). Factors affecting the relationship between the timing of psychiatric consultation and general hospital length of stay. *Psychosomatics, 45*(6), 470–476.

Koocher, G. P., Curtiss, E. K., Pollin, I. S., & Patton, K. E. (2001). Medical crisis counseling in a health maintenance organization: Preventive intervention. *Professional Psychology: Research and Practice, 32*(1), 52–58.

Kronenberger, W. G., Carter, B. D., & Thomas, D. (1997). Assessment of behavior problems in pediatric inpatient settings: Development of the Pediatric Inpatient Behavior Scale (PIBS). *Children's Health Care, 26,* 211–232.

Meltzer, L. J., & Mindell, J. A. (2009). Pediatric sleep. In M. C. Roberts and R. G. Steele (Eds.), *Handbook of pediatric psychology* (4th ed., pp. 491–507). New York: Guilford Press.

Novotney, A. (2010). Lights, camera, action: Children with chronic illness star in their own videos thanks to this pediatric psychologist. *American Psychological Association Monitor, 65*(4), 58–60.

Powers, S. W., Jones, J. S., & Jones, B. A. (2005). Behavioral and cognitive-behavioral interventions with pediatric populations. *Clinical Child Psychology and Psychiatry, 10*(1), 65–77.

Reynolds, C. R., & Kamphaus, R. W. (2012). *Behavior Assessment System for Children* (2nd ed.). San Antonio, TX: Pearson.

Silverman, W. K., & Pina, A. A. (2008). Psychosocial treatments for phobic and anxiety disorders. In R. G. Steele, T. D. Elkin, & M. C. Roberts (Eds.), *Handbook of evidence-based therapies for children and adolescents: Bridging science and practice* (pp. 65–82). New York: Springer.

Society of Hospital Medicine. (2009). *Board of the Society of Hospital Medicine.* Retrieved from *www.hospitalmedicine.org.*

Spirito, A., & Kazak, A. E. (2006). *Effective and emerging treatments in pediatric psychology.* New York: Oxford University Press.

CHAPTER 6

Pediatric Psychology Practice in Primary Care Settings

TERRY STANCIN

LYNNE STURM

LISA Y. RAMIREZ

The medical setting that most children in the United States and Europe visit is not a hospital or specialty clinic but an outpatient primary care office or clinic. The primary care setting serves as the "medical home" for a child, with activities that focus on prevention of illness (e.g., vaccines, screening), health and wellness (e.g., developmentally targeted anticipatory guidance), and consequences of chronic health conditions. In the United States, primary care providers (PCPs) for children and adolescents are usually general pediatricians and family medicine physicians or advanced practice nurses, nurse practitioners, and physician assistants. In the medical home framework, the PCP serves as the health care coordinator of all the care that the patient receives, including behavioral health (Stancin, Perrin, & Ramirez, 2009; Stancin & Perrin, in press).

For a variety of reasons, including the adoption of the medical home model, there is growing interest in provision of behavioral health services in primary care settings. First, child behavior and developmental problems are prevalent and represent some of the most common concerns of parents seeking pediatric care. Yet most behavioral health problems and some developmental problems are not identified, and even those that are referred are unlikely to ever reach a mental health professional when referrals are made to outside providers. Because children are seen routinely in primary care, there are ample opportunities to screen and intervene early, often before problems become more severe. The primary care setting may be a less stigmatizing setting for some families who are otherwise reluctant to seek mental health services. Moreover, there is emerging evidence that behavioral health services that are coordinated with medical care can improve health outcomes and reduce costs (Stancin & Perrin, in press).

Imagine a pediatric primary care clinic and the following concerning case scenarios:

> While in the waiting room, the mother of a 24-month-old boy completes a general developmental screening checklist and an autism questionnaire, and results suggest possible communication and autistic-spectrum concerns. However, the pediatrician suspects that the mother misunderstood the autism questions and takes a "watch-and-wait" approach, recommending rescreening in 3 months to see whether language skills have improved.

> During a well-child visit for siblings ages 3 and 5 years, the older brother begins hitting and threatening to bite his sister when she wants to play with his toy. The single father reports that he has a difficult time controlling his son at home and appears to be stressed and exhausted as he describes feeling overwhelmed by the boy's behaviors. The pediatrician provides the father with a phone number to the hospital's outpatient child behavioral health clinic, where the wait for an intake appointment is typically 6–8 weeks.

> A 14-year-old girl is seen by her pediatrician for concerns related to poor sleep habits. The teenager has difficulty falling asleep, is difficult to wake in the morning, and feels tired throughout the day. She feels less energy to do the things she used to like to do, including playing with friends and eating dinner with the family. The physician recommends 3 milligrams of melatonin before her typical bedtime. As the family is leaving, the girl mentions to her physician that she feels sad and worried at night as she thinks about school the next day and the group of girls that frequently make fun of her for being overweight. Unsure of how to respond and under pressure to see the next patient, her physician suggests making a follow-up appointment in 6 weeks to discuss the girl's concerns.

The cases outlined here represent examples of missed opportunities for interventions in primary care. They are pulled from our personal experiences and are not uncommon, likely because there are few psychologists or other behavioral health providers in most pediatric primary care clinics

(Stancin et al., 2009). Parents often express willingness to meet with a psychologist during pediatric clinic visits but are less likely to follow through with referrals to outside agencies (Kolko, Campo, Kilbourne, & Kelleher, 2012).

The purpose of this chapter is to review models of collaborative practice and to provide examples of how pediatric psychologists can provide "value-added" services in primary care. Case examples of direct psychological services to families and consultation services to health care providers complement discussion of psychologists' potential roles at the macrosystems and clinic levels. The latter include program development and quality improvement projects, as well as establishment of clinical service protocols, research collaboration, and outcome evaluations. A theme throughout the discussion is how the unique training of pediatric psychologists positions the profession to assume leadership roles in health care service model development, in addition to the more familiar, and highly valued, role of clinical service provision.

MODELS OF
COLLABORATIVE/INTEGRATED PRACTICE

Behavioral health services in primary care can vary considerably in terms of the level of integration and collaboration (Collins, Hewson, Munger, & Wade, 2010). At the least integrated level, primary care and behavioral health practices have separate and distinct services and treatment plans. Basic collaborative models involve colocated but separate services: separate treatment plans but with some routine sharing of information about patient matters. Colocation signifies proximity of mental health providers but does not necessarily include integration. For example, a psychologist who is located in the same building or office suite with a primary care practice can offer greater accessibility to families but have a completely separate practice. This may mean that families can schedule a behavioral health appointment before they leave their medical visit instead of having to call a separate division. Additionally, families may feel more comfortable returning to a familiar clinic instead of having to navigate a different department.

Collaborative care models imply a greater degree of interdisciplinary and coordinated patient care, usually directed toward children with behavioral or developmental needs and/or chronic health conditions, with providers who may or may not be part of the same office staff. Collaboration may occur without colocation as long as it involves accessible and ongoing communication between providers. Families often report feeling comforted and supported knowing that their various providers are able to communicate with each other and contribute to ongoing treatment planning. Interdisciplinary collaboration and coordination are especially helpful in cases in which there are complex and bidirectional medical and social issues to be addressed. One example is that of a school-age child diagnosed with a degenerative muscle disorder who was struggling with toilet training. During this child's primary care visit, the team of physicians and a consulting psychologist worked together to create a reasonable toilet training plan based on developmental and medical needs.

Fully integrated care implies that mental health services are a component of primary care, offered to children with and without mental health diagnoses. Behavioral health providers are part of the professional staff, writing notes in the same medical record, participating in staff meetings, and benefiting from full staff support for scheduling, billing, and so forth. A fully integrated practice is one in which all services are merged: one reception area, one appointment system, one visit to address all needs, and one treatment plan. There is integrated funding, one governing board, and a fully integrated health record. Psychologists in integrated practices tend to have larger client loads than in traditional practices, offset by more flexible time limits, briefer treatments, and open-ended treatment plans (i.e., treatment as needed over time). In this model, many barriers to accessing mental health care are alleviated, and families will often see medical staff and psychologists during the same visit to address ongoing problems. At times, two providers, such as a pediatrician and a psychologist, will conduct joint interviews or family interventions. For example, a preschool-age child diagnosed with failure to thrive may be seen in a single visit by the PCP, a nutritionist, and a psychologist who is working with the family on behavioral interventions to introduce healthy foods.

Pediatric psychologists have specialized training that bridges gaps between child and adolescent psychosocial assessment and intervention and health/medical issues and disorders. They are trained to understand the bidirectional influences of psychosocial stress and health and to intervene at the appropriate individual or familial level. Examples include stress-induced insomnia and weight loss, decline of adherence to medical regimens during adolescence, delayed toilet training, stress-induced or -exacerbated gastrointestinal pain, food aversions, medical-procedure-related trauma, and lead-exposure-related neurocognitive deficits. In addition, pediatric psychologists appreciate the importance of prevention and early intervention with subthreshold symptoms that may not yet meet the level of a psychiatric diagnosis.

INTEGRATED CARE MODELS

Health care reform legislation provides for expanded health care coverage and new opportunities for integrated primary care while preserving mental health parity and coverage. Reform approaches embrace patient-centered medical home (PCMH) and accountable care organization (ACO) models that emphasize interprofessional practice. In fact, PCMH and ACO models carry with them the potential for increased demand for pediatric psychologists due to the expectation for behavioral health care services (Hunter & Goodie, 2010; Rozensky & Janicke, 2012). The American Psychological Association (APA) is represented on the executive committee of the Patient-Centered Primary Care Collaborative and encourages the integration of evidence-based, culturally appropriate behavioral health into primary care (American Psychological Association, 2011).

When psychologists are part of the primary care team, there is less demand on the medical provider to actively consult a separate service for behavioral health concerns. One example is a young girl diagnosed with phenylketonuria (PKU; a rare chronic metabolic disorder) who was not adhering to vital dietary restrictions. The psychologist helped the parents create a behavior management plan focused on mealtime and followed up with the family at every visit to adjust the plan. The parents, who had not been willing to seek outpatient psychological help in the past, felt supported and less stigmatized by the recommendations when the psychological support was delivered in the context of their daughter's medical care.

EXPERTS IN
PROVIDER–PATIENT/FAMILY COMMUNICATION

The best designed patient-centered medical care plans can go awry unless patients and providers jointly identify nondisease factors that might derail them (Peek, 2010). Pediatric psychologists' familiarity with health communication research and motivational interviewing techniques (Naar-King & Suarez, 2011) position them to consult with providers about how to explore potential interferences to desired behavioral change, such as unaddressed patient ambivalence and concrete, real-life obstacles to fulfilling a medical plan.

Consider the following case. The pediatric psychologist was asked to assist with a pediatric appointment with an overweight Hispanic teen that was not going well. The pediatrician was encouraging behavioral changes, including significant dietary modifications and daily activity. However, the family—and the teen in particular—reported feeling overwhelmed by what the pediatrician was "prescribing." The psychologist encouraged the family to discuss barriers to the proposed behavior changes and worked to create a manageable plan that the family believed they could implement. Specifically, the family felt that they could focus initially on eliminating junk food with success and asked to postpone implementing daily activity. At a return visit 3 weeks later, both the family and the pediatrician agreed they were making progress, and the family did not feel overwhelmed by being asked to make multiple changes at one time. This example highlights pediatric psychologists' unique ability to help affect behavior changes in medical settings by working with families rather than following a traditional medical model in which families are prescribed medications and treatments. Psychologists understand ambivalence and can help providers work with their patients to address this barrier.

MAXIMIZING DEVELOPMENTAL AND BEHAVIORAL SCREENING

Central to primary care is an emphasis on prevention and early identification of conditions leading to morbidity and dysfunction; therefore, developmental and behavioral screening activities are integral in pediatric primary care settings (Stancin et al., 2009). Pediatricians have embraced the use of standardized screening methods, armed with knowledge that they enhance the detection of developmental delays and result in increased referrals to early intervention and mental health providers. With their considerable expertise in psychometrics, pediatric psychologists are ideally suited to lead the medical home team to identify and monitor children at risk for developmental and behavioral problems and to address less-than-acceptable rates of follow-up evaluation and treatment (Kavanagh, Gerdes, Sell, Jimenez, & Guevara, 2012).

For example, psychologists in a primary care setting serving mostly low-income families led the development of a two-step developmental screening program that included brief universal screening at well-child visits with standardized tools, followed by more focused but brief secondary screening when problems were suspected. During one visit, a young, pregnant, African American mother attended a well-child visit with her 20-month-old son and 4-year-old daughter. The overwhelmed mother reported that the toddler was becoming increasingly aggressive toward his 4-year-old sister, including scratching her face and pushing her down when he was upset. During the pediatric visit, the child exhibited these aggressive behaviors toward his sister. The PCP was concerned with the mother's strategies for managing his behavior, which included yelling and yanking him away from his sister in a rough manner. In addition to the behavior concerns, this toddler was not gaining weight at a satisfactory rate, and the developmental screening test was positive for possible speech delays.

The psychologist was invited by the health care provider to join the visit to discuss some adaptive behavior management techniques with the mother and to explore further the developmental concerns. During the visit, the mother reported feeling frustrated and burdened by her son's behavior, her pregnancy-related fatigue and nausea, and her living situation, which included extreme poverty and a dangerous neighborhood. The psychologist modeled basic behavior management strategies, including positive reinforcement of prosocial behaviors and ignoring negative behaviors. As the young boy responded well to the in vivo strategies, his mother's mood appeared to brighten. She expressed interest in learning more strategies but wanted to include the children's father. The psychologist provided the mother with a broad-based behavior rating scale and agreed to see the family for a follow-up visit the following week. When the family returned, the mother reported that she had noticed improvement in her son's behavior but was still frustrated with his refusal to eat and his temper tantrums. The psychologist provided additional behavior management strategies, specifically focused on feeding and mealtime, and reinforced the parents for exhibiting motivation to help their child regulate his behaviors. Results of the standardized rating scales indicated that the boy had more behavioral problems and withdrawn behaviors than were typically reported for boys his age and confirmed that his language development was delayed.

On the basis of the behavior and developmental screeners and the interventions initiated, the psychologist referred the child for speech therapy and early intervention services but continued to work with the family and PCP on managing his behavior and weight gain. Despite several attempts to transition the family to outpatient psychology services, the parents could not keep their intake appointments and were placed on a long-term waiting list. However, with the support they received in the clinic, they were able to help their son decrease his disruptive behaviors and began receiving in-home early intervention services for his speech delay.

BRIEF, PROBLEM-FOCUSED COUNSELING WITH PARENTS AND/OR CHILDREN

Often, a child will present in primary care with a mild problem that does not appear severe enough to warrant overcoming barriers to reaching a mental health provider but would nonetheless benefit from brief, focused psychological intervention. In one case, a foster parent brought a 6-year-old typically developing Caucasian child to the PCP to address the recent onset of enuresis. The child had been involved in a motor vehicle accident with his biological father within the preceding month. Since the accident, the child had nightmares, did not like to be alone in his room, and urinated on himself during the day. The pediatrician suspected that the child was suffering from posttraumatic stress disorder (PTSD) and suggested that the collaborating psychologist meet with the family.

The psychologist interviewed the caregiver and agreed that the child was exhibiting symptoms of a stress reaction. However, when the psychologist interviewed the child, it became evident that the child's stress was not due to the experience of the recent accident per se but was the result of having witnessed his father being handcuffed and arrested afterward for driving without a license. The child had not spoken with his father since the incident and was convinced that his father was still "locked up." Further, it was believed that the child had witnessed violence or traumas prior to the accident as well that may have exacerbated the stress response. The psychologist worked with the foster parent to facilitate a visit between the child and his father so that the child could be reassured that his father was no longer in jail. Additionally, the psychologist modeled and practiced several relaxation techniques (e.g., deep breathing and bubble blowing, guided imagery) with the child and his caregiver to be implemented as part of the child's bedtime routine. Lastly, the caregiver was instructed to devise a reward chart and to give the child a sticker when he informed his caregiver that he needed to use the restroom. When the foster family returned for the follow-up visit, the child had met with his father, and all reports of nightmares and fear of sleeping alone had remitted. Additionally, the child had stopped exhibiting enuresis. The caregiver expressed her satisfaction with the effectiveness of the intervention and requested further education about using behavior charts in other situations. The psychologist followed up with the family, and the child continued to function at his preaccident level. Because the case stimulated interest among the medical staff about PTSD, the psychologist provided an in-service seminar about child anxiety at a subsequent staff meeting.

It is important to note that although the child in the preceding example did not meet criteria for a diagnosis of PTSD, the prompt intervention he received in one visit likely prevented further functional impairment. This illustrates both the substantial benefits to the family and the cost effectiveness within the health care delivery system of providing early intervention with subthreshold symptoms, rather than waiting for a child to meet criteria for a "disorder."

PARENT PSYCHOEDUCATION GROUPS

Increasingly, group intervention models are being adapted for primary care, ranging from group well-child visits (Saysana & Downs, 2012) to parent education and clinical intervention (Stancin & Perrin, in press). Parent groups have been shown to be particularly effective when working with children with attention-deficit/hyperactivity disorder (ADHD) and disruptive behavior problems. However, intensive group interventions may not be necessary to produce positive effects in primary care. For example, written handouts given to parents in primary care settings have been shown to reduce negative behaviors in some cases (Berkovitz, O'Brien, Carter, & Eyberg, 2010; Lavigne et al., 2008).

In one clinic, a pediatric psychologist collaborated with senior staff pediatricians, the clinic's colocated behavioral health providers, fitness and wellness staff, and the clinic nurse manager to develop a program for providing group well-child visits for children ages 8–11 with a diagnosis of ADHD and their parent(s). During the planning stage, the psychologist reviewed models from other medical centers and participated in planning activities that included pediatric residents, wellness/fitness experts, and staff from a parent educational resource center into the parent educational sessions and child activity groups. She developed the parent satisfaction survey to document impact of the project on parent knowledge about ADHD. When a pediatrician in a separate clinic within the practice network decided to implement a series of group well-child care visits, the psychologist provided technical assistance.

FACILITATING EFFECTIVE REFERRALS TO COMMUNITY-BASED RESOURCES

Many children have behavioral health needs beyond what can be addressed by brief interventions in the primary care clinic. However, providing initial support and reinforcement of the need for additional services can help families ultimately receive the help they need.

For example, a psychologist was consulted after a pediatrician screened a typically developing 6-year-old Caucasian boy for ADHD following his mother's report of his problems at school and at home. The boy's home environment was chaotic due to his parents' recent separation. The pediatrician was having difficulty determining to what extent his symptoms were due to ADHD versus changes in his environment. The pediatrician requested the psychologist's help in determining whether the next step should be a trial of ADHD medication or a referral to psychology.

The psychologist joined the visit as the pediatrician began to interview the family about precipitating factors and triggers of the boy's negative behaviors. As the interview progressed, it was apparent that the boy was having an especially difficult time regulating his behaviors and emotions following visits with his father. He was more prone to fighting with peers and voiced passive, and sometimes active, suicidal thoughts to his mother. As she discussed her concerns about the recent changes in her son, the mother became more distraught and requested support to manage her son's behaviors and negative moods. The child then met with the psychologist alone and reported his anger toward his father. The boy reported that during visits with his father he often spent hours watching television or playing video games while his father seemed to ignore him. He denied having suicidal intent but acknowledged that he sometimes thought hurting himself would get his father's attention. Both the mother and child denied any concerns about physical or sexual abuse, but both acknowledged that the father did not have much quality time with his son.

The psychologist reviewed this information with both the mother and son, provided support to both, and suggested coping strategies for dealing with stress and negative emotions. The psychologist and family agreed on a plan to ensure the boy's safety, and the psychologist referred the family to a local community mental health agency for ongoing psychological support. All agreed that he did not meet criteria for ADHD. Because the wait list at the mental health center was 3–4 weeks, the psychologist offered to see the family until an intake could be completed. By the second visit, the mother felt that she better understood the source of her son's negative behaviors, and the boy's suicidal ideations had disappeared. However, he still experienced significant feelings of resentment toward his father. Once the family was assigned to an intake worker at the mental health agency, the psychologist obtained a release of information to share information with the agency staff, and the family was successfully transitioned to long-term therapy.

CONSULTATION TO FAMILIES AND PCP

Sometimes the psychologist's intervention is by consultation to the pediatrician and supportive guidance to the family. Illustrative of this point is the case of a 14-year-old African American boy whose family reported increasing oppositional behavior, especially when he was told to do his schoolwork. The family had recently relocated from another state and were concerned that he had become more withdrawn as well. The pediatrician had discussed with the parents behavior management techniques to increase his homework productivity but was feeling ineffectual at helping the family with problem solving around the child's negative attitude at home. The pediatrician requested help generating ideas from the psychologist, who encouraged the pediatrician to explore the boy's avoidance of schoolwork. Subsequently, the boy shared that he felt "stupid" and did not learn as quickly as other students. Academic expectations in his new school were more advanced than at his old school, and he was afraid that he could not do the work. The teen reported that he often forgot much of what he had learned earlier in the day in school and that struggling through his home-work made him angry and embarrassed. The parents were surprised to hear that he was struggling in school and were not aware that he felt that he was doing poorly in his classes.

The psychologist encouraged the parents to request a meeting with and progress reports from their son's teachers to monitor his progress and also to request a formal academic evaluation. The pediatrician and the psychol-ogist provided guidance for parents in assisting him with his homework and frustration. Additionally, the parents were discouraged from applying negative consequences for incomplete homework until they were able to get clarification from the school on their son's functioning. Following the psy-chologist's recommendation, the pediatrician scheduled a follow-up visit and offered to help the family request a school evaluation. After the family left, the pediatrician reported feeling satisfied with the advice he was able to give the family and expressed appreciation for his consultation with the psychologist.

IDENTIFICATION OF COMMUNITY RESOURCES

In addition to providing direct intervention, primary care psychologists can help direct patients to appropriate community resources or coordinate pediatric care with colocated services. For instance, a mother new to the region arrived to the clinic for a primary care visit with her 8-year-old son with autism. He had had an established individualized education plan at his former school, but the mother had been unsuccessful at having accom-modations reinstated in the new school. Additionally, her son's behavioral challenges at home had increased in severity, and this mother felt over-whelmed by his daily needs. The psychologist first referred the family to the hospital's onsite medical-legal service for assistance in obtaining edu-cational services. She then consulted the colocated representative from the local board serving children with developmental conditions, who met with the family to determine eligibility and enrolled the family in their in-home therapy program and school-based support services.

NON-SERVICE ROLES OF PEDIATRIC PSYCHOLOGISTS IN SYSTEMS OF PRIMARY CARE

In addition to direct service to families and consultation with fellow team members about psychosocial aspects of child health, psychologists can serve in important capacities related to program evaluation and collabora-tive research.

Continuous Quality Improvement

Psychologists can play important roles in the quality-improvement (QI) requirement of the patient-centered medical home model, including design and evaluation of behavioral health and developmental care programs in primary care. Psychologists bring unique research skills, interest in the use of technology to deliver care (e.g., text messaging, electronic medical record reminders), and ability to function on collaborative research teams (Nash, McKay, Voget, & Masters, 2012). For example, a psychologist served as one of two nonphysician members of an advisory team for a pediatric learning collaborative on developmental screening for a practice network. This learning collaborative conducted monthly phone conferences to support community pediatricians' integration of recommended screening into office practices. The psychologist collaborated with project staff to survey practice changes enacted during the collaborative, as well as longer term impact on physician behavior.

Collaboration in Clinic–Based Research

There is increasing awareness of the need for research on effective interventions to address family psychosocial issues, as well as child behavior problems, in primary care settings (Stancin & Perrin, in press). For example, a pediatric psychologist offered to serve as a liaison from a primary care clinic to a children's health service research team. During weekly research review meetings, the psychologist drew on her expertise and familiarity with the clinic culture to play a key role in instrument development, article preparation, and communication between the research team and clinic staff. In a second example, a pediatric psychologist served as coinvestigator on an education project that colocated professionals from community-based organizations within continuity clinics to teach residents and faculty members about community resources. The psychologist's prior experience as a nonphysician preceptor in resident continuity clinics allowed her to support the community professionals' acclimation to the unfamiliar primary care culture. The psychologist also helped disseminate the project's educational approach through regional and national presentations and a publication (Sturm, Shultz, Kirby, & Stelzner, 2011).

PROFESSIONAL CONSIDERATIONS

To meet the substantial need for behavioral health services in primary care, some primary care practices may look to community mental health (CMH) professionals and agencies for assistance. Despite the appeal of this notion, the training and orientation of pediatric psychologists differ from that of most community behavioral health professionals in substantive ways. For example, behavioral health providers in CMH clinics have training in traditional psychological models that do not typically focus on the influence of health on psychosocial functioning, and vice versa. Many CMH providers see patients who meet diagnostic criteria for a "disorder" in a regular outpatient setting with weekly, biweekly, or even monthly appointments aimed at improving psychosocial functioning. Pediatric psychologists based in pediatric clinics are prepared to consult with pediatricians or other health care providers who may want expert input on behavior, mood, or educational issues in an expedited manner for complicated cases but also for subthreshold symptoms. Further, psychologists are more likely to be considered coequal partners with physicians than are non-doctoral-level counselors, who most often staff CMH agencies. One caveat to the preference for doctoral-level psychological providers is the issue of billing and reimbursements. Although psychologists have doctoral degrees, reimbursement rates for services are often similar to those of social workers or non-doctoral-level counselors. Due to limited reimbursement rates and inconsistent ability to bill for services provided, it is important that pediatric psychologists communicate clearly the breadth of clinical services and professional collaborations and the intensity of intervention that their training allows. Many pediatric psychologists based in primary care settings will seek to enhance their base salaries with grant-supported activities and other forms of supplemental support.

An important issue for primary care psychologists is protecting themselves from getting overwhelmed and "burned out" in the clinic setting. In primary care settings, consultations can range from simple behavioral interventions to intervening with crisis concerns about psychosis and suicidality. Psychology providers should make it clear to the pediatric health care providers what types of cases they are willing to see and what cases should be triaged to another mental health service. Additionally, many primary care clinics may have social workers and child life personnel embedded within their staffs. It is important for psychologists to differentiate how psychology differs from both of these disciplines, both to prevent over- or underutilization of their services due to confusion of roles and to allow for complementary consultation and support between the disciplines.

One method for addressing frequent use of the psychology provider is educating the medical providers about brief and effective interventions. For example, pediatricians are well suited to provide basic behavior management guidance, but they may not feel comfortable or prepared to do so. Psychologists can assist physicians by joining their sessions or engaging in a role play to allow the provider to gain confidence in their abilities to intervene with appropriate cases. Greater skill and confidence by physician providers will free up the psychology provider for more complex consultations and ensures that the pediatricians are comfortable providing basic guidance, especially when the psychologist is not available.

Klonoff (2012) identified challenges for health psychologists in this era of "transdisciplinary practice." She argued that although psychologists offer unique and important contributions to leaders in other disciplines (research, health care, and education), we have not articulated a clear vision about what we do. She cautions that "If we continue down this path, over time we will have educated and disseminated ourselves out of existence, as myriad other health-related fields are happy to define what they do to include aspects of our skill set" (p. 2). The challenge for pediatric psychologists who adopt integrated care models may be how to strengthen the behavioral health skills of medical providers while claiming the expertise to handle complex consultation and the leadership to develop and evaluate innovative services in the areas of behavioral and developmental health.

CONCLUDING COMMENTS

Considering the rapidly changing landscape of health care, pediatric psychologists have an opportunity to play an important role in primary care settings. With training in research, program development, and clinical and health psychology, psychologists are uniquely equipped to navigate multiple settings and roles while offering clinical support and evidence-based intervention to children, families, and medical staff. Challenges to psychologists' presence in pediatric primary care settings include establishing a distinct professional identity within the clinic, providing justification for psychology services, and limited reimbursement and fees. In addition, primary care psychologists would do well to expand their professional identity beyond the individual clinic or academic health center to encompass roles in macrolevel health policy development that have impact on pediatric psychology in primary care. This could include involvement in advisory boards to state offices of Medicaid policy and planning and serving on federal grant review panels related to integrated behavioral health. Returning to the cases that introduced this chapter, imagine how much more attention, support, and potential intervention each health care provider and family could have received if the expertise and training of pediatric psychologists were available to them those days during their clinic visits.

REFERENCES

American Psychological Association. (2011, Fall). Health care reform proceeds toward an uncertain future. *Good Practice*, 2–5.

Berkovitz, M. D., O'Brien, K. A., Carter, C. G., & Eyberg, S. M. (2010). Early identification and intervention for behavior problems in primary care: A comparison of two abbreviated versions of parent–child interaction therapy. *Behavior Therapy, 41*, 375–387.

Collins, C., Hewson, D. L., Munger, R., & Wade, T. (2010). *Evolving models of behavioral health integration in primary care*. New York: Millbank Memorial Fund.

Hunter, C. L., & Goodie, J. L. (2010). Operational and clinical components for integrated collaborative behavioral healthcare in the patient-centered medical home. *Families, Systems, and Health, 28*, 308–321.

Kavanagh, J., Gerdes, M., Sell, K., Jimenez, M., & Guevara, J. (2012). SERIES: An integrated approach to supporting child development. *PolicyLab Evidence to Action*. Retrieved from *222.research.chop.edu/policylab*.

Klonoff, E. (2012). Why buy the cow when you can get the milk for free? *Health Psychologist, 34*, 1–3.

Kolko, D. J., Campo, J. V., Kilbourne, A. M., & Kelleher, K. (2012). Doctor–office collaborative care for pediatric behavior problems: A preliminary model. *Archives of Pediatrics and Adolescent Medicine, 166*, 224–231.

Lavigne, J. V., Lebailly, S. A., Gouze, K. R., Cicchetti, C., Jessup, B. W., Arend, R., et al. (2008). Treating oppositional defiant disorder in primary care: A comparison of three models. *Journal of Pediatric Psychology, 33*, 449–461.

Naar-King, S., & Suarez, M. (2011). *Motivational interviewing with adolescents and young adults*. New York: Guilford Press.

Nash, J. M., McKay, K. M., Voget, J. B., & Masters, K. S. (2012). Functional roles and foundational characteristics of psychologists in integrated primary care. *Journal of Clinical Psychology in Medical Settings, 19*, 93–104.

Peek, C. J. (2010). Building a medical home around the patient: What it means for behavior. *Families, Systems, and Health, 28*, 322–333.

Rozensky, R. H., & Janicke, D. M. (2012). Commentary: Healthcare reform and psychology's workforce: Preparing for the future of pediatric psychology. *Journal of Pediatric Psychology, 37*, 359–368.

Saysana, M., & Downs, S. M. (2012). Piloting group well child visits in pediatric resident continuity clinic. *Clinical Pediatrics, 51*(2), 134–139.

Stancin, T., & Perrin, E. C. (in press). Psychologists and pediatricians: Opportunities for collaboration in primary care. *American Psychologist*.

Stancin, T., Perrin, E. C., & Ramirez, L. (2009). Pediatric psychology and primary care. In M. C. Roberts & R. G. Steele (Eds.), *Handbook of pediatric psychology* (4th ed., pp. 630–646). New York: Guilford Press.

Sturm, L. A., Shultz, J., Kirby, R., & Stelzner, S. (2011). Community partners as co-teachers in resident continuity clinics. *Academic Medicine, 12*, 1–7.

CHAPTER 7

Pediatric Multidisciplinary and Interdisciplinary Teams and Interventions

CAITLIN CONROY
DEIRDRE E. LOGAN

Pediatric psychologists often work in the context of multidisciplinary and interdisciplinary teams. This model has proliferated in pediatric health care since the 1980s and is now frequently used in the treatment of many complex conditions in pediatric health care, including feeding disorders (Kerwin, 1999; Rommel, De Meyer, Feenstra, & Veereman-Wauters, 2003), weight management (Skelton, DeMattia, & Flores, 2008), chronic pain (Eccleston, Malleson, Clinch, Connell, & Sourbut, 2003; Logan et al., 2012), chronic illness such as diabetes (Beck et al., 2004), and physical rehabilitation (Chevignard, Toure, Brugel, Poirier, & Laurent-Vannier, 2010). The model is also being increasingly employed in primary care and preventive medicine settings (Campo et al., 2005; Kazak, 2006). Psychological interventions are empirically supported and cost-effective components of comprehensive care for many physical health conditions (Levant et al., 2001), making psychologists key members of multidisciplinary health care teams.

In pediatric health care, a multidisciplinary team (MDT) involves several health specialists (e.g., medicine, psychology, nursing, social work, physical, and occupational therapies) working toward an agreed-upon set of health outcomes with varying degrees of collaboration and coordination. Typically, each professional conducts an assessment of the child and family and develops a treatment plan that emphasizes the skills they can offer based on their professional training. Ideally, the information and treatment plans of each discipline are integrated into a cohesive and comprehensive plan of care. Often, the term *interdisciplinary* is used to denote a team that is not just composed of members of multiple professions but is one in which these disciplines work toward a shared set of treatment goals, frequently creating some fluidity of professional boundaries as team members collaborate to help patients achieve these goals. For example, pediatric treatment teams focused on encouraging symptom self-management (e.g., in the treatment of diabetes or chronic pain rehabilitation) are typically interdisciplinary in nature, because all team members may employ cognitive-behavioral motivational techniques to help children and families enhance their self-management skills. For the purposes of this chapter, we use the term *multidisciplinary* to encompass interdisciplinary approaches as well. In their description of multidisciplinary pain rehabilitation, Townsend, Bruce, Hooten, and Rome (2006) provide a useful definition of the multidisciplinary treatment approach:

> Multidisciplinary treatment . . . requires more than the presence of multiple disciplines that occupy a common clinical environment. Rather, multidisciplinary care entails concurrent treatment by multiple disciplines, often including physicians, psychologists and mental health therapists, nurses, physical therapists, occupational therapists [and others] who contribute expertise to the actual treatment planning, implementation, and follow-up care for every patient throughout the course of treatment. (p. 1435)

Navigating the complexities of specialized health care can be extremely challenging to families of children and adolescents with a chronic illness. The advantages of MDT approaches for these families include enhanced coordination and communication among health care providers, as well as a reduction in duplication of services, often resulting in increased cost efficiency (Shute, 1997; Townsend et al., 2006). In the age of family-centered health care, parents and other family members are typically considered core members of the pediatric patient's MDT (Rosen, Stenger, Bochkoris, Hannon, & Kwoh, 2009).

THEORETICAL ORIGINS
OF THE MULTIDISCIPLINARY MODEL

The concept of MDT-based pediatric health care is intertwined with the biopsychosocial model (Engel, 1980). According to the biopsychosocial model, an individual's experience of illness includes biological, psychological, and social dimensions. To treat an illness or constellation of symptoms adequately, therefore, requires health care professionals to address each of these central components of the illness experience.

The organizational psychology literature offers several other theoretical models that also inform the MDT approach to health care, such as cognitive resource theory and social identity/social categorization theory. Cognitive resource theory (Fay, Borrill, Amir, Haward, & West, 2006; Williams & O'Reilly, 1988) highlights the advantages of multidisciplinary approaches. This theory essentially holds that increasing the multidisciplinarity of a team results in an increasingly broad set of knowledge, skills, and abilities (or "cognitive resources"), resulting in better performance and innovation through cross-fertilization of ideas and practices. In contrast, theories of social identity or social categorization (Fay et al., 2006; Tajfel, Flament, Billig, & Bundy, 1971) reveal potential pitfalls that frequently plague MDTs. These theories highlight the inherent human tendency to identify with one's own group and to affirm one's own identity by distancing this "ingroup" from other groups (which become viewed as "outgroups"). Applying this model to multidisciplinary health care teams, these theories suggest that members of MDTs sometimes hold onto their identities as members of their professional discipline (e.g., psychology) at the expense of identifying themselves primarily as members of a specific MDT. When social categorization exerts a strong pull, it can threaten the integrity of the team, ultimately stifling collaboration and innovation in clinical care.

MDTs IN PRACTICE

To create an effective MDT, team members must possess several important skills. They must hold sufficient expertise in their own disciplines to make valuable individual contributions to the team. They must have or quickly obtain adequate knowledge of and expertise in the areas that represent the team's collaborative focus; for example, a psychologist on an MDT for children with diabetes must have a competent working knowledge of the illness and the aspects of diabetes care that cut across discipline-specific treatments. Finally, an effective MDT member must be committed to the team and have the requisite social skills necessary to facilitate ongoing communication with team members (Armstrong, 2009). In addition to individual team member attributes, there are a number of key components that characterize a well-functioning MDT (Liberman, Hilty, Drake, & Tsang, 2001; Nicholson, Artz, Armitage, & Fagan, 2000; Williams & O'Reilly, 1998). These include:

- Shared vision and goals: A unified, often transdisciplinary set of goals or patient outcomes.
- Integration: Sharing physical space, holding allegiance to a single program versus having team members who provide limited consultation or liaison to numerous programs. On a well-integrated MDT, individuals see themselves primarily as members of this team, with their own disciplinary allegiance secondary to this membership.
- Frequent interaction: Regular team meetings and other opportunities to exchange information related to clinical care and to promote team building.
- Trust and reflection: Good communication norms across disciplines, time and willingness to reflect back on both successes and failures in team-based care.
- Appropriate structure: Similar reporting structures across disciplines, healthy boundaries between team members, clear role definition, cross-disciplinary similarities in level of expertise and degree of commitment to the team.
- Competent leadership: A leader who can facilitate productive communication, adjudicate conflicts fairly, engender respect and trust, and provide strong leadership to the MDT.

In the current health care environment, there are a number of challenges to effective MDT functioning. External challenges include economic hurdles to offering coordinated MDT care, such as developing appropriate cost structures and obtaining insurance coverage for bundled services (e.g., Levant et al., 2001). This issue particularly affects the provision of psychological services in the context of multidisciplinary health care, given that mental health benefits are often "carved out" of patients' medical insurance coverage. Models of bundled charges have been developed in attempts to navigate this financial barrier to MDT care. The growing use of health and behavior codes in pediatric psychology (e.g., Claar, Kaczynski, Lyons, & Lebel, 2011) may also help address this barrier. There are also challenges that commonly arise within the team itself. For example, coordinating team members' input and negotiating conflicts around treatment goals or plans of care can pose challenges to effective MDT care. A strong and effective leader who models respect for all team members is crucial for effectively negotiating these challenges. Psychologists are often well equipped to provide leadership to MDTs given their skills in conflict negotiation, group dynamics, and other relevant areas of interpersonal interactions.

Another set of challenges lies in the realm of respecting boundaries and individual members' roles within the team context. Sometimes team members overstep boundaries and attempt to provide care that may be better provided by another team member. It is important for teams to communicate well in order to identify each member's role on the team and to be aware of areas in which there may be overlap in the provision of care. Team roles and contributions can also be challenged by real or perceived power imbalances within a multidisciplinary team. Traditional medical settings are typically very hierarchical in nature; in some MDT settings these traditional hierarchies can hinder effective team functioning.

THE ROLE OF THE PSYCHOLOGIST ON THE MDT

In the context of the multidisciplinary pediatric health care team, the psychologist can make multiple contributions. Perhaps foremost, the psychologist plays a lead role in assessing and treating emotional and behavioral factors that influence or arise from the child's health condition. This focus can take a number of forms in practice, including a comprehensive initial assessment of psychological functioning tailored to the presenting problem, assessments of behavioral change through the course of treatment, and periodic reevaluation (e.g., at discharge from an intensive program or at specified follow-up time points in ongoing care settings). In certain multidisciplinary health care team settings, such as pediatric organ transplant programs, psychologists' assessments play the central role in determining whether a patient is suitable for a particular type of health care procedure or intervention.

Psychologists on MDTs typically design and implement psychological or behavioral interventions to treat both coexisting psychological problems and psychological reactions to physical health issues (e.g., illness beliefs and coping responses). For example, a psychologist on an MDT for children with juvenile diabetes might implement interventions to facilitate adherence to a diabetes care regimen. Treatment might incorporate contingency management, as well as addressing anxiety, depressive symptoms, family conflicts, and/or other psychological factors that might contribute to nonadherence. Psychological treatment in the context of the MDT may occur through less traditional routes as well. For example, a psychologist and a speech-language pathologist might cotreat a child with feeding difficulties to address simultaneously both physical and emotional/behavioral hurdles (e.g., anxiety) to proper feeding techniques.

Beyond the obvious roles of psychological assessment and intervention, psychologists are uniquely poised to serve other important team functions. With their training background, many pediatric psychologists are well suited for roles in administration, program design, and program evaluation (Levant et al., 2001). Psychologists are uniquely well-trained researchers among clinical health care professionals and are thus usually qualified to assume a lead role in clinical outcome studies and other research endeavors in the multidisciplinary health care context.

RESEARCH SUPPORT FOR THE EFFECTIVENESS OF MDTs IN PEDIATRIC HEALTH CARE

A growing body of research supports the effectiveness of the MDT approach across a range of pediatric health conditions, as well as in the primary and preventive care settings (e.g., Campo et al., 2005; Kazak, 2006). Positive outcomes, such as reductions in cholesterol levels and body mass, have been documented following involvement in a multidisciplinary pediatric weight management program (Skelton et al., 2008). An MDT approach to pediatric functional constipation resulted in high levels of parent satisfaction and reductions in constipation and related bowel symptoms over a 16-month period (Poenaru et al., 1997). Multidisciplinary feeding programs show positive outcomes for a range of feeding and swallowing difficulties in young children (Rommel et al., 2003). Studies have shown reductions in pain and improvements in functional ability following comprehensive multidisciplinary pediatric chronic pain assessment (Simons, Logan, Chastain, & Cerullo, 2010) and with coordinated outpatient multidisciplinary treatment (Lee et al., 2002). Multiple studies document significant improvement in physical and psychological functioning after participation in intensive inpatient or day hospital multidisciplinary pediatric pain management programs (Eccleston et al., 2003; Hechler et al., 2009; Logan et al., 2012). Overall, a solid evidence base supports the utility of the MDT approach to pediatric health care for a diverse range of child health conditions.

CASE EXAMPLE: MULTIDISCIPLINARY TREATMENT OF AN ADOLESCENT WITH COMPLEX REGIONAL PAIN SYNDROME

Presenting Problem and Evaluation

Robin was a 12-year-old Caucasian female with a diagnosis of complex regional pain syndrome (CRPS) in her right leg. CRPS is a chronic pain condition characterized by persistent pain, typically in the extremities, as well as other specific features, including increased sensitivity of the skin, color and temperature changes of the affected area, swelling, and/or motor impairments. Robin's symptoms developed following an injury to her right ankle while playing soccer. Initial medical assessment did not reveal any fractures or tissue damage, and she was instructed to rest, avoid weight bearing through the use of crutches, and to ice her ankle as needed. She was prescribed narcotic pain medication by her local providers to use as needed. Despite these interventions, Robin's pain and sensitivity continued to worsen. School absences increased, and the family grew frustrated by the lack of improvement.

After a period of 2 months without symptom resolution, the family was referred by local providers to a tertiary care multidisciplinary pediatric chronic pain clinic, where Robin underwent a comprehensive evaluation by a pain physician, a physical therapist, and a pediatric pain psychologist. The clinic applies a biopsychosocial framework to evaluating a child's pain experience, taking into account the physiological, psychological, and social contexts of the child's pain complaints, and provides a similar framework for the treatment of chronic pain. Both discipline-specific goals (e.g., muscle strengthening with physical therapy) and interdisciplinary patient- and family-centered goals (e.g., increasing the child's ability to self-manage pain, improving school functioning) are considered in treatment planning. Following individual disciplinary evaluations and a team conference, the team members then meet with the parents and child to reflect the results of the assessment and discuss the treatment plan, which includes input from parents and children when appropriate.

Robin's medical evaluation was consistent with the diagnosis of CRPS. Her physical therapy evaluation noted muscle atrophy and weakness, heightened sensitivity, and intolerance to touch or weight bearing. She was using a walking boot and crutches to ambulate, further contributing to muscle loss and weakness and reduced range of motion in her ankle. During her examinations, Robin was compliant but tearful, with many behaviors indicative of pain. Robin's psychological evaluation described a previously high-functioning child with an anxious temperament. Since the onset of her pain, Robin's mood had become increasingly irritable, and her parents had observed increased anxiety about attending school, socializing with peers, or participating in her recreational activities due to fear of exacerbating her pain. Robin had no previous significant mental health history and no history of prior psychological treatment. She lived with both parents and a younger sibling, all of whom were medically and psychologically healthy.

As discussed in the chapter "Chronic and Recurrent Pain" in the fourth edition of the *Handbook of Pediatric Psychology* (Dahlquist & Nagel, 2009), there are a variety of treatment strategies to ameliorate the pain experience and restore functioning in children with chronic pain. Many children with CRPS, for example, respond to intensive outpatient physical therapy (PT) in combination with weekly cognitive-behavioral therapy with emphasis on increasing functioning and learning effective coping strategies for pain (Lee et al., 2002; Wilder, 2006). Given that Robin had not previously tried outpatient physical or psychological therapies, she was initially referred for PT multiple times per week and for weekly psychological counseling in her community. The combination of separate intensive outpatient therapies offered Robin the least restrictive treatment environment, which gave her the potential to continue attending school and to engage in peer and family activities.

After 3 months of outpatient treatments, Robin was seen for a pain clinic follow-up visit. Despite adherence to her outpatient regimen, she continued to struggle with intense pain and sensitivity, was not ambulating independently, and was unable to tolerate wearing a sock and shoe for more than a 10-minute time period. Robin had difficulty engaging fully in outpatient PT due to her anxiety about painful activity and her tearfulness during treatment. Because of limited availability, Robin was unable to find a local psychologist with expertise in pain management. She also expressed some resistance to engaging in psychological treatment, indicating a belief that her pain disorder was a medical issue and that she was not "crazy." Thus, despite a comprehensive outpatient plan, Robin's overall functioning was declining, and she was referred to the hospital's multidisciplinary day hospital program for children with chronic pain and associated disability.

Multidisciplinary Treatment Course

The multidisciplinary day treatment program offered daily individual physical therapy, occupational therapy, and psychological intervention, as well as group-based treatments, family counseling, and parenting support. A pain physician provided medication management and oversight of medical issues. Daily nursing support addressed wellness behaviors (e.g., diet, sleep habits) and provided case management. During a child's stay in the program, the overall treatment focus across disciplines is to facilitate a return to normal functioning across multiple domains of the child's life, including physical functioning, emotional functioning, school, recreation, and socialization. Related psychology-specific goals for the child include learning effective coping strategies for managing pain, adoption of an identity of wellness versus disability, and successful transition back to school; the goal for parents is to develop responses to their child's pain that facilitate adaptive pain management. To achieve these goals, psychologists play many roles within the treatment model. They provide individual cognitive-behavioral therapy and function as group therapy leaders, family therapists, and parenting coaches, all in collaboration with their multidisciplinary colleagues to achieve common treatment goals. It is in this last case that Robin's treatment differed significantly from her previous, discipline-specific outpatient treatments.

Robin was admitted for 4 weeks to the pain rehabilitation program, in which she attended five 8-hour days a week. Her days consisted of a combination of individual, group, and family-based treatment in physical, occupational, and psychological therapies. Robin initially presented with severe pain (9 on a 0–10 scale when moving) and significant deficits in muscle strength, muscle bulk, and tolerance to bearing weight or wearing appropriate footwear (sock and shoe). On her admission day, empirically validated psychological measures were used to assess Robin's physical, psychological, and family functioning, as well as her perceptions about her own capabilities and readiness to engage in a self-management approach to pain treatment. Her parents also completed psychological measures to assess their responses to their child's pain and readiness to engage in treatment. These measures allow the multidisciplinary team to shape the treatment of the child, as well as to collect information on treatment outcomes. Robin's psychological measures indicated elevated levels of anxiety; however, the levels were below the threshold of clinical significance. She endorsed high levels of pain-related fear and a self-perception of being disabled. Robin's parents also endorsed high levels of anxiety about their daughter being in pain and subjectively reported difficulty with observing their daughter's struggles. Their responses to their child's pain behaviors indicated a high level of protectiveness, a pattern that has been found to inadvertently reinforce pain behaviors (Walker & Zeman, 1991).

The course of Robin's treatment in the pain-rehabilitation program highlights the valuable role of pediatric psychologists on an MDT. During her individual psychology sessions, Robin learned cognitive-behavioral techniques for pain management and anxiety, including specific relaxation techniques (supported by biofeedback training), cognitive restructuring, exposure-based techniques, and behavioral reinforcement models. During family therapy sessions, treatment focused on specific parenting strategies, particularly reinforcement of positive behaviors and implementation of coping strategies, shifting focus away from pain complaints and pain assessment toward the child's functioning and progress and encouraging independence and self-management of pain in the child. Parents had the opportunity to rehearse these skills each evening when they assisted their child in completing their nightly home physical and occupational therapy exercise programs.

Despite Robin's initial hesitation about engaging in psychological treatment, she participated fully throughout her admission and progressed in her ability to implement psychological strategies for pain management. The inclusion of psychological treatment within a multidisciplinary model allows children and families to view psychologists as part of their medical treatment and has the potential for reducing the stigma of engaging in psychological counseling for what may be perceived as a solely medical problem. The inclusion of psychology also challenges the dualistic notion of chronic pain as either of organic *or* psychological origin and focuses on the complex interplay between the mind and body. The collaboration among the multiple disciplines actively demonstrates the biopsychosocial philosophy and the team approach to accomplishing common goals.

One of the many benefits of the MDT model in this case was the opportunity to rehearse coping skills in vivo in the presence of supportive clinicians. The success of this model can be found in one of Robin's more significant challenges with treatment: her ability to wear her sock and shoe. Robin had not been able to make effective progress on this goal with her outpatient provider and initially continued to struggle with this task during her multidisciplinary treatment. When asked to put on her sock and shoe, Robin would start crying and refuse to participate in the activity. The physical therapist working with Robin approached the psychologist on the treatment team for consultation, as this activity was a primary treatment goal and the first step in making other functional gains. The psychologist addressed the issue with Robin during an individual session in which she expressed her anxieties about the expectation to wear her sock and shoe for the entire day and her fear that she would be unable to succeed in reaching this goal due to increased pain.

The psychologist and physical therapist engaged Robin in a collaborative discussion about possible solutions to this problem, having Robin contribute her own ideas to the pace of a shoe-wearing progression. The psychologist added a behavioral reinforcement plan (see Figure 7.1) that rewarded Robin for her efforts with time spent in a preferred activity, such as playing a game, and introduced Robin to a basic diaphragmatic breathing technique to use during times of increased pain and anxiety. The collaboration among the physical therapist, the psychologist, the patient, and the parents (responsible for carrying out the behavior plan during the evening) led to a successful intervention.

Additionally, because the team engaged in frequent communication in the form of daily team meetings and shared space, the psychologist was able to act as a coach during Robin's physical therapy sessions for both this and subsequent challenges, assisting Robin with use of her coping skills in vivo and providing the physical therapist with extra staff support during her session for challenging patient-pain behaviors. Robin's parents also benefited from this form of collaboration. Parental presence during physical or occupational therapy sessions allowed Robin's parents to observe

	Monday (min) (pts)		Tuesday (min) (pts)		Wednesday (min) (pts)		Thursday (min) (pts)		Friday (min) (pts)	
8:00	10	1	10	1	15	1.5	60	6	60	6
9:00	0		10	1	15	1.5	30	3	60	6
10:00	0		0		30	3	30	3	60	6
11:00	0		0		0		0		0	
12:00	0		0		0		0		0	
1:00	10	1	10	1	0		60	6	60	6
2:00	0		0		30	3	30	3	60	6
3:00	0		10	1	15	1.5	30	3	60	6
BONUS		2		2		4		5		6
Total	20	4	40	6	105	14.5	240	29	360	42

FIGURE 7.1. Robin's sock- and shoe-wearing plan.
min, minutes spent wearing a sock and shoe; pts, points earned, at a rate of 1 for each 10 minutes. Points can be banked and traded in for minutes of a preferred activity (e.g., playing a video game, watching a favorite TV program, going online). Bonus points are added for utilizing a coping strategy during the sock-and-shoe time.

positive modeling of adult responses to the child's pain, such as the physical therapist's encouraging Robin to use active pain coping strategies. Her parents were also provided with the opportunity to assist Robin in her PT activities in the presence of her physical therapist and psychologist, who provided active coaching in positive parental responses.

During her 4-week admission, Robin's treatment team met daily to discuss progress toward goals in each discipline and overall treatment goals. Frequent communication and interaction of team members encourages cross-disciplinary education and collaboration. Each team member has received specific training in the treatment of chronic pain and operates under the same philosophy that the focus of treatment is increasing functioning in the child through active management of pain. Each team member reinforces this message by providing education as well as modeling during therapies through infrequent assessment of pain, reinforcement of use of coping strategies, and encouragement of positive coping statements. For example, physical and occupational therapists may ask a child to reframe a negative thought expressed about pain, as they have been educated about cognitive restructuring by team psychologists.

Upon discharge, Robin had made excellent physical functioning gains and was able to use coping skills independently to manage pain. She had gradually weaned off of the narcotic medications she had previously been prescribed to manage her pain. The treatment team participated in a school reentry conference call that provided the school staff with education from each discipline about how to help Robin attend school for the full day and manage her pain effectively in the school environment. The school staff was provided with specific plans for how to respond should Robin present to the nurses' or guidance office with pain complaints. She was discharged from the day treatment program with a comprehensive home exercise program designed to assist her in maintaining her gains and a self-management plan for managing any increases in her pain in the future. Robin continued to report some pain and sensitivity at discharge, but her functioning had improved greatly. On a measure of perceived functional disabilities, Robin's scores improved from a perception of herself as functioning at 38% of total ability at admission to functioning at 79% of her full ability at discharge. Clinically, Robin was endorsing fewer symptoms of anxiety, and her parents had demonstrated excellent improvement in their overall distress tolerance and reduction of protective parenting behaviors.

Although the multidisciplinary approach to Robin's treatment was successful in accomplishing Robin's treatment goals, the collaboration was not without challenges. At times, team members held disparate expectations for the pace of the child's progress. For example, Robin made excellent and rapid progress in her physical rehabilitation, achieving her physical functioning goals in a short period of time. Robin's achievement of psychological goals, however, was slower to progress, given the time needed to establish rapport and to learn and rehearse new coping skills before using them effectively. Communication among team members was essential in negotiating goals for Robin's continued stay in the program. Ultimately, success lay in formulating transdisciplinary goals, such as having Robin demonstrate consistent use of coping strategies while engaging in exercise tasks during physical therapy sessions and independently in the home setting.

Postdischarge and Follow-Up Course

Robin returned for a multidisciplinary follow-up appointment 8 weeks postdischarge that consisted of four 1-hour evaluations with team members from PT, occupational therapy, psychology, and medicine. Assessment measures administered at admission and discharge were repeated for ease of clinical comparison and data collection for research purposes. Each discipline evaluated Robin's progress and updated her treatment plan accordingly.

Following discharge, Robin was able to return to full school days and reported that she used her pain management plan effectively on a number of occasions, allowing her to manage her pain and remain in school full time. Apprehensively at first, Robin returned to playing her sports, implementing a gradual, exposure-based transition plan to help build her confidence and prevent injury. She also reported engaging in more social events since discharge, reporting greater confidence in her ability to manage her pain during social functions. Robin reported average pain scores of 3/10, and her perceived functional ability score improved to a perception of herself as functioning at 91% of her total ability. At the conclusion of Robin's follow-up visit, team recommendations included discontinuing the structured home exercise program due to excellent maintenance of her physical gains, continuing age-appropriate recreational activities, and utilizing her pain management plan for any episodes of pain. Robin was encouraged to continue using her active coping strategies for any further pain episodes, and her parents expressed confidence in their ability to maintain their own gains in providing positive reinforcement of her functioning.

One year postdischarge, Robin again presented for a multidisciplinary follow-up evaluation. She no longer suffered from CRPS pain in her ankle and was not restricted physically in any way. She and her family were pleased with their progress. Robin's perceived physical functioning was now at 100%. Robin had developed new symptoms of anxiety, however, and her parents discussed their concerns with the psychologist at this visit. Robin's anxiety had decreased with the reduction in her pain and improvements in her functioning at the previous follow-up visit. Since that time, however, Robin had developed worries about the health and safety of her family, and her parents reported frequent checking of the doors and locks in recent months. The therapeutic relationship between Robin and her treating psychologist that developed during her chronic pain treatment provided a positive model for the benefit of psychological services for other challenges. Robin and her parents were open to the recommendation that Robin attend outpatient counseling for her new symptoms of anxiety.

CONCLUSIONS

The case presented highlights the valuable and challenging role of the pediatric psychologist on MDTs, particularly the potential for interdisciplinary collaboration and the necessity of effective and frequent team communication. As demonstrated, the psychologist on an MDT must fulfill a variety of functions and possess effective communication skills to aid the patient and the team in achieving common goals. This can be a difficult challenge given the pressures of brief treatment, the necessity of maintaining role boundaries, and the importance of negotiating differences in treatment approaches, pace, and training levels across collaborating disciplines. As the use of multidisciplinary approaches to medical treatment continues to expand, pediatric psychologists have growing opportunities to collaborate with other specialists to treat a variety of pediatric health conditions. These valuable opportunities should encourage pediatric psychologists to implement their clinical skills across a range of settings and to hone additional skills to effectively collaborate and lead these innovative health care teams.

REFERENCES

Armstrong, F. D. (2009). Individual and organizational collaborations: A roadmap for effective advocacy. In M. C. Roberts & R. G. Steele (Eds.), *Handbook of pediatric psychology* (4th ed., pp. 774–784). New York: Guilford Press.

Beck, J. K., Logan, K. J ., Hamm, R. M., Sproat, S. M., Musser, K. M., Everhart, P. D., et al. (2004). Reimbursement for pediatric diabetes intensive case management: A model for chronic diseases? *Pediatrics, 113*(1), e57–e50.

Campo, J. V., Shafer, S., Strohm, J., Lucas, A., Cassesse, C. G., Shaeffer, D., et al. (2005). Pediatric behavioral health in primary care: A collaborative approach. *Journal of the American Psychiatric Nurses Association, 11*(5), 276–282.

Chevignard, M., Toure, H., Brugel, D. G., Poirier, J., & Laurent-Vannier, A. (2010). A comprehensive model of care for rehabilitation of children with acquired brain injuries. *Child: Care, Health and Development, 36*(1), 31–43.

Claar, R. L., Kaczynski, K. J., Lyons, M. M., & Lebel, A. A. (2011). Commentary: Health and behavior codes in a pediatric headache program: Reimbursement data and recommendations for practice. *Journal of Pediatric Psychology, 37*(5), 509–513.

Dahlquist, L. M., & Nagel, M. S. (2009). Chronic and recurrent pain. In M. C. Roberts & R. G. Steele (Eds.), *Handbook of pediatric psychology* (4th ed., pp. 153–170). New York: Guilford Press.

Eccleston, C., Malleson, P. N., Clinch, J., Connell, H., & Sourbut, C. (2003). Chronic pain in adolescents: Evaluation of a programme of interdisciplinary cognitive behaviour therapy. *Archives of Disease in Childhood, 88*(10), 881–885.

Engel, G. L. (1980). The clinical application of the biopsychosocial model. *American Journal of Psychiatry, 137*(5), 535–544.

Fay, D., Borrill, C., Amir, Z., Haward, R., & West, M. A. (2006). Getting the most out of multidisciplinary teams: A multi-sample study of team innovation in health care. *Journal of Occupational and Organizational Psychology, 79*, 553–567.

Hechler, T., Dobe, M., Kosfelder J., Damschen, U., Hubner, B., Blankenburg, M., et al. (2009). Effectiveness of a 3-week multimodal inpatient pain treatment for adolescents suffering from chronic pain: Statistical and clinical significance. *Clinical Journal of Pain, 25*(2), 156–166.

Kazak, A. E. (2006). Pediatric psychosocial preventative health model (PPPHM): Research, practice, and collaboration in pediatric family systems medicine. *Families, Systems, and Health, 24*(4), 381–395.

Kerwin, M. E. (1999). Empirically supported treatments in pediatric psychology: Severe feeding problems. *Journal of Pediatric Psychology, 24*, 193–214.

Lee, B. H., Scharff, L., Sethna, N. F., McCarthy, C. F., Scott-Sutherland, J., Shea, A. M., et al. (2002). Physical therapy and cognitive-behavioral treatment for complex regional pain syndromes. *Journal of Pediatrics, 141*(1), 135–140.

Levant, R. F., Reed, G. M., Ragusea, S. A., DiCowden, M., Murphy, M. J., Sullivan, F., et al. (2001). Envisioning and accessing new roles for professional psychology. *Professional Psychology: Research and Practice, 32*(1), 79–87.

Liberman, R. P., Hilty, D. M., Drake, R. E., & Tsang, H. W. H. (2001). Requirements for multidisciplinary teamwork for psychiatric rehabilitation. *Psychiatric Services, 52*, 1331–1342.

Logan, D. E., Carpino, E. A., Chiang, G., Condon, M., Firn, E., Gaughan, V. J., et al. (2012). A day-hospital approach to treatment of pediatric complex regional pain syndromes: Initial functional outcomes. *Clinical Journal of Pain, 28*(9), 766–774.

Nicholson, D., Artz, S., Armitage, A., & Fagan, J. (2000). Working relationships and outcomes in multidisciplinary collaborative practice settings. *Child and Youth Care Forum, 29*(1), 39–73.

Poenaru, D., Roblin, N., Bird, M., Duce, S., Groll, A., Pietak, D., et al. (1997). The pediatric bowel management clinic: Initial results of a multidisciplinary approach to functional constipation in children. *Journal of Pediatric Surgery, 32*(6), 843–848.

Rommel, N., De Meyer, A., Feenstra, L., & Veereman-Wauters, G. (2003). The complexity of feeding problems in 700 infants and young children presenting to a tertiary care institution. *Journal of Pediatric Gastroenterology and Nutrition, 37*, 75–84.

Rosen, P., Stenger, E., Bochkoris, M., Hannon, M. J., & Kwoh, C. K. (2009). Family-centered multidisciplinary rounds enhance the team approach in pediatrics. *Pediatrics, 123*(4), e603–e608.

Shute, R. H. (1997). Multidisciplinary teams and child health care: Practical and theoretical issues. *Australian Psychologist, 32*(2), 106–113.

Simons, L. E., Logan, D. E., Chastain, L., & Cerullo, M. (2010). Engagement in multidisciplinary interventions for pediatric chronic pain: Parental expectations, barriers, and child outcomes. *Clinical Journal of Pain, 26*(4), 291–299.

Skelton, J. A., DeMattia, L. F., & Flores, G. A. (2008). Pediatric weight management program for high-risk populations: A preliminary analysis. *Obesity, 16*, 1698–1701.

Tajfel, H., Flament, C., Billig, M. G., & Bundy, R. P. (1971). Social categorization and intergroup behaviour. *European Journal of Social Psychology, 1*, 149–178.

Townsend, C. O., Bruce, B. K., Hooten, M., & Rome, J. D. (2006). The role of mental health professionals in multidisciplinary pain rehabilitation programs. *Journal of Clinical Psychology, 62*(11), 1433–1443.

Walker, L. S., & Zeman, J. L. (1991). Parental response to child illness behavior. *Journal of Pediatric Psychology, 17*(1), 49–71.

Wilder, R. T. (2006). Management of pediatric patients with complex regional pain syndrome. *Clinical Journal of Pain, 22*(5), 443–448.

Williams, K. Y., & O'Reilly, C. A. (1998). Demography and diversity in organizations. In B. M. Staw & R. M. Sutton (Eds.), *Research in organizational behavior* (pp. 77–140). Stamford, CT: JAI Press.

CHAPTER 8

School Reintegration

Providing Consultation to Schools and Families

MELISSA A. ALDERFER
MARY T. ROURKE

Child development occurs through bidirectional exchanges between the child and others in the various social environments that surround the child (Bronfenbrenner, 1977). Second to the family home, children spend most of their time in the school environment, and schools are the major venue for the acquisition and growth of academic skills and for the development of social, emotional, and behavioral functioning. However, approximately 20% of children (Weiner, Hoffman, & Rosen, 2009)—those with chronic medical conditions—may be removed from the school environment for an extended amount of time or for repeated brief time periods over the course of their school-age years. These children face specific challenges associated with loss of instruction and the normative social experience of school. Children with medical conditions often require some special consideration at the time of diagnosis or of their initial entry to school, and a good number of these children will have evolving needs for school-based intervention as new cognitive, social, and emotional challenges related to their health history emerge.

CASE EXAMPLE 1: NOAH

Noah is a 7-year-old first grader recently diagnosed with a posterior fossa brain tumor. Only 2 months into his first-grade year, he has missed 5 weeks of school because of his symptoms, the diagnostic process, and surgical resection of his tumor. To finish treatment, Noah will need to return to the hospital 4–5 days per week over the next 8 weeks to receive craniospinal radiation and approximately 1 day per week for the next 15 months to receive chemotherapy.

CASE EXAMPLE 2: JORDAN

Jordan, an 11-year-old girl in the fifth grade, is a long-term survivor of acute lymphoblastic leukemia (ALL). She was diagnosed as an infant, treated with intensive chemotherapy, including high doses of intrathecal methotrexate, and, at the age of 2, after a relapse, received total body irradiation and a bone marrow transplant (BMT). Nine years later, Jordan has developed various medical late effects associated with her treatment and sees medical specialists every month. Jordan began kindergarten 1 year late due to her protracted medical treatment. During first grade, she had difficulties with attention, impulsivity, following multistep directions, and learning to read. Jordan began to hate and refuse school. Her mother opted to homeschool Jordan beginning in second grade. Now, near the end of fifth grade, Jordan's mother is having difficulty with the homeschooling process and feels challenged to understand and meet Jordan's unique learning needs. She believes it is time to transition Jordan back to school.

CASE EXAMPLE 3: BILLY

Billy is a 15-year-old in 10th grade in a small, private school. He has relapsed osteosarcoma, first diagnosed when he was 9. Billy's cancer has not responded to treatment, and cure is very unlikely. The focus of treatment is now palliative, and Billy and his family understand this. Billy has always enjoyed school and feels well supported by his school community. Billy has missed several weeks of his sophomore year but is eager to return to school and attend as frequently as possible for as long as possible.

CASE EXAMPLE 4: ROBIN

Robin is a 13-year-old girl who is currently being treated for non-Hodgkin's lymphoma. Her treatment is largely outpatient, requiring a weekly visit to clinic. Robin's response to treatment has been good, and aside from hair loss and some intermittent fatigue, she feels relatively well. She has been encouraged to continue attending school, with appropriate modifications and supports, and wants to do this but is feeling very self-conscious about her physical changes.

Effective family–school partnerships have long been cited as important contributors to child success (Pelco, Jacobson, Ries, & Melka, 2000). That partnership is complicated by the medical, social, emotional, cognitive, and practical issues that arise when children have significant health-related needs. The two-way family–school partnership must be replaced by a three-way family–school–health care team partnership, which requires communication, collaboration, and coordination to ensure a continuity of care that fosters the child's success in all realms. This effort is not just good clinical practice; it is mandated by law. Federal legislation entitles children with chronic illness to an education that is responsive to their individual needs through the Individuals with Disabilities Act (IDEA) and Section 504 of the Rehabilitation Act of 1973 (Public Law 93-112). Additionally, the Preventive Health Amendments of 1992 (Public Law 102-531) require coordination among health care and school systems in preparing educators for reentry of children with chronic health conditions into school.

Finding ways to successfully integrate and reintegrate children with medical conditions into the school environment as part of a multidisciplinary team spanning the family, school, and hospital is a role that pediatric psychologists are well positioned to assume (DuPaul, Power, & Shapiro, 2009). The aim of this chapter is to illustrate the process of school reintegration by incorporating the current evidence base regarding this practice with case examples. For coherence, case examples in this chapter are limited to children with cancer. Although some issues are specific to pediatric oncology treatment, the general principles of school reintegration are applicable across the broad array of most chronic or serious childhood illnesses.

THE PURPOSE OF SCHOOL REINTEGRATION

The experience of school, with its focus on education and child development, is an important complement to the medical care that children with chronic illnesses require to foster their health and well-being. School reintegration programs aim to coordinate smooth transitions between the health care and school systems in order to maximize the degree to which the basic developmental needs of a child with a chronic medical condition can be met.

Chronic illness presents several barriers to school return, however, and absences are common. Children with cancer, for example, miss an average of 40 days of school during their first year of treatment (Lansky,

Cairns & Zwartjes, 1983). Absences from school may be due to hospitalizations, medical appointments, and feeling physically unable to attend. Parental concerns about the school's ability to meet their children's medical needs, monitor their symptoms, protect them from possible infections, and handle potential medical emergencies can also influence school attendance (Shapiro & Manz, 2004). Sometimes the children's concerns about their academic abilities and the ways in which their classmates might receive them can result in missed school days. Further, schools may be reluctant to welcome back a seriously ill child.

The primary goal of school reintegration programs is to surmount these barriers and get the child attending school to the greatest extent possible. Both the medical and school systems strongly believe that getting a child back into the classroom environment reestablishes routines and restores a sense of normalcy, hope, and healing for all involved (Weiner et al., 2009). Indeed, in a qualitative study of 8- to 17-year-old childhood cancer survivors, involvement in education during treatment was described as "extremely important" and valued because it was something familiar and productive and made survivorship seem more likely. Over 50% of these survivors reported positive feelings about school attendance during their illness, with fewer than 20% reporting negative feelings (Bessell, 2001).

CASE EXAMPLE 1: NOAH

Noah's parents and the medical team are eager to preserve a sense of normalcy and routine in Noah's life and want his academic schooling—which had just begun—to start off on the right track. They have questions, however, about when and how much he should attend school given his risk for infection and treatment-related cognitive fatigue. Noah is not feeling well, but he frequently expresses sadness over not being able to see his friends regularly. The lack of daily routine is causing its own complications, and Noah's behavior is deteriorating. It is clear to Noah's parents, and to Noah, that attending school is important to his development, now and moving forward.

CASE EXAMPLE 2: JORDAN

As Jordan approached middle school, her mother became aware that she was no longer able to provide the level of instruction that Jordan needed. It also became apparent that Jordan's nonparticipation in school had resulted in missed social learning opportunities. At larger social events, for example, Jordan typically withdrew and was not able to forge connections with other children her age nor to ask for assistance from adults. Jordan's mother recognized that getting Jordan back to school was an urgent priority for both academic and social/developmental reasons.

Despite the challenges it brings, a return to school can be an important element of a child's recovery and continued development. For each child with a chronic illness, the larger goal of getting back to school requires a focus on three objectives: (1) identifying and meeting the individual needs of the child; (2) preparing school professionals to meet the child's educational and illness-related needs; and (3) working to ease the social aspects of transition back to school.

Various school reintegration programs have been described in the literature. Most are multicomponent programs outlining a series of steps or important elements to include in a comprehensive school reintegration program (e.g., McCormick, 1986; Sachs, 1980). Typically these approaches are based on theory and clinical experience (e.g., Worchel-Prevatt et al., 1998), and with few exceptions (e.g., Katz, Rubenstein, Hubert, & Blew, 1988; Katz, Varni, Rubenstein, Blew, & Hubert, 1992) they have not been subject to efficacy or effectiveness trials. Because of the variability inherent in each child's individual and illness-related needs and their family, school, and hospital environments, having a general process to guide reentry is more appropriate than proposing standardized content. Toward that end, we present a core set of components that are common to school reentry paradigms (Shaw & McCabe, 2008) and, using the pediatric literature as our guide, suggest a process that may support each component.

STEPS IN THE PROCESS
OF SCHOOL REINTEGRATION

Build a Connected, Collaborative
Family–School–Hospital Reintegration Team

It is critical to start the process of school reentry planning by building a collaborative family–school–hospital team. The team should be multidisciplinary, span the family, school, and hospital, and be capable of attending to the interrelated educational, social, and medical needs of the child (Power, DuPaul, Shapiro, & Kazak, 2003). Parents should be included as part of the family team, as should the child (at levels appropriate to his or her level of development). School team members may include the principal, school psychologist, guidance counselor, school nurse, classroom teacher, special education teacher, school social worker, and others. Finally, the hospital team should include a physician or nurse practitioner familiar with the child's medical needs, as well as a hospital-based psychologist and/or social worker. Hospital-based psychologists are well poised to lead such teams, and the roles and responsibilities of all team members should be clear. Further, the composition of the team should be stable, and mechanisms for how and how often team members will contact each other, as well as how often a child's progress will be monitored, should be specified. This process is very similar to the individualized education plan (IEP) process mandated by federal law and currently executed by public school districts.

CASE EXAMPLE 1: NOAH

As Noah's return to school began, the school nurse suggested that members of the hospital team be identified for collaboration purposes. Noah's parents were then supported, both by school personnel and by the hospital-based psychologist, in developing a team to plan their son's school reentry. The team members included the school principal, the school psychologist, Noah's teacher, the school nurse, a hospital-based psychologist, a nurse practitioner from Noah's medical treatment team, and Noah's parents. An individual in each system was designated as a point person, and it was agreed that communications would be circulated by e-mail copied to all members of the team.

Assessment: Identify the Specific Needs and Resources of the Child, Family, and School

A potentially successful school reentry plan relies on careful and comprehensive assessment of the child, the family, and the school environment.

The Child

Identifying the specific neurocognitive strengths and weakness of children with medical conditions requires a comprehensive awareness of the wide array of variables that will affect academic and developmental success. Certainly, assessing physical health, effects of disease, and treatment variables is important; gathering this information directly from the medical team will ensure accuracy. Neuropsychological assessment—particularly using measures that can be administered repeatedly over the course of the illness—can provide a standardized map to guide a team's understanding of a child's academic needs, though the feasibility of completing testing must be explored relative to the child's medical status.

Assessment should also include the specific social and emotional needs of the child as he or she makes the important transition back to school. Using observations and interviews, the team should collect information about the child's school history (e.g., levels of achievement, place in the social network, feelings about school before getting sick) and current feelings about returning. Understanding the child's current abilities (e.g., fatigue/endurance, physical abilities, cognitive abilities) and how they may differ from his or her own personal history and that of the peer group is part of this process. The opportunities for creatively and collaboratively gathering assessment information are supported by involvement of the larger family–school–hospital team.

CASE EXAMPLE 2: JORDAN

Jordan's school psychologist was concerned that the school, although expert at identifying more typical learning disabilities, did not have the resources to identify and understand the types of learning changes associated with Jordan's cancer treatment. A critical element of Jordan's reentry plan, then, was fostering a family–school–hospital collaboration to design, administer, and interpret a thorough neurocognitive, psychoeducational, and social-emotional assessment battery. The hospital-based psychologist conducted tests of cognitive, memory, and executive functioning and provided the school psychologist with information on the cognitive and social "late effects" of cancer treatment. The school psychologist conducted a thorough evaluation of Jordan's current psychosocial status and academic achievement. The two psychologists worked together to interpret the results and find interventions to match Jordan's current academic and social needs and her predicted trajectory given her illness and treatment experience.

CASE EXAMPLE 3: BILLY

Billy was very eager to return to school, and his parents and the school team were confident they could map out a plan to meet Billy's changing medical and educational needs. Of more concern to everyone was how to address Billy's emotional needs. He was working hard to stay connected to the people and things most important to him, while also moving toward saying goodbye. Effective assessment therefore included naming a team member (in Billy's case, the hospital-based psychologist, who collaborated closely with the school counselor) responsible for interviewing Billy and his family to assess their needs, concerns, and resources and for gathering information from the school team regarding needs and resources in that environment. The final planning for this portion of the reentry plan included a collaborative meeting of the school principal and counselor, the hospital-based psychologist, and Billy and his parents to put all of the information together and list the needs that an effective plan would address.

The Family

Uncovering a family's ideas about when a child might return to school and what that return might be like are critical to uncovering expectations that might influence school reintegration. Understanding parents' perceptions of support in the school environment, their current relationships with teachers and administration, and their specific questions and concerns will help focus portions of the school reentry plan. This information can be gathered by careful interview and should include assessment of a family's level of distress. Understanding sibling concerns may be an integral part of this assessment phase (Alderfer & Hodges, 2010).

CASE EXAMPLE 2: JORDAN

As the assessment phase of Jordan's school reentry plan unfolded, her parents shared that Jordan's sister, Tina, 1 year older than Jordan and a student at the school that Jordan would attend, was feeling uncomfortable about the transition. In a meeting with her parents and the hospital-based psychologist, Tina expressed concern that she and Jordan might be teased because of Jordan's visible medical issues and that her worries about how Jordan was doing would weigh on her mind during school hours. To address these concerns, the reentry plan included an assessment by the school team of Tina's needs and the identification of school resources to meet those needs (the school counselor would check in with Tina weekly in an unobtrusive way).

The School

Assessment must also include a consideration of the school team's needs, concerns, and resources. Though federal law requires public schools to be responsive to the needs of children with chronic illness, tremendous diversity remains in the resources available to individual school districts to accomplish this mandate. Additionally, private or independent schools are not subject to the same requirements as public schools and may be more variable in their approach to specialized education. In assessing the school environment it is important to know: (1) which school personnel (e.g., nurses, counselors) will be available to the child and how often; (2) the team's knowledge of and experience with children with similar medical needs; and (3) what form and level of ongoing support the school may need (and want) to support the family.

CASE EXAMPLE 3: BILLY

Although Billy's school-based team was eager to help and agreed to provide a creative and extensive array of accommodations, they were quite nervous about the course of Billy's illness. How long would he be well enough to attend school? How should they talk to each other, to their students, to Billy, and to Billy's family about Billy's impending death? A meeting at school among Billy (for part of the meeting), his parents, the school team, and the hospital-based psychologist was held. The psychologist facilitated a conversation to identify the school

team's concerns and to start to develop a plan and an increased sense
of comfort about how to manage Billy's needs.

Identify Appropriate Mechanisms for Intervention and Develop Tailored Plans

Once the team has been built and the needs of the child, the family, and the
school have been identified, the family–school–hospital team must begin
the process of matching interventions to a child's specific areas of need.
Although most often it is incumbent on the school team to take a leadership role in identifying available mechanisms, the process should be largely
informed by active and ongoing consultation among the family, school, and
hospital team members.

There are multiple intervention plan formats available to children with
special needs.

Individualized Health Plan

An individualized health plan (IHP) is a written plan of care that is developed by the school nurse, in collaboration with a child's medical team.
The goal of an IHP is to minimize any negative effects that a child's health
condition may have on his or her academic performance (Betz & Nehring,
2007). IHPs have no standard format but typically include health-related
accommodations that children may need in the classroom, processes to
deliver necessary nursing care and to monitor a child's medical status, and
a mechanism for the school nurse (or designee) to function as an informational liaison between the hospital and the school teams. IHPs typically
include considerations related to medication taking, special equipment,
environmental needs, participation in field trips or gym class, and so forth.
The best IHPs are organic documents that change with changes in a child's
medical condition and offer specific and informed guidelines for maximizing a student's ability to participate in academic activities. A well-planned
IHP is a necessary part of school reentry for all children with serious illness.

Emergency Action Plan

An emergency action plan (EAP) is often part of an IHP and is a protocol
that identifies action steps that school staff, faculty, and administrators
should take to respond to potential emergencies until emergency medical
personnel arrive at the scene. The list of potential emergencies (e.g., faint-
ing, anaphylaxis, asthma attack, extreme hypoglycemia), as well as the
medical/nursing responses, should be co-constructed by the nurse and the

hospital team, with input from the family, the larger school-based team, and the hospital teams.

Section 504 Plan

Based on antidiscrimination provisions of Section 504 of the Rehabilitation Act of 1973, a 504 plan lists accommodations necessary to help students with medical illness or other disabilities participate fully in academic programming and school activities. A 504 plan does not include specific goals for a child but instead documents how a school might make the regular curriculum and activities more accessible to students (e.g., use of elevator, extra time to walk to class, extra time on tests or assignments). To promote coherence and collaborations, 504 plans can include IHP goals (Betz & Nehring, 2007).

Individualized Education Plan

An IEP, mandated by IDEA for children with specific disabilities, is an individualized plan that sets educational goals for children and documents interventions that the school will deliver in order to help students meet these goals. Children for whom chronic illness interferes with cognition or learning may qualify for an IEP under the "Other Health Impairment" criterion. IEPs are evolving documents that assist school-based teams in addressing educational needs that are now different because of a child's health condition. Given the frequent lack of knowledge about medical issues among school-based teams (Barraclough & Machek, 2010; Kaffenberger, 2006), the standard school-based IEP team must be part of a larger family–school–hospital collaboration. This kind of collaboration also allows IHPs to be subsumed into IEP goals (Betz & Nehring, 2007).

Prepare School Professionals to Reintegrate the Child with a Chronic Illness

Although expert in the education of children, school personnel are not necessarily well informed about specific chronic illnesses. In one survey, 99% of school teachers reported knowing at least one student with a chronic illness; however, only about one-third reported receiving formal education about working with such children (Clay, Cortina, Harper, Cocco, & Drotar, 2004). Surveys of school counselors and school psychologists suggest that more than 70% indicate a need for more training specific to chronic illnesses to aid in their roles related to schooling children with these conditions (Barraclough & Machek, 2010; Kaffenberger, 2006). The types of information these school personnel require includes the educational needs of the child with the chronic medical condition, the medical aspects of the condition, its treatment, and the possible consequences of both. The best developed reentry plan, however, will fail to support a student if the school-based team implementing that plan is not fully prepared and supported to deliver it. Preparation should extend beyond the child's classroom teachers, nurse, and counselors. Administrative assistants, food service personnel, and maintenance workers, depending upon their role with the child and amount of contact, often play important roles in a child's transition back to school and need to feel prepared and supported to intervene and assist the returning child (Badger, 2008).

Information alone is unlikely to be enough to prepare school staff for the child's reentry. Staff/faculty preparation should include opportunities for real-time discussion, in which educators can ask questions, discuss resources available in the school for child and parents, and share their concerns (and their support for each other) regarding the child's reintegration. Providing ongoing supports for staff, including regular assessments of how the integration is going and what additional information or support staff members need, is an important element of the plan.

CASE EXAMPLE 1: NOAH

As the reentry team began planning for Noah's return, the school suggested homebound instruction. Noah's parents were worried about his safety at school but also felt concerned that homebound instruction would not provide their son with the social experience, structure, and routine of school. A teleconference was set up, and the nurse practitioner, hospital social worker, school nurse, and parents worked together to find ways to address school-based concerns about Noah returning to the classroom and to brainstorm staff education mechanisms. Potential medical emergencies were addressed, and appropriate responses were outlined. The nurse practitioner and the school nurse arranged for an ongoing regular weekly e-mail to share information and address issues related to Noah's medical care. The school nurse was also given a direct way to contact the nurse practitioner if questions arose that could not wait for the weekly check-in. Finally, a time was set for a nurse at the hospital and the hospital social worker to come to a faculty meeting to educate the team on the items of concern.

Prepare Classmates for the Child's Return

The return to school can be anxiety-provoking for all involved; effectively helping a child enter a school community can depend on working with peers to promote acceptance and to reduce misconceptions. Children with chronic illness are prone to social functioning difficulties; however, such difficulties appear to be minimal (Pinquart & Teubert, 2012). The misperceptions of classmates about the child and the illness, however, can influence peer relationships (Prevatt, Heffer, & Lowe, 2000). For example, fears of contagion and physical differences can lead to avoidance, neglect, pity, teasing, or rejection (Shapiro & Manz, 2004). Preparing classmates of the child with a chronic medical condition prior to the child's school return is an important step in school reintegration.

School reentry presentations typically include a combination of general information about the child's condition and also individualized information about the child's specific experience and needs. Effective presentations address the issues of concern to children with illness and their peers: handling changes in and reactions to changes in physical appearance, coaching social responses and how to engage the returning child in activities, and information on the disease and treatment process, including concerns about contagion and prognosis. Many videos and programs have been developed (see Badger, 2008, for examples). Using developmentally appropriate materials, reentry preparation can take several formats (individual, small group, parent–child meetings, school assembly) and should provide a framework in which children can ask questions and staff can address possible emotional reactions of classmates.

CASE EXAMPLE 4: ROBIN

Robin had no academic concerns, minimal absences from school, and strong peer connections, but two issues complicated her reentry to school. First, Robin's peers began expressing worries to school staff and to their parents about how to interact with Robin when she came back. They worried about Robin's prognosis, her changed appearance, and how to support her. Although a common school reentry intervention—a psychoeducational presentation to Robin's class or grade about her illness, return to school, and recovery—would have been a clear answer to this issue, Robin developed considerable anxiety and self-consciousness about her illness and refused to allow a standard reentry presentation for her peers. The hospital–school–family team met to try to formulate a creative solution to the dilemma, and a three-part plan was developed. First, the school nurse presented a standard reentry inservice to school staff, who were coached on how to prepare Robin's peers for her return. Second, Robin engaged in individual work aimed at giving her tools to manage her worry and distress and become more comfortable having information shared with her peers. Third, as her comfort grew, Robin worked with her oncology outpatient child life specialist to videotape a day in the oncology outpatient clinic from her perspective. Robin worked to edit the video and then presented it to her class. Although she was still worried about returning to school, she was able to do so with some confidence and mastery, while adequately preparing her peers.

FACTORS INFLUENCING
SCHOOL REINTEGRATION PLANS

Developmental Level of the Child

For all children, childhood and adolescence are times of enormous developmental change. The effects of the chronic illness on the child and the family, therefore, must be considered within a developmental context, and so, too, must the approach to school reintegration. Both the content and the delivery of the school reintegration plan should be tailored to the issues and learning process most relevant to the developmental stage of the child and his or her classmates. For example, younger classmates may have misperceptions about the cause of the illness and contagion and may react to the physical changes they see in the child returning to school, whereas an adolescent with chronic illness may have concerns about how the illness and its treatment may affect his or her participation in social pursuits and activities (e.g., dating, driving), and his or her classmates may have concerns about prognosis that are not evident at younger ages. These types of developmental differences need to be considered when developing a reintegration plan.

Phase of the Illness

Illnesses, too, have developmental courses (Rolland, 2003) resulting in varying illness-related needs and considerations. School reintegration is a process that should begin at the diagnosis phase of an illness, as soon as it is known that the child will be missing school (Badger, 2008; Weiner et al., 2009), and progress through the phases of the illness (Madan-Swain, Fredrick, & Wallander, 1999), taking different forms and meeting different needs. Shortly after diagnosis, for example, friends, classmates, and teachers from school may help children adjust to health issues through letters, e-mails, visits, videos, and Web-based communication, or the child may take part in a portion of the school day through a webcam. This can help set the social stage for the child's reentry into the classroom. In terms of academics, if admitted to the hospital, most children will be enrolled in a hospital-based school program that allows a child to continue to participate in the educational process. Once out of the hospital, the child may continue contact with the school and receive homebound services through which certified teachers come out to the home on a regular basis to ensure that the child keeps up with schoolwork. When the child is physically able, partial day attendance at school with accommodations may be the next viable step until full attendance is possible. After reintegration into school, it is important to modify the reintegration plan as needed and address any newly emerging issues for the child, while also ending interventions that are no longer necessary.

Specific Characteristics of the Medical Condition

Medical conditions vary in many ways and can result in vast fluctuations in both the child's needs at school and the way in which those in the school environment must be configured to respond to the child. The onset of a condition may be acute or gradual and may occur before or during the child's school-age years, allowing some families and teams to prepare for the child's entry into the school system (e.g., children with cerebral palsy, spina bifida), while requiring others to make urgent accommodations (e.g., children with cancer, traumatic injuries, diabetes; Wade & Walz, 2010). The course of a child's condition may be stable, may show a progressive decline in functioning, or may be variable with fluctuations in functioning (Rolland, 2003), and this must be considered during reintegration planning. The degree of incapacitation of the child, including physical abilities such as mobility and fatigue, and the degree of cognitive-behavioral impairment varies from one illness to another. Finally, the degree of uncertainty surrounding the illness, its course, and its prognosis may influence school reintegration planning. For example, traumatic brain injury poses a particular challenge because the symptoms are ambiguous and the course and recovery trajectory may be uncertain and extremely variable, with rapid initial recovery followed by plateaus, fluctuations in abilities, and, in some cases, emerging deficits as new skills are required (Wade & Walz, 2010). A successful reintegration plan needs to consider these issues.

Evolving Health Care Trends

Medical care is moving toward increased outpatient service delivery, and this may make programming for transition back to school more complex (Shaw & McCabe, 2008). Rather than a 2- to 4-week hospital stay, for example, a child with cancer may have a brief admission followed by 6–10 outpatient clinic visits over that 2- to 4-week period (Blank & Burau, 2004). That child will have no access to hospital-based school services and may have less access to hospital psychosocial staff to aid in transition to school (Shaw & McCabe, 2008). Further, children are returning home and intermittently to the classroom with ongoing medical needs and more compromised functioning than in the past. The parameters of the child's medical care need to be carefully considered when developing a reintegration plan.

SUMMARY AND CONCLUSION

Systematic efforts to support school reintegration have been developed for children with a wide range of chronic health problems, but most of the published work regarding such programs has involved children with cancer and brain injury. Generally the empirical support for school reintegration programs is limited, and concerns have been raised about the effectiveness of these approaches in improving child outcomes (Power et al., 2003). Comprehensive, multicomponent programs, targeted to the specific needs of the child, family, and school system, show the greatest promise (Madan-Swain, Katz, & LaGory, 2004). These programs typically include the following components: family support to maintain strong parent–child relationships and prepare the family for school entry or reentry; education of school staff regarding the child's illness and effective school-based approaches to intervention; peer education and support programs; and sustained follow-up to monitor progress and adjust the educational plan as needed. With a developmentally informed process that includes these elements, multidisciplinary family–school–hospital teams can create organic and flexible reentry plans that allow students full developmental engagement in the important activity of going to school.

REFERENCES

Alderfer, M. A., & Hodges, J. A. (2010). Supporting siblings of children with cancer: A need for family-school partnerships. *School Mental Health, 2,* 72–81.

Badger, K. (2008). School reentry for the elementary school child with an altered physical appearance as a result of injury or illness. *School Social Work Journal, 32,* 87–102.

Barraclough, C., & Machek, G. (2010). School psychologists' role concerning children with chronic illnesses in the schools. *Journal of Applied School Psychology, 26,* 132–148.

Bessell, A. G. (2001). Children surviving cancer: Psychosocial adjustment, quality of life, and school experiences. *Exceptional Children, 67,* 345–359.

Betz, C. L., & Nehring, W. M. (2007). *Promoting health care transitions for adolescents with special health care needs and disabilities.* Baltimore, MD: Brookes.

Blank, R. H., & Burau, V. (2004). *Comparative health policy.* London: Macmillan.

Bronfenbrenner, U. (1977). Toward an experimental ecology of human development. *American Psychologist, 32,* 513–531.

Clay, D. L., Cortina, S., Harper, D. C., Cocco, K. M., & Drotar, D. (2004). School teachers' experiences with childhood chronic illness. *Children's Health Care, 33,* 227–239.

DuPaul, G. J., Power, T. J., & Shapiro, E. S. (2009). Schools and integration/

reintegration into schools. In M. Roberts & R. Steele (Eds.), *Handbook of pediatric psychology* (4th ed., pp. 689–702). New York: Guilford Press.

Kaffenberger, C. J. (2006). School reentry for students with a chronic illness: A role for professional school counselors. *Professional School Counseling, 9,* 223–230.

Katz, E. R., Rubenstein, C. L., Hubert, N. C., & Blew, A. (1988). School and social reintegration of children with cancer. *Journal of Psychosocial Oncology, 6,* 123–140.

Katz, E. R., Varni, J. W., Rubenstein, C. L., Blew, A., & Hubert, N. (1992). Teacher, parent, and child evaluative ratings of a school reintegration intervention for children with newly diagnosed cancer. *Children's Health Care, 21, 69–75.*

Lansky, S. B., Cairns, N. U., & Zwartjes, W. (1983). School attendance among children with cancer: A report from two centers. *Journal of Psychosocial Oncology, 1, 75–82.*

Madan-Swain, A., Fredrick, L. D., & Wallander, J. (1999). Returning to school after a serious illness or injury. In R. T. Brown (Ed.), *Cognitive aspects of chronic illness in children* (pp. 312–332). New York: Guilford Press.

Madan-Swain, A., Katz, E. R., & LaGory, J. (2004). School and social reintegration after a serious illness or injury. In R. T. Brown (Ed.), *Handbook of pediatric psychology in school settings* (pp. 637–655). Mahwah, NJ: Erlbaum.

McCormick, D. (1986). Social acceptance and school reentry. *Journal of the Association of Pediatric Oncology Nurses, 3, 13–25.*

Pelco, L. E., Jacobson, L., Ries, R., & Melka, S. (2000). Perspectives and practices in family–school partnerships: A national survey of school psychologists. *School Psychology Review, 29, 235–250.*

Pinquart, M., & Teubert, D. (2012). Academic, physical and social functioning of children and adolescents with chronic physical illness: A meta-analysis. *Journal of Pediatric Psychology, 37, 376–389.*

Power, T. J., DuPaul, G. J., Shapiro, E. S., & Kazak, A. E. (2003). *Promoting children's health: Integrating school, family, and community.* New York: Guilford Press.

Prevatt, F. F., Heffer, R. W., & Lowe, P. A. (2000). A review of school reintegration programs for children with cancer. *Journal of School Psychology, 38,* 447–467.

Rolland, J. S. (2003). Mastering family challenges in illness and disability. In F. Walsh (Ed.), *Normal family processes* (3rd ed., pp. 460–489). New York: Guilford Press.

Sachs, M. B. (1980). Helping the child with cancer go back to school. *Journal of School Health, 50,* 328–331.

Shapiro, E. S., & Manz, P. H. (2004). Collaborating with schools in the provision of pediatric psychological services. In R. T. Brown (Ed.), *Handbook of pediatric psychology in school settings* (pp. 49–64). Mahwah, NJ: Erlbaum.

Shaw, S. R., & McCabe, P. C. (2008). Hospital-to-school transition for children with chronic illness: Meeting the new challenges of an evolving health care system. *Psychology in the Schools, 45,* 74–87.

Wade, S. L., & Walz, N. C. (2010). Family, school, and community: Their role in the rehabilitation of children. In R. G. Frank, M. Rosenthal, & B. Caplan,

Handbook of rehabilitation psychology (2nd ed., pp. 345–354). Washington, DC: American Psychological Association.

Weiner, P. L., Hoffman, M., & Rosen, C. (2009). Child life and education issues: The child with a chronic illness or special healthcare needs. In R. H. Thompson (Ed.), *Handbook of child life: A guide for pediatric psychosocial care* (pp. 310–326). Springfield, IL: Thomas.

Worchel-Prevatt, F. F., Heffer, R. W., Prevatt, B. C., Miner, J., Young-Saleme, T., Horgan, D., et al. (1998). A school reentry program for chronically ill children. *Journal of School Psychology, 36*, 261–279.

CHAPTER 9

The Role of Pediatric
Psychology in Health Promotion
and Injury Prevention

KERI J. BROWN KIRSCHMAN
BRYAN T. KARAZSIA

The value of pediatric psychology in health promotion and injury prevention efforts is duly noted (Black, 2002; Tercyak, 2008). Pediatric psychologists are uniquely positioned to understand the cognitive, behavioral, and environmental factors involved in maintaining optimal health (see Brown Kirschman, Mayes, & Perciful, 2009, and Wilson & Lawman, 2009, for a full review of injury prevention and health promotion). Alongside medical personnel, epidemiologists, health services administrators, biostatisticians, and environmental health scientists, pediatric psychologists work to identify, assess, prevent, and remediate illness, injury, and associated sequelae. Pediatric psychologists in a multitude of settings have opportunities to engage in health-promoting activities with children, their families, and their communities. In this chapter, a theoretical framework for exploring the role of pediatric psychology in the provision of health promotion and injury prevention services across different locations is presented. Within this framework, examples of health promotion efforts that can be fulfilled by pediatric psychologists are identified. Where available, these examples are based on published literature. The chapter concludes with a sample case study of injury prevention work by a pediatric psychologist.

THEORIES OF HEALTH PROMOTION

Health promotion and illness prevention initiatives are often classified using the framework created by Gordon (1983). In this framework, the target population defines the level of a given initiative as universal, selective, or indicated. Universal programs are pitched at a population level with the primary aim of preventing what would be future incidences of the target problem. Selective programs utilize evidence-based risk factors to target subpopulations or specific groups known to be at a higher risk of a disease or injury. Indicated programs are geared toward individuals following onset of the target problem with the goal of preventing progression and secondary symptoms.

When considering specific avenues of prevention, professionals often utilize Bronfenbrenner's ecological systems theory (e.g., Bronfenbrenner, 1979) as a heuristic (see Steele & Aylward, 2009, for a discussion of systems theory in the context of pediatric psychology research and practice). This theory organizes level of influence according to the proximity to a child. When considering roles of pediatric psychologists in health promotion and injury prevention, it may be helpful to integrate Gordon's (1983) levels of prevention with Bronfenbrenner's theory. Doing so creates a matrix that organizes prevention efforts along two axes: target populations (prevention level) and agents of influence (ecological levels). The result is 12 cells that represent distinct opportunities for promoting health and preventing injuries. This matrix is presented in Figure 9.1, with representative examples of evidence-based prevention programs in corresponding cells, where available. Please note that this is not intended to be an exhaustive list.

INTEGRATIVE PREVENTION FRAMEWORK: IDENTIFYING OPPORTUNITIES OF INFLUENCE

Microsystemic Influence (Cells 1–3)

In the current U.S. health care system, the preponderance of work among pediatric psychologists, as well as most health care providers, has been devoted to the treatment of individual children following onset of a disorder, disease, or injury event (e.g., Black, 2002; Patterson, Scherger, & Smith, 2010). Pediatric psychologists who work in hospital settings with medical care teams in such areas as burn, orthopedics, intensive care, emergency, and rehabilitational medicine routinely provide microindicated (cell 1) psychological services to children following an injury. Further, pediatric psychologists throughout the health care system contribute to indicative health promotion via those roles traditionally in their bailiwick, such as promoting adherence, reducing pain, and promoting adjustment during the

Ecological Level	Prevention Levels		
	Indicated	Selective	Universal
Microsystem	*Cell 1* Preventing future injuries among youth presenting with an injury; preventing or reducing psychological sequelae following medical trauma (Kazak et al., 2009)	*Cell 2* Reducing disparities in home safety practices (Kendrick, Mulvaney, & Watson, 2009); improving driving behaviors of teens with ADHD ("STEER" program; Fabiano et al., 2011)	*Cell 3* School-based efforts to prevent spinal cord injury (Richards, Hendricks, & Roberts, 1991) and bike injury (McLaughlin & Glang, 2010)
Mesosystem	*Cell 4* Collaborations between medical teams, schools, and families to promote healthy eating and activity levels for obese teens	*Cell 5* Collaborations in primary care to provide early intervention to promote health; enhancing parental understanding of preschoolers' risk of home injury (Brown, Roberts, Mayes, & Boles, 2005)	*Cell 6* Collaborations between pediatric psychologists and schools for benefit of all children in the school ("Stamp in Safety" Program; Schwebel, Summerlin, Bounds, & Morrongiello, 2006)
Exosystem	*Cell 7* Area for novel approaches	*Cell 8* Targeting at-risk communities (Schwarz, Grisso, Miles, Holmes, & Sutton, 1993)	*Cell 9* Community-based injury prevention programs (Klassen et al., 2000); mass-media antismoking campaigns (Flynn et al. 1994)
Macrosystem	*Cell 10* New regulations for post-concussion management (Zackery Lystedt Law)	*Cell 11* Graduated Drivers Licensing legislation (Chen, Baker, & Li, 2006)	*Cell 12* Public policy and legislative initiatives (traffic laws, creation of safe roadways; Peden et al., 2008); bicycle helmet laws (Karkhaneh et al., 2006)

FIGURE 9.1. An integrative prevention matrix: Illustrative examples of roles for pediatric psychologists. *Note.* Bronfenbrenner also proposed the chrono-system, which considers the dimension of time and to a large extent is outside the focus of this chapter.

course of an illness or injury treatment. For example, there is a well-defined literature to guide pediatric psychologists in the identification, reduction, and treatment of pediatric traumatic medical stress (PTMS; National Child Traumatic Stress Network, 2004) that may occur subsequent to an injury or illness event. For children experiencing PTMS, remediation of these symptoms can promote short- and long-term physiological and psychological well-being (see Kazak, Schneider, & Kassam-Adams, 2009, for a review).

Work on these outcomes and in these settings, however, typically involves rehabilitation or treatment of injury or illness that has already occurred. As suggested by Aujoulat, Simonelli, and Deccache (2006), the concept of promoting the total health of children and adolescents who are in hospital settings is also important. Such health promotion initiatives extend beyond rehabilitating a previous ailment. Such initiatives include health promotion across the lifespan, promoting parent–child interactions to promote future health and well-being within the family, supporting reintegration into school systems, and promoting healthy lifestyles.

Selective intervention aimed at children and families (cell 2) who are at increased risk of disease or injury due to known risk factors is also fertile ground for the practicing pediatric psychologist, particularly those located in primary care settings (Roberts & Brown, 2004; Stancin, Sturm, & Ramirez, Chapter 6, this volume). Talmi and Fazio (2012) noted that "These settings are ideally suited to promote optimal development and well-being through the provision of expanded services that address parental concerns, developmental tasks, psychosocial factors, and behavioral health issues in the context of a trusting relationship with familiar providers" (p. 496). Pediatric psychologists in primary care settings are well situated to identify struggling families and to provide early intervention services for issues that may become more pronounced if left untreated. However, documenting that prevention occurred and getting paid for selective prevention work—even for those patients who present with risk factors that are associated with later psychological and/or physical health problems—can be problematic. For example, billing by psychologists for health promotion work via health and behavior codes often yields low reimbursement (see Roberts & Brown, 2004, and Talmi & Fazio, 2012, for discussions of barriers to behavioral health delivery in pediatric primary care).

Opportunities to engage in universal prevention within the microsystem (cell 3) include involvement in health promotion initiatives such as school-based exercise and nutrition programs. In general, universal health programs at the microsystemic level that are theory-driven with well-defined anticipated outcomes, that are tailored to specific developmental levels of the target children, and that are comprehensive with multiple approaches to teaching behaviors are most effective in achieving long-term change (Nation et al., 2003).

Mesosystemic Influence (Cells 4–6)

Across all prevention levels in this section of the matrix (cells 4–6), pediatric psychologists can engage in health promotion by working directly with central figures within the child's microsystem (e.g., parents, schools, physicians) or by facilitating communication and integration of efforts among those individuals who have direct interaction with the child. Indeed, work at the mesosystemic level has been described primarily as consultative in nature (Sheridan & Cowan, 2004). For pediatric psychologists, work to improve communication among school, health care, and home in regard to children's health issues is likely to improve health outcomes for all children.

Steele and Aylward (2009) conceptualized the health care system itself as part of the mesosystem. For example, Pisani, Berry, and Goldfarb (2005) detailed a collaborative effort to provide all families in a primary care practice with behavioral health checks while waiting for well-child appointments. Families were receptive to this approach, with 25% of families asking questions or expressing concerns that were then addressed by a pediatric psychology intern. Concerns were communicated to the physician and referrals were made as needed. This level of collaborative care normalizes developmental and behavioral health questions and has the potential to enhance a child's overall well-being by developing interconnections within the mesosystem (cells 5, 6).

While work within the mesosystem may be a powerful way to promote the health of children, these interactions are difficult to operationally define and systematically study outside of a research setting. However, health promotion interventions that target multiple relationships within the microsystem (e.g., child–parent, child–teacher) tend to be most effective in promoting behavioral change (Nation et al., 2003).

Exosystemic Influence (Cells 7–9)

Settings in the exosystem usually do not include a child, so opportunities for pediatric psychologists to promote health and prevent injury at this level likely do not fall within the traditional models of health care. However, as discussed by Steele and Aylward (2009), pediatric psychologists can and do have roles at this level, including facilitating parent support groups and cultivating support from extended family. Applying the framework presented in Figure 9.1, it is perhaps most challenging to identify roles of pediatric psychologists at the intersection of the exosystem and indicated prevention (cell 7). In the current health care system, it can be difficult to bill for services without direct patient contact (Lines, Tynan, Angalet, & Pendley, 2012). Accordingly, there is a lack of empirical research regarding indicated prevention efforts at the level of the exosystem. However, it is not hard to imagine possibilities for roles of pediatric psychologists at this level, and it is likely that many clinicians actively perform these roles (e.g., developing parent support groups that emphasize health promotion).

Published examples of prevention efforts at the exosystem do exist for selective and universal prevention. For selective prevention at the exosystem level (cell 8), prevention efforts often rely on findings from epidemiology to target neighborhoods with higher rates of injuries. For example, the Harlem Hospital Injury Prevention Program targeted high-risk urban neighborhoods with a variety of prevention efforts, including establishing safe play areas, organizing positive peer groups for modeling safe play behavior, and implementing educational efforts. Over a 3-year period (1988–1991), the area targeted by the prevention program showed a decrease in injuries resulting in fewer hospital admissions than in areas not targeted (Davidson et al., 1994). Selective prevention efforts at the exosystem level have also been documented in low-income communities in South Africa. Schwebel, Swart, Hui, Simpson, and Hobe (2009) empowered and mobilized paraprofessionals from communities with very high risks and incidences of kerosene-related injuries. The paraprofessionals, in turn, distributed prevention messages to the local communities. Using random assignment that compared an intervention group with a control group, the intervention group demonstrated significant increases in knowledge about kerosene, adoption of prevention practices, and decreases in injury risk.

Represented by cell 9, universal injury prevention programs also exist at the level of the exosystem. In such programs, at-risk communities are not targeted specifically. Rather, these programs may be useful to any and all communities. This is important because, even when risk for injury is relatively low, the risk is still greater than zero. A review of community-based programs concluded that these programs could be effective in enhancing safety practices, such as adoption of car seats and utilization of bicycle helmets (Klassen, MacKay, Moher, Walker, & Jones, 2000). Programs demonstrating the most promise include those that are grounded in behavior change theory, are integrated with and tailored to specific communities and their needs, and achieve buy-in from community stakeholders. Community-based interventions often do not include outcome data about actual injuries, however. Thus opportunities exist for psychologists to design program evaluations that more thoroughly examine the evidence base for these universal community initiatives.

Macrosystemic Influence (Cells 10–12)

Published literature regarding macrosystem influences at the levels of indicated and selective interventions is lacking. The dearth of such research is due, in part, to methodological challenges with operationalizing and assessing community-level constructs (Steele & Aylward, 2009). Thus cells 10 and 11 represent novel opportunities for pediatric psychologists to engage in health promotion work that would have a unique impact. At the intersection of the macrosystem and indicated prevention, pediatric psychologists may be able to play an important role in cultivating macrolevel cultures in which health promotion becomes the norm among individuals who have incurred an injury or whose health is compromised (such as individuals who develop type 2 diabetes). Such efforts would be consistent with the view of health as being more than the absence of disease but rather an ongoing process by which an individual continually strives for well-being (World Health Organization, 1948). Where the macrosystem intersects with selective prevention, at-risk communities or cultures might be targeted with campaigns to change attitudes and/or with legislation geared toward safety and health. For example, psychologists have been involved in pediatric sports-related concussion research (e.g., Kirkwood, Yeates, & Wilson, 2006), legislative, and advocacy efforts that have led to evidence-based guidelines that emphasize the health and safety of athletes—that is, "when in doubt, sit them out" (Giza et al., 2013). These multidisciplinary efforts have likely affected the culture of youth sports by changing the attitudes and behaviors of coaches, parents, and players regarding the severity of concussions and the risks associated with postconcussive play.

Documented effectiveness of universal prevention efforts at the level of the macrosystem (cell 12) do exist in peer-reviewed literature and typically involve evaluations of public policy or laws geared toward preventing injuries. For example, careful planning in the creation of roads, in the establishment of driving laws, and in the careful execution of these laws can protect children from deaths involving motor vehicles (e.g., Peden et al., 2008). More specifically, there is evidence to suggest that bicycle helmet laws are effective in increasing adoption of bicycle helmets (Karkhaneh, Kalenga, Hagel, & Rowe, 2006). Although these efforts obviously include roles outside the realm of psychology, it is important for pediatric psychologists to be involved in advocacy and the evaluation of interventions designed to reduce child injury rates (Tremblay & Peterson, 1999). A timely example is the rapidly growing evidence demonstrating increased risks of injuries when cellular phones are utilized in unsafe manners. Although this body of literature is quite interdisciplinary, pediatric psychologists are playing important roles in developing this evidence base (e.g., Stavrinos, Byington, & Schwebel, 2009).

BARRIERS AND FUTURE DIRECTIONS

The matrix presented in this chapter highlights health promotion and injury prevention initiatives and identifies roles for pediatric psychologists. Efforts by pediatric psychologists to populate the matrix have been constrained by four main issues. First, health promotion and injury prevention work has not been emphasized in training. Mackner, Swift, Heidgerken, Stalets, and Linscheid (2003) found that less than 35% of pediatric psychology internship programs offer students opportunities in alcohol, injury, obesity, or substance-use prevention. Further, limited training in public policy and advocacy, 46 and 57% of programs, respectively, may deter pediatric psychologists from becoming involved in macrosystemic activities. Second, reimbursement issues for prevention work, particularly for work that does not directly involve the child or for which there is no formal diagnosis (the cells outside of 1, 2, 4, and 5, most probably), are of concern. Although the use of health and behavior codes to bill for health promotion work is promising (Noll & Fischer, 2004), the full potential of these codes has not yet been actualized (Lines et al., 2012). Psychologists must continue to strive toward documenting the cost savings for preventive initiatives so that this may be less of a concern in the future (Rozensky & Janicke, 2012). Third, patients may not be interested in these initiatives. This lack of interest, particularly in adolescents, may work against clinicians' efforts (e.g., Tercyak, Donze, Prahlad, Mosher, & Shad, 2006). Fourth, even when interested, children "age out" of what is preventively trained, and additional health promotion efforts will be needed as their risk profiles change with age.

As has been echoed throughout this chapter, a significant barrier to health promotion and injury prevention work by pediatric psychologists is the limited empirical research base to guide clinical practice. Relatively few articles published in the *Journal of Pediatric Psychology* have taken a prevention or public health perspective (Brown, 2007). As with the limited scope of training regarding health promotion (e.g., Mackner et al., 2003), the limited scope of research initiatives may also be related to a lack of training among pediatric psychology trainees at macrosystemic levels. Rozensky and Janicke (2012) encourage collaborations with public health colleagues, who routinely engage in population-level work, in order to engage in a "meeting of the minds" (p. 6) to develop effective solutions for health promotion at the population level.

CASE EXAMPLE: MICROINDICATED INJURY PREVENTION

Children and their families do not typically present with concerns regarding "prevention" or "health promotion," and therefore identifying representative case studies for this work is challenging. At the same time, however, preventive work is and arguably should be done by nearly all pediatric psychologists in every setting. Presented here is a brief case study of injury prevention at the microindicated level (cell 1).

Andy, a 7-year-old Caucasian male, sustained a third-degree burn injury to his hand while igniting tissue paper with a cigarette lighter "for fun." At the time of the injury, Andy's mother was at work, and a 13-year-old neighbor was watching the children. Following an inpatient hospital stay, Andy's injuries necessitated weekly follow-up appointments in the pediatric burn clinic. The surgeon reported that the burn was consistent with the mother's account of the injury event. As part of the multidisciplinary burn team, a pediatric psychologist was charged with assessing Andy's coping and identifying individual and familial factors that would put Andy at risk for additional injuries.

Andy lived at home with his mother and two younger siblings (ages 2 and 4). He had infrequent and irregular contact with his biological father. Andy was in second grade, with no medical or developmental concerns noted by his mother. Andy had not received any previous psychological assessment or treatment. Andy had received treatment in the emergency department for two previous injuries: He had sustained lacerations due to running into a glass patio door (age 6) and a fractured arm as a result of a fall from playground equipment (age 5). In addition, Andy's mother reported that he was discovered playing with matches on two prior occasions. Andy's mother said that he was an affectionate child but that he could be disruptive at home and school and that he engaged in problematic behaviors, such as "disappearing" in stores. This report was substantiated by observations of Andy in the exam room. For example, he had difficulty sitting still and continued to touch the medical equipment in the room despite his mother's direction not to do so. Andy's mother believed that the burn injury would "teach him a lesson" and that Andy would not play with fire again. A formal psychological evaluation was conducted. Andy met criteria for attention-deficit/hyperactivity disorder (ADHD), combined subtype.

Case Conceptualization

Individual and environmental factors that increased Andy's risk for future injury were identified. First, children with behavioral disorders have been found to have an increased risk of injury (Schwebel & Gaines, 2007). Treatment of Andy's underlying and previously undiagnosed ADHD might help prevent risk behaviors—such as impulsivity and inattention—that could result in a subsequent injury. Second, maternal attitudes regarding injury (e.g., that Andy would be "once burned twice shy") are not substantiated by research (Jaquess & Finney, 1994). In fact, these attitudes might prohibit the mother from engaging in effective parental injury prevention tactics, such as safety-proofing her home or increasing supervision levels. Third, the adequacy of the supervision that Andy and his younger siblings receive while their mother is at work should come into question. For young children, close supervision is related to decreased injury risk (Morrongiello, Ondejko, & Littlejohn, 2004). Supervision by adolescent caregivers has not been well studied but is generally thought to increase risk of injury when compared with supervision by adult caregivers. Given these factors, a comprehensive plan to decrease future risk for Andy and his siblings was developed.

Treatment consisted of increasing maternal knowledge of injury risk and child development. This included psychoeducation regarding the role of impulsivity, inattention, and behavior problems in injury risk (Schwebel & Gaines, 2007). Next, the psychologist assisted the family *and* teachers in problem solving to identify and employ developmentally appropriate passive (e.g., ensuring a safe play environment) and active (e.g., enhancing supervision and finding more appropriate babysitters) injury prevention strategies. Behavioral reinforcements for safe play were also established for Andy. To decrease injury risk for the younger siblings, home safety equipment and safety-proofing instruction was provided by the local Safe Kids USA® chapter. The family was referred to a child psychologist in their community (about an hour drive from the hospital) for ongoing ADHD treatment. Routine consultation with the community clinician allowed reinforcement of treatment goals during Andy's pediatric burn care appointments. As of 6 months postinjury, Andy had not had any injuries that warranted medical attention.

SUMMARY AND CONCLUSIONS

As illustrated in the conceptual framework and examples of applications, pediatric psychologists contribute to health-promoting and injury-preventing activities with children. The field has much to offer the improvement of children's health status through various settings and modalities.

REFERENCES

Aujoulat, I., Simonelli, F., & Deccache, A. (2006). Health promotion needs of children and adolescents in hospitals: A review. *Patient Education and Counseling, 61,* 23–32.

Black, M. M. (2002). Society of Pediatric Psychology presidential address: Opportunities for health promotion in primary care. *Journal of Pediatric Psychology, 27,* 637–646.

Bronfenbrenner, U. (1979). *The ecology of human development: Experiments by nature and design.* Cambridge, MA: Harvard University Press.

Brown, K. J., Roberts, M. C., Mayes, S., & Boles, R. (2005). Effects of parental viewing of children's risk behavior on home safety practices. *Journal of Pediatric Psychology, 30,* 571–580.

Brown, R. T. (2007). *Journal of Pediatric Psychology* (JPP), 2003–2007: Editor's vale dictum. *Journal of Pediatric Psychology, 32,* 1165–1178.

Brown Kirschman, K. J., Mayes, S., & Perciful, M. S. (2009). Prevention of unintentional injury in children and adolescents. In M. C. Roberts & R. G. Steele (Eds.), *Handbook of pediatric psychology* (4th ed., pp. 587–602). New York: Guilford Press.

Chen, L., Baker, S. P., & Li, G. (2006). Graduated driver licensing programs and fatal crashes of 16-year-old drivers: A national evaluation. *Pediatrics, 118,* 56–62.

Davidson, L. L., Durkin, M. S., Kuhn, L., O'Connor, P., Barlow, B., & Heagarty, M. C. (1994). The impact of the Safe Kids/Healthy Neighborhoods Injury Prevention Program in Harlem, 1988 through 1991. *American Journal of Public Health, 84,* 580–586.

Fabiano, G. A., Hulme, K., Linke, S., Nelson-Tuttle, C., Pariseau, M., Gangloff, B., et al. (2011). The Supporting a Teen's Effective Entry to the Roadway (STEER) program: Feasibility and preliminary support for a psychosocial intervention for teenage drivers with ADHD. *Cognitive and Behavioral Practice, 18,* 267–280. Retrieved from *http://dx.doi.org/10.1016/j.cbpra.2010.04.002*

Flynn, B. S., Worden, J. K., Secker-Walker, R. H., Pirie, P. L., Badger, G. J., Carpenter, J. H., et al. (1994). Mass media and school interventions for cigarette smoking prevention: Effects 2 years after completion. *American Journal of Public Health, 84,* 1148–1150.

Giza, C. C., Kutcher, J. S., Ashwal, S., Barth, J., Getchius, T. S., Gioia, G. A., et al. (2013). Summary of evidence-based guideline update: Evaluation and management of concussion in sports. *Neurology, 80*(24), 2250–2257.

Gordon, R. S. (1983). An operational classification of disease prevention. *Public Health Reports, 98*(2), 107–109.

Jaquess, D. L., & Finney, J. W. (1994). Previous injuries and behavior problems predict children's injuries. *Journal of Pediatric Psychology, 19,* 79–89.

Karkhaneh, M., Kalenga, J. C., Hagel, B. E., & Rowe, B. H. (2006). Effectiveness of bicycle helmet legislation to increase helmet use: A systematic review. *Injury Prevention, 12,* 76–82.

Kazak, A. E., Schneider, S., & Kassam-Adams, N. (2009). Pediatric medical traumatic stress. In M. C. Roberts & R. G. Steele (Eds.), *Handbook of pediatric psychology* (4th ed., pp. 205–215). New York: Guilford Press.

Kendrick, D., Mulvaney, C., & Watson, M. (2009). Does targeting injury prevention towards families in disadvantaged areas reduce inequalities in safety practices? *Health Education Research, 24,* 32–41.

Kirkwood, M. W., Yeates, K. O., & Wilson, P. E. (2006). Pediatric sport-related concussion: A review of the clinical management of an oft-neglected population. *Pediatrics, 117,* 1359–1371.

Klassen, T. P., MacKay, J. M., Moher, D., Walker, A., & Jones, A. L. (2000, Spring/Summer). Community-based injury prevention interventions. *Future of Children, 10,* 83–110.

Lines, M. M., Tynan, W. D., Angalet, G. B., & Pendley, J. S. (2012). Commentary:

The use of health and behavior codes in pediatric psychology: Where are we now? *Journal of Pediatric Psychology, 37,* 486–490.

Mackner, L. M., Swift, E. E., Heidgerken, A. D., Stalets, M. M., & Linscheid, T. M. (2003). Training in pediatric psychology: A survey of predoctoral internship programs. *Journal of Pediatric Psychology, 28,* 433–441.

McLaughlin, K. A., & Glang, A. (2010). The effectiveness of a bicycle safety program for improving safety-related knowledge and behavior in young elementary students. *Journal of Pediatric Psychology, 35,* 343–353.

Morrongiello, B. A., Ondejko, L., & Littlejohn, A. (2004). Understanding toddlers' in-home injuries: II. Examining parental strategies, and their efficacy, for managing child injury risk. *Journal of Pediatric Psychology, 29,* 433–446.

Nation, M., Crusto, C., Wandersman, A., Kumpfer, K. L., Seybolt, D., Morrissey-Kane, E., et al. (2003).What works in prevention: Principles of effective prevention programs. *American Psychologist, 58,* 449–456.

National Child Traumatic Stress Network. (2004). *Pediatric medical traumatic stress toolkit.* Retrieved July 13, 2012, from *www.nctsnet.org*

Noll, R. B., & Fischer, S. (2004). Commentary. Health and behavior CPT codes: An opportunity to revolutionize reimbursement in pediatric psychology. *Journal of Pediatric Psychology, 29,* 571–578.

Patterson, J., Scherger, J. E., & Smith, A. M. (2010). Primary care and prevention. In J. Suls, K. W. Davidson, & R. M. Kaplan (Eds.), *Handbook of health psychology and behavior medicine* (pp. 340–353). New York: Guilford Press.

Peden, M., Oyegbite, K., Ozanne-Smith, J., Hyder, A. A., Branche, C., Rahman, A. K. M., et al. (2008). *World report on child injury prevention.* Geneva, Switzerland: World Health Organization.

Pisani, A. R., Berry, S. L., & Goldfarb, M. (2005). A predoctoral field placement in primary care: Keeping it simple. *Professional Psychology: Research and Practice, 36,* 151–157.

Richards, J. S., Hendricks, C., & Roberts, M. (1991). Prevention of spinal cord injury: An elementary education approach. *Journal of Pediatric Psychology, 16,* 595–609.

Roberts, M. C., & Brown, K. J. (2004). Primary care, prevention, and pediatric psychology: Challenges and opportunities. In B. G. Wildman & T. Stancin (Eds.), *Treating children's psychosocial problems in primary care* (pp. 35–60). Greenwich, CT: Information Age.

Rozensky, R. H., & Janicke, D. M. (2012). Commentary: Healthcare reform and psychology's workforce: Preparing for the future of pediatric psychology. *Journal of Pediatric Psychology, 37,* 359–368.

Schwarz, D. F., Grisso, J. A., Miles, C., Holmes, J. H., & Sutton, R. L. (1993). An injury prevention program in an urban African-American community. *American Journal of Public Health, 83,* 675–680.

Schwebel, D. C., & Gaines, J. (2007). Pediatric unintentional injury: Behavioral risk factors and implications for prevention. *Journal of Developmental and Behavioral Pediatrics, 28,* 245–254.

Schwebel, D. C., Summerlin, A. L., Bounds, M. L., & Morrongiello, B. A. (2006). The Stamp-in-Safety program: A behavioral intervention to reduce behaviors that can lead to unintentional playground injury in a preschool setting. *Journal of Pediatric Psychology, 31*, 152–162.

Schwebel, D. C., Swart, D., Hui, S.-K. A., Simpson, J., & Hobe, P. (2009). Paraffin-related injury in low-income South African communities: Knowledge, practice, and perceived risk. *Bulletin of the World Health Organization, 87*, 700–706.

Sheridan, S. M., & Cowan, R. J. (2004). Consultation with school personnel. In R. T. Brown (Ed.), *Handbook of pediatric psychology in school settings* (pp. 599–616). Mahwah, NJ: Erlbaum.

Stavrinos, D., Byington, K., & Schwebel, D. C. (2009). Effect of cell phone distraction on pediatric pedestrian injury risk. *Pediatrics, 123*, e179–e185.

Steele, R. G., & Aylward, B. S. (2009). An overview of systems in pediatric psychology research and practice. In M. C. Roberts & R. G. Steele (Eds.), *Handbook of pediatric psychology* (4th ed., pp. 649–655). New York: Guilford Press.

Talmi, A., & Fazio, E. (2012). Commentary: Promoting health and well-being in pediatric primary care settings: Using health and behavior codes at routine well-child visits. *Journal of Pediatric Psychology, 37*, 496–502.

Tercyak, K. P. (2008). Editorial: Prevention in child health psychology and the *Journal of Pediatric Psychology. Journal of Pediatric Psychology, 33*, 31–34.

Tercyak, K. P., Donze, J. R., Prahlad, S., Mosher, R. B., & Shad, A. T. (2006). Identifying, recruiting, and enrolling adolescent survivors of childhood cancer into a randomized controlled trial of health promotion: Preliminary experiences in the Survivor Health and Resilience Education (SHARE) program. *Journal of Pediatric Psychology, 31*, 252–261.

Tremblay, G. C., & Peterson, L. (1999). Prevention of childhood injury: Clinical and public policy challenges. *Clinical Psychology Review, 19*, 415–434.

Wilson, D. K., & Lawman, H. G. (2009). Health promotion in children and adolescents: An integration of the biopsychosocial model and ecological approaches to behavior change. In M. C. Roberts & R. G. Steele (Eds.), *Handbook of pediatric psychology* (4th ed., pp. 603–617). New York: Guilford Press.

World Health Organization. (1948). Preamble to the Constitution of the World Health Organization as adopted by the International Health Conference, New York, 19–22 June, 1946; signed on 22 July 1946 by the representatives of 61 States (Official Records of the World Health Organization, no. 2, p. 100) and entered into force on 7 April 1948.

CHAPTER 10

The Use of Technology
in Pediatric Psychology Practice

BRANDON S. AYLWARD
CHRISTOPHER C. CUSHING
TIMOTHY D. NELSON

There has been a burgeoning use of technology within health care to facilitate the measurement of health-related behaviors, to assess outcomes, and to deliver therapeutic interventions, including within the field of pediatric psychology (Palermo, 2008). More specifically, technology can play a critical role in (1) assessing health behaviors remotely, (2) determining the efficacy of various interventions, (3) serving as a proxy for clinicians in educational and/or behavioral treatment delivery, and (4) providing support for health prevention and self-management in the home environment (Cushing & Steele, 2010). These measurement methods can use technology that includes, but is not limited to, patient Internet portals, mobile sensors, smartphone and other handheld applications, virtual reality, and electronic event monitors, all used for the provision of medical care (Palermo, 2008).

The current chapter provides an introduction to the types of technologies used in pediatric psychology, discusses ways to utilize individual data from technology at the point of care, and highlights potential challenges associated with seamlessly integrating technology into practice. Given the diverse disciplines involved in health care technology (e.g., clinicians, programmers, venture capitalists, designers), as well as the seemingly rapid emergence and adoption of new technologies, we recognize that this chapter cannot be an exhaustive review of health technology devices and factors associated with integration into clinical practice.

TECHNOLOGY DEVICES

There are a wide range of technology devices that can be of use in the clinical practice of pediatric psychology. However, the practicing clinician (and even the dedicated observer) may quickly find him- or herself overwhelmed by the rapidly changing digital technology landscape. To protect against this problem, we provide a conceptual rather than a device-specific approach to organizing and understanding health care technology. This conceptual approach is based on the methodology and types of data that can be captured in a clinical setting and includes (1) ecological momentary assessment or experience sampling methodology, (2) continuous data collection, and (3) dynamic feedback loop technologies. A brief overview of each of these methodologies, their application to clinical practice, and a few commercially available exemplars are detailed in the following.

Ecological Momentary Assessment

Ecological momentary assessment (EMA) involves asking questions of patients outside of the clinical setting using some triggering event (e.g., a time-based alarm, a bout of physical activity, or a family meal). For example, as part of a weight management intervention, patients in the Healthy Pokes Program at Oklahoma State University monitor their mood and behavior using a time-based EMA application designed for the Android operating system that can be customized based on the treatment session content for the week. Questions are added to monitor specific clinical features such as mood when weekly sessions focus on emotional eating and are changed to monitor the adolescent's perception of praise when sessions focus on increasing family praise for positive health behavior. Responses are then reviewed in session to tailor the intervention.

Although EMA is commonly performed using some form of digital technology such as a palmtop computer or smartphone, it is important to note that the technique should not be thought of as reliant on any particular device (e.g., paper and pencil measures completed following a watch alarm could also represent an EMA approach). However, use of technology for EMA can provide time-stamped information on responses that can aid in examining the antecedents, behaviors, and consequences centered around a particular phenomenon of interest. The key advantages of EMA are that (1) data can be collected as patients go about their lives, (2) data are reported "in the moment," removing recall bias and retrospective reporting, (3) assessments can follow a clinically meaningful pattern (e.g., when the child is scheduled to take a medication) or at random intervals (to capture patterns that may be difficult to hypothesize a priori), and (4) the technique allows for multiple observations of the same participant, which is more consistent with the idiographic approach to clinical care (Shiffman, Stone, & Hufford, 2008). The central features required for EMA are the ability to prompt a response (alarm), the ability to deliver a question, and the ability to record the response for later review. If a data acquisition approach includes these features, it can be thought of as EMA.

Continuous Data Collection

As the field moves toward a better understanding of psychophysiology and the effect of behavior on physical health, variables such as physical activity performed in real time, sleep, and even heart rate variability as a proxy for psychological stress can add value to clinical assessment and intervention within pediatric psychology. Modern body sensor technologies allow truly continuous capture of these physiological and behavioral variables. A common example is the use of accelerometry, which collects information about movement and which can apply algorithms to determine measures of physical activity, sedentary time, and sleep. For example, Actigraph is a commercial manufacturer of accelerometers that also provides data management support through proprietary software. Actigraph's products are reliable and valid for estimating physical activity in children (Puyau, Adolph, Vohra, & Butte, 2002; Yang & Hsu, 2010). Additionally, these devices have been validated against polysomnography (i.e., comprehensive physiological sleep assessment), with the Actigraph performing relatively well; however, the device has been found to overestimate sleep efficiency and total sleep time and also to demonstrate poor identification of wakefulness (Montgomery-Downs, Insana, & Bond, 2012).

Dynamic Feedback Loop Technologies

In some cases it may be advantageous to both assess and intervene using digital technology outside of the clinical suite. In this case, practitioners may choose to use a body sensor or EMA application that also provides feedback to the user. Many commercial products are available for such functions, and most are built on sound behavioral self-regulation principles (e.g., self-monitoring, goal setting, and feedback) that have been shown to work in the eHealth intervention context (Cushing & Steele, 2010; Cushing, Jensen, & Steele, 2011).

When considering a dynamic intervention, we encourage practitioners to recall Carver and Scheier's (1982) control theory model. Briefly, the model states that a person's moment-to-moment behavior is governed by the following process: (1) An individual holds a goal in mind (either prescribed by a practitioner or personally derived); (2) the person then compares his or her current behavior with the goal; (3) if there is a discrepancy, a behavior is performed to decrease the discrepancy; (4) this behavior has an impact on the environment, which is monitored by the patient; and (5) the process repeats. Within this model, technology can be used to help the individual set goals (step 1) and to self-monitor (step 2), as well as to provide feedback regarding goal attainment (step 4). The evidence is relatively clear that these techniques are effective for promoting and maintaining health behavior in pediatric populations (Kahana, Drotar, & Frazier, 2008) and translate well to an eHealth context (Cushing & Steele, 2010). Many devices for creating these feedback systems are commercially available (e.g., Nike+ FuelBand, Fitbit, and others). However, there have been limited controlled trials examining these devices. Therefore, we recommend that the practitioner be familiar with the control theory model and use informed clinical judgment regarding selection of commercially available devices for intervention and assessment.

USE OF TECHNOLOGY IN CLINICAL PRACTICE

Many behaviors often examined in pediatric psychology (e.g., daily medication adherence, dietary intake, emotional functioning, sleep) operate in a temporal fashion; that is, they can fluctuate day to day and thus single, "snapshot" measures of these variables may not truly capture individual trends in health behaviors (e.g., daily pain). Moreover, summary scores ignore the day-to-day variation of health behaviors and may introduce recall bias (Kikuchi et al., 2006). As a result, various types of technology are increasingly being used in the field of pediatric psychology to better assess behavioral data and symptoms at a more granular level (e.g., daily, continuously). Several methodologies exist to harness these data and use the full information at the point of care; these are discussed subsequently.

Data Analysis with Technology

Technology can provide clinicians with a wealth of individual health behavior data useful for care. Although group-aggregate data may provide an evidence base to inform clinical practice, they may not always be applicable to the individual patient. The time-ordered variation in health variables can provide insight into important clinical processes (Kotagal & Nolan, 2010). As a result, various individual time-series charts are being increasingly used to evaluate health care processes, to make the course of treatment more "visible," and to examine individual data as trends rather than in a static or summary view.

Single-case designs are symbiotic with technology-based assessment and intervention methods and can capitalize on the repeated, unobtrusive assessment of health-related behaviors gathered from technology devices (Dallery, Cassidy, & Raiff, 2013). For clinical assessment and/ or intervention purposes, a number of single-case designs exist to utilize technology-derived data in assessing behavior change and providing preliminary efficacy testing for technology interventions. These designs can include reversal, multiple-baseline, alternating-treatment, factorial, and/ or changing-criterion designs and can permit inferences about causal relations between independent and dependent variables useful for assessing the effectiveness of clinical interventions (see Dallery et al., 2013, for further description of analytic techniques).

The evaluation of data in single-case designs is largely done using visual inspection, which prioritizes clinically significant changes in health behaviors. Visual analysis is recommended as the first step in evaluating treatment outcomes, and clinical relevance of findings should be based on visual inspection, subject matter experience, and scientific judgment (Dallery et al., 2013; Wilkinson and the Task Force on Statistical Inference, 1999). Typically, statistical analyses are used to augment visual interpretations and can include the conservative dual-criteria (CDC) method and nonoverlap techniques (see Dugard, File, & Todman, 2012, and Satake, Jagaroo, & Maxwell, 2008, for further review of statistical analysis of time-series data). It should be noted that there is no consensus on best practices for statistical analyses for single-case designs and that these approaches do not control for autocorrelation.

In addition to the analytical techniques just described, statistical control charts can also be utilized to assess variation in clinical processes (e.g., daily mood, frequency of symptom events) for assessment and intervention purposes. Similar to other time-series charts, a statistical control chart allows providers to (1) view baseline assessments with high resolution to provide better insight into developing treatment plans; (2) examine the effectiveness of individualized treatment plans over time in an easily viewable format; and (3) evaluate clinical processes using statistically derived decision rules. Using these charts and probability-derived decision rules, clinicians can evaluate daily or weekly variables of interest in a distinguishable fashion for those parameters that represent significant changes in care (signal or special cause variation; e.g., significant improvement or decline in functioning) versus those that are random noise (routine or common-cause variation; e.g., ebb and flow of daily pain ratings). For a more detailed explanation of variation and charts, the reader is referred to Neuhauser, Provost, and Bergman (2011) and Perla, Provost, and Murray (2011).

Case Example in Pediatric Psychology

Within the pediatric psychology literature, Cushing and colleagues (2011) utilized a multiple-baseline design to examine the impact of a mobile device with automated software to increase adherence to self-monitoring of dietary intake and physical activity levels for a pediatric weight management intervention. Self-monitoring is an integral component to positive behavioral treatment outcomes and can potentially be enhanced by the use of technology, which is very appealing to youth and which allows participants to provide information in their own environment (Atienza, Stone, Shiffman, & Nebeling, 2007; Cushing et al., 2011). In the study, three adolescents, all above the 90th percentile on body mass index (BMI) based on age and gender, enrolled in a 10-week family-based intervention. Participants were provided with paper notebooks to record weekly dietary consumption and participation in physical activity during a baseline phase. Individual daily self-monitoring goals were identified by participants, and therapists examined the percentage of goal attainment for each week of the program. In the second phase of the study, participants were given an Apple iPod Touch device preloaded with commercially available software to track dietary intake and physical activity information. All participants evidenced an increase in the attainment percentage of self-monitoring goals with the introduction of the electronic device compared with baseline.

POTENTIAL CHALLENGES WITH INTEGRATING TECHNOLOGY INTO PRACTICE

Despite the multibillion dollar investments and attention surrounding the use of technology for health care issues, there are several challenges related to the use of technology in clinical assessment and intervention. First, access to health technologies may present a challenge, and the cost of certain devices may be prohibitive in some settings. Even if a clinician is inclined to employ an existing technology in treatment, the upfront investments required to purchase and support the technology, as well as limited opportunity to recoup these costs, could prove a powerful disincentive. Second, it is incumbent upon practitioners to ensure that client confidentiality is not compromised by the introduction of new technologies. Data entered electronically—whether online or using a variety of mobile devices—must be protected and transferred using secure means (e.g., data encryption). Third, clinical technologies must be reliable, because device malfunction or other technical errors can result in the loss of valuable clinical data and frustration on the part of both patients and clinicians.

Fourth, new technologies must be designed to maximize functionality within the particular clinical context. That is, every aspect of the application or program, from patient interface to clinician accessing of the data, should be developed in a way that supports easy and efficient use for clinical practice. Data entry interfaces need to be "user-friendly" to promote consistent patient adherence, and the data collected must capture clinically relevant and useful information. For educational components of technology-based interventions, the way information is presented (e.g., developmental level of material, interactive format) can be crucial in facilitating patient learning and retention, and considerable forethought is needed to develop these elements in ways that will optimize their impact. It is also essential that data can be accessed and displayed by clinicians in a way that facilitates data-informed clinical decision making. Technology often allows for the collection of tremendous amounts of data, but ensuring that those data can be summarized quickly and clearly is key to enhancing services. Currently, the ability for data from technology devices to be directly integrated with the electronic medical record is limited. For all of these challenges, clinical providers must work closely with information technology (IT) specialists to develop and refine technologies for maximum benefit.

A final challenge presented by new clinical technologies can be found in the rapid proliferation of new applications that may have limited or no evidence to support their effectiveness. Recently, there has been a shift from eager acceptance of the abundant proof-of-concept projects for health care to a "call for evidence" of improvements in health care systems and patient outcomes (Labrique, Vasudevan, Chang, & Mehl, 2013; World Health Organization, 2011). New technologies appear almost daily, claiming to "revolutionize" how a particular problem is treated and making all previous interventions obsolete. The reality, however, is that many, or even most, of these new approaches lack the rigorous evaluation or even basic empirical evidence that is at the foundation of sound evidence-based pediatric practice (Breton, Fuemmeler, & Abroms, 2011). Yet-to-be-validated technologies may be aggressively marketed, particularly when the potential for profit is considerable, further complicating the decisions practitioners must make about what to use in clinical care. Responding to this issue, the

Food and Drug Administration (FDA) has developed guidelines for regulating mobile medical applications, yet will only police those classified as high risk (Mobile Medical Applications, 2013).

RECOMMENDATIONS FOR PRACTICE

As others have highlighted (i.e., Chakrabarti, 2012; Palermo, 2008), we suggest that clinicians maintain an open mind to new technologies that may enhance their interventions, but also that they maintain a healthy scientific skepticism regarding new applications that have yet to be appropriately validated. "Show me the evidence" has been a sort of mantra for pediatric psychologists for decades, and we see no reason to abandon our tried-and-true principles of basing clinical decisions on a combination of research evidence, clinical expertise, and client characteristics (Nelson & Steele, 2009). In fact, to adopt new technologies simply for the sake of using technology would betray the core of evidence-based practice and could compromise clinical care. Conversely, integrating well-designed and well-validated applications into pediatric practice has the potential to strengthen services by improving access, facilitating engagement, or enhancing ecological validity. Perhaps most promising are applications that build on existing evidence-based treatments and mechanisms, seeking to apply technology to make these interventions more powerful, feasible, and efficient. Along these lines, Cushing and Steele (2010) found that eHealth interventions that employed well-validated behavioral components (e.g., self-monitoring with feedback, goal setting, contingency management) were most likely to produce positive outcomes. When established treatment strategies are incorporated within new and exciting technological platforms, the field can move forward with a strong foundation of effective interventions delivered in innovative ways.

Although most pediatric psychologists would agree that the integration of technology into clinical care should be based on rigorous research, practitioners are faced with a daunting task of keeping up with the rapidly expanding literature in this area. To help facilitate the dissemination of high-quality clinical technologies, periodic reviews summarizing the evidence base for various applications would be valuable. Such reviews could focus on the most promising applications of technology, especially those that seek to use technology to improve the delivery of already established interventions. The *Journal of Mobile Technology in Medicine* is one outlet that was recently launched to disseminate peer-reviewed articles that document developments in health care technology (Perera, 2012). Similarly, the Society of Pediatric Psychology (SPP) recently announced a task force on eHealth interventions, with one of its stated goals being to provide an updated review of the eHealth literature (Rapoff, 2013). Further, regulation by the FDA or other government agencies could also be helpful in limiting false claims of effectiveness and separating evidence-based applications from the countless unsupported programs on the market.

CONCLUSIONS AND FUTURE DIRECTIONS

The field of pediatric psychology is an interdisciplinary field devoted to promoting "the health and psychological well-being of children, youth, and their families" (Palermo, 2012, p. 1). The integration of technology into pediatric psychology practice can provide additional avenues for multidisciplinary collaboration in the delivery of effective clinical care. There has been a proliferation of health technology, and the integration of this technology into care is not without some challenges. Nonetheless, pediatric psychologists can provide insight on behavioral methods to empower and engage patients with technology (Wang & Huang, 2012), as well as provide empirical support and validation for various innovative technologies for use in clinical practice. Health technology is a rapidly growing enterprise with many stakeholders (e.g., venture capitalists, insurance companies, technology start-up companies, health care industry), and pediatric psychologists are well positioned to prove the "worth" of these devices for prevention, assessment, and intervention activities with children and adolescents with chronic illness.

REFERENCES

Atienza, A. A., Stone, A. A., Shiffman, S., & Nebeling, L. (2007). Introduction. In A. A. Stone, S. Shiffman, A. A. Atienza, & L. Nebeling (Eds.), *The science of real-time data capture: Self-reports in health research* (pp. xi–xiv). New York: Oxford University Press.

Breton, E. R., Fuemmeler, B. F., & Abroms, L. C. (2011). Weight loss—there is an app for that! But does it adhere to evidence-informed practices? *Translational Behavioral Medicine, 1*(4), 523–529.

Carver, C. S., & Scheier, M. F. (1982). Control theory: A useful conceptual framework for personality-social, clinical, and health psychology. *Psychological Bulletin, 92*, 111–135.

Chakrabarti, R. (2012). The need for an evidence base in mobile technology in medicine. *Journal of Mobile Technology in Medicine, 1*, 3–4.

Cushing, C. C., Jensen, C. D., & Steele, R. G. (2011). An evaluation of a personal electronic device to enhance self-monitoring adherence in a pediatric weight management program using a multiple baseline design. *Journal of Pediatric Psychology, 36*, 301–307.

Cushing, C. C., & Steele, R. G. (2010). A meta-analytic review of eHealth interventions for pediatric health promoting and maintaining behaviors. *Journal of Pediatric Psychology, 35*(9), 937–949.

Dallery, J., Cassidy, R. N., & Raiff, B. R. (2013). Single-case experimental designs to evaluate novel technology-based health interventions. *Journal of Medical Internet Research, 15*, 1–17.

Dugard, P., File, P., & Todman, J. (2012). *Single-case and small-n designs: A practical guide to randomization tests* (2nd ed.). New York: Taylor & Francis.

Kahana, S., Drotar, D., & Frazier, T. (2008). Meta-analysis of psychological interventions to promote adherence to treatment in pediatric chronic health conditions. *Journal of Pediatric Psychology, 33*, 590–611.

Kikuchi, H., Yoshiuchi, K., Miyasaka, N., Ohashi, K., Yamamoto, Y., Kumano, H., et al. (2006). Reliability of recalled self-report on headache intensity: Investigation using ecological momentary assessment technique. *Cephalalgia, 26*, 1335–1343.

Kotagal, U., & Nolan, T. (2010). Commentary: The application of quality improvement in pediatric psychology: Observations and applications. *Journal of Pediatric Psychology, 35*, 42–44.

Labrique, A., Vasudevan, L., Chang, L. W., & Mehl, G. (2013). Letter to the editor: H_pe for mHealth: More "y" or "o" on the horizon? *International Journal of Medical Informatics, 82*, 467–469.

Mobile Medical Applications. (2013, September 25). *Guidance for industry and Food and Drug Administration Staff.* Retrieved from http://www.fda.gov/downloads/MedicalDevices/DeviceRegulationandGuidance/GuidanceDocuments/UCM263366.pdf

Montgomery-Downs, H. E., Insana, S. P., & Bond, J. A. (2012). Movement toward a novel activity monitoring device. *Sleep and Breathing, 16*(3), 1–5.

Nelson, T. D., & Steele, R. G. (2009). Evidence-based practice in pediatric psychology. In M. C. Roberts & R. G. Steele (Eds.), *Handbook of pediatric psychology* (4th ed., pp. 99–113). New York: Guilford Press.

Neuhauser, D., Provost, L., & Bergman, B. (2011). The meaning of variation to healthcare managers, clinical and health-services researchers, and individual patients. *BMJ Quality and Safety, 20*(Suppl. 1), i36–i40.

Palermo, T. M. (2008). Editorial: Section on innovations in technology in measurement, assessment, and intervention. *Journal of Pediatric Psychology, 33*, 35–38.

Palermo, T. (2012, October). The president's message. *Society of Pediatric Psychology Progress Notes, 36*(3), 1–2.

Perera, C. (2012). The evolution of e-health: Mobile technology and mHealth. *Journal of Mobile Technology in Medicine, 1*, 1–2.

Perla, R. J., Provost, L. P., & Murray, S. K. (2011). The run chart: A simple analytical tool for learning from variation in healthcare processes. *BMJ Quality and Safety, 20*, 46–51.

Puyau, M. R., Adolph, A. L., Vohra, F. A., & Butte, N. F. (2002). Validation and calibration of physical activity monitors in children. *Obesity Research, 10*, 150–157.

Rapoff, M. A. (2013). The president's message: Updates on mentoring and promotions of eHealth interventions. *Progress Notes, 37,* 1.

Satake, E., Jagaroo, V., & Maxwell, D. L. (2008). *Handbook of statistical methods: Single subject design.* San Diego, CA: Plural.

Shiffman, S., Stone, A. A., & Hufford, M. R. (2008). Ecological momentary assessment. *Annual Review of Clinical Psychology, 4,* 1–32.

Wang, C. J., & Huang, A. T. (2012). Integrating technology into health care: What will it take? *Journal of the American Medical Association, 307,* 569–570.

World Health Organization (WHO). (2011, September). *Call to action on global eHealth evaluation: Consensus statement of the WHO Global eHealth Evaluation Meeting, Bellagio.* Available from: *http://ghdonline.org/uploads/The_Bellagio_eHealth_Evaluation_Call_to_Action-Release.docx*

Wilkinson, L., & the Task Force on Statistical Inference. (1999). Statistical methods in psychology journals: Guidelines and explanations. *American Psychologist, 54,* 594–604.

Yang, C. C., & Hsu, Y. L. (2010). A review of accelerometry-based wearable motion detectors for physical activity monitoring. *Sensors, 10,* 7772–7788.

PART III

PEDIATRIC CONDITIONS AND THE ROLE OF THE PSYCHOLOGIST

CHAPTER 11

Infants Born Prematurely
and/or at Biological Risk

GLEN P. AYLWARD

Pediatric psychologists may assume various roles in the care of children born prematurely or at other medical–biological risks. Services could be provided in neonatal intensive care units (NICUs), NICU follow-up clinics, developmental diagnostic clinics, outpatient pediatric psychology clinics, or even schools (Aylward, 2009a). The services provided often overlap with developmental, neuropsychological, school, or clinical child psychology. The range of activities includes developmental assessment, involvement in infant stimulation programs, family consultation, serial neurodevelopmental follow-up, addressing psychological components of subsequent health-related issues (e.g., asthma, motor impairment, feeding problems, epilepsy), or identification and treatment of later high-prevalence–low-severity dysfunctions such as cognitive, academic, neuropsychological, and behavioral concerns (Aylward, 2005; 2009a). Different roles depend on the child's age, specific precipitating factors (prematurity, central nervous system [CNS] injury, environmental risk), and the concerns of the family. It is important to note that major disabilities in these children are often identified during infancy; more subtle, high-prevalence–low-severity dysfunctions are not evident until school entry or later, when increasing situational demands make previously latent problems more obvious.

The emergence of disabilities is influenced by two factors: (1) *disruption* of normal developmental processes and (2) *insult* to the infant's CNS.

This is sometimes referred to as the "two-hit" hypothesis. With regard to disruption, because of preterm birth, the development of the infant's brain is altered in terms of timing, architecture, and connectivity (Aylward, 2005). Phases of brain development that normally would occur in utero now happen postnatally, affected by qualitatively different sensory experiences (tactile, visual, auditory, nociceptive). Moreover, there is a fourfold increase in cortical volume from 28 to 40 weeks, and 35% of the infant's brain weight is gained over the last 6 weeks of gestational age. In response to early disruption, there are brain *reorganization* processes and "catch-up." Although not universally accepted, catch-up is reflected in the practice of correction for prematurity, which typically is applied over the first 24 months. (Degree of prematurity is subtracted from the child's chronological age to produce a corrected or conceptional age. For example, if a child's chronological age is 9 months but she was born 3 months prematurely, the corrected age would be 6 months.) In response to damage or insult (e.g., intraventricular hemorrhage [IVH], hypoxic–ischemic encephalopathy [HIE], or similar conditions; see Aylward, 2009a), the infant's brain may compensate via a second process, namely, *recovery* (plasticity). Here, compensatory "rewiring" of the brain occurs in response to deficits in areas that have been damaged. The combination of reorganization and recovery functions in response to disruption and injury can best be conceptualized using a Venn diagram: One circle indicates disruption, a second indicates insult, and a third, overlapping circle identifies those infants who have both processes occurring simultaneously and who may manifest what is termed *encephalopathy of prematurity*. These children have sustained both disruption and insult and will experience compensatory reorganization and recovery. These compensatory processes occur against a backdrop of environmental, genetic, nutritional, and experiential influences, explaining the conundrum of prediction in any given child.

Similarly, there are corresponding stages of parental concern for children born at biological risk. Initially, the prime concern is survival or viability, which primarily falls under the purview of neonatologists, particularly in the case of an infant born extremely preterm (EPT; less than 28 weeks gestational age). The second phase of concern involves presence of a major disability, with parents worried about cerebral palsy (CP), significant intellectual disability (ID), visual–auditory impairment, or epilepsy. The next constellation of concern is focused on more specific, less severe developmental delays that may or may not improve with intervention (e.g., fine motor, speech–language, gross motor function). As the child ages, school performance and the possibility of high-prevalence–low-severity dysfunctions (learning disabilities, lower IQ, executive dysfunction, neuropsychological deficits, attention-deficit/hyperactivity disorder [ADHD], or behavioral problems) becomes an issue. Subsequently, social adjustment and future vocation are the focus of concern. Each of these stages of parental concern requires different services from pediatric psychologists. This process is exemplified in the following case scenario.

CASE EXAMPLE: JENNY

Neonatal/Postnatal Course

Jenny was born at 24 weeks' gestational age, weighing 610 grams, and had a fairly complicated perinatal–postnatal course. She was born average for gestational age (AGA), had a 5-minute Apgar of 5, sustained a Grade III IVH, and had respiratory distress syndrome (RDS) requiring ventilator assistance, hyperbilirubinemia, and Stage III retinopathy of prematurity (ROP). She remained in the NICU for 162 days after delivery and was discharged on oxygen. The family lived several hours away from the tertiary care NICU, and they periodically stayed at the Ronald McDonald House. Jenny's parents were both college graduates, and her father was an executive and her mother an elementary school teacher. Her parents called Jenny their miracle baby, her birth following two previous miscarriages.

Commentary

Given Jenny's gestational age of 24 weeks and birthweight of 610 grams, she fell into the extremely preterm/extremely low birth weight (EPT/ELBW) range. The age of viability is 22–25 weeks (with 23–24 weeks cited frequently). Of these infants, 59% survive. In preterm infants, emphasis has now shifted from birthweight to gestational age, as previously birthweight was a proxy for gestational age because, in part, it was easier to measure (Aylward, 2009a). Extremely preterm is considered to be less than 28 weeks, very preterm less than 32 weeks, and moderately preterm 32–36 weeks (although the late preterm classification is 34–36 weeks). In infants born EPT/ELBW, 20–34% have major handicaps; 70+% have high-prevalence–low-severity dysfunctions. Of children with Grade III IVH, 35–55% have neurodevelopmental disabilities, and risk is further increased by concomitant respiratory problems and hyperbilirubinemia. There is a "gradient of sequelae"—the younger and smaller the baby, the greater likelihood of disability—and as many as 50% of children born at less than 1000 grams have neurocognitive (intellectual/neuropsychological) deficits at school age. There are also early risks of a potential "vulnerable child syndrome" (Green, 1986)—these being prematurity, long hospitalization, the chance that the child might die, and a previous history of miscarriages. Parents displaying this syndrome have difficulty with separation, are overprotective, and are hypervigilant with respect to medical concerns.

The last issue is exacerbated because the infant continues to be medically fragile. At this time, the pediatric psychologist could work with the family, nursing staff, and allied health professionals to address questions about infant stimulation, discuss concerns regarding outcome, encourage use of early intervention (EI) services postdischarge, and probe the potential vulnerable-child syndrome indicators, intervening if necessary.

Six–Month Follow–Up

Jenny was subsequently seen for routine follow-up in the NICU Developmental Continuity Clinic (DCC) at the corrected age of 6 months (10 months chronological age). She had just been taken off supplemental oxygen but still had frequent wheezing. Jenny had been referred for EI services and was receiving developmental therapy, occupational and physical therapy, and speech–language therapy two times per month on average. On the Bayley Infant Neurodevelopmental Screener (BINS; Aylward, 1995), administered by the DCC pediatric psychologist, Jenny scored in the moderate to high risk range. There was increased truncal (axial) tone, brisk deep tendon reflexes, poor head control, and tightness of the lower extremities. She tended to keep her hands fisted. No imitative skills, precursory appreciation of object permanency, or vocalizations were observed. Clinic staff recommended continued increased EI services. A hearing evaluation was also recommended. The parents reported some feeding difficulties, and they continued to have the infant sleep in a bassinet next to their bed, rather than in her own room. Her mother indicated that she took a leave of absence from teaching in order to care for Jenny.

Commentary

There are many follow-up protocols, and selected ages at time of evaluation differ (Sherman, Aylward, & Shoemaker, 2011; Vohr, Wright, Hack, Aylward, & Hirtz, 2004). The age of 6 months was chosen because severe disabilities can be identified and because this age allows continuity with the family and also helps to ensure that EI services are in place. Findings can also be reported to the child's coordinating primary care physician (PCP) vis-à-vis the medical home concept. The impact of medical–biological issues (e.g., supplementary oxygen) decreases; however, recovery from medical conditions still can affect neurodevelopmental assessments at this age. The utility of an earlier assessment is arguable, although a lower level follow-up, such as a telephone interview by a clinic nurse, might be sufficient at 3 months' corrected age. At 6 months, tone, neurosensory function (hearing, vision), gross and fine motor abilities, vocalizations and interactive capacities could also be evaluated. Some cognitive processes, reflecting integration of neural networks, can also be assessed. Serial, longitudinal follow-up is critical, and this would be the first step in that regard. Age is corrected for prematurity (Aylward, 2009a), as this is considered to help differentiate transient maturational issues from more persistent deficits. Jenny displayed what has been termed *transient dystonia of prematurity*, characterized by increased extensor tone of the trunk, tightness in the lower extremities, head lag, and persistence of some primitive reflexes (e.g., hands fisted). This occurs in 21–36% of preterm infants and peaks at approximately 7 months; these findings disappear between 8 and 12 months in 80%, with the remaining 20% being at risk for CP. Transient dystonia also increases the risk of other neurocognitive delays. Continued concern regarding the vulnerable-child syndrome is raised by the parents' fear of separation (e.g., keeping the bassinet in the parents' bedroom).

At this stage the pediatric psychologist can perform evaluations, participate in discussion regarding findings, and work with the family regarding the continuing possibility of the vulnerable-child syndrome. The need for serial assessment should be emphasized, as should the fact that nothing is definitive at this point and that, with regard to later developmental outcome, Jenny would "tell us over time." Care should be taken to emphasize her areas of strength as well, so as to provide some positive feedback.

Twelve-Month Follow-Up

Jenny was again seen at the corrected age of 12 months (16 months chronological age). She had continued involvement in EI services. In the interim, Jenny was evaluated by a pediatric neurologist and was diagnosed with mild cerebral palsy (spastic diplegia). On the BINS she again scored in the high-risk range. She did not receive optimal scores on any cognitive-processes items, was not ambulating independently, did not point to indicate wants, and said "dada" and "mama" inconsistently. Jenny could cruise around furniture if she was placed upright next to a chair or other stationary object; she could not get to the upright position on her own. Her parents have not yet allowed anyone to babysit Jenny, including her grandparents, who live in close proximity.

Commentary

By 12 months' corrected age, biomedical issues, such as oxygen supplementation for chronic lung disease, typically have resolved. Environmental factors are not strongly influential yet. A more varied behavioral repertoire can be assessed, including emerging language and cognitive processes. Nonetheless, cognitive and motor functions still are highly intertwined (and do not diverge until later ages), and this period of rapid developmental acquisition is also a time of variability in skills (Vohr et al., 2004). Some neurodevelopmental abnormalities that have been identified earlier may disappear or become dormant in what is referred to as a "silent period," whereas others may worsen over time. Children born EPT have an increased risk of CP, and spastic diplegia makes up 40–50% of CP diagnoses. Moreover, 20–30% of those born EPT/ELBW will have severe motor delays (not CP), whereas 30–40% have cognitive deficits, and these two areas of disability often co-occur. The risk for CP is increased because of potential damage to the descending motor tracts due to the Grade III IVH. In Jenny's case, it appeared that disabilities were found in various areas of development and that these concerns are global. Fear of separation and overprotectiveness are evident in the parents' not using any babysitter (even close relatives) to watch Jenny even for a short period of time.

Many of the activities performed by the pediatric psychologist at the 6-month evaluation are still applicable at 12 months' corrected age. Discussion of the pattern of findings becomes more imperative, and the fact that the findings thus far indicate global delays should also be addressed. Developmental and/or behavioral strengths should also be underscored. Separation issues should be explored more aggressively, because this may have increasingly negative effects on the spouse subsystem.

Twenty-Four-Month Follow-Up

At the corrected age of 24 months, Jenny once again scored in the high-risk range on the BINS. Gross motor problems were evident in terms of difficulty running, jumping, kicking a ball, and motor overflow. Although she was able to identify pictures and body parts of a doll, she could not name pictures or objects. She still received EI services. The Modified Checklist for Autism in Toddlers (M-CHAT; Robins, Fein, Barton & Green, 2001) was also administered, and Jenny received a critical score of 3 and an overall score of 6. These scores exceeded the threshold for both developmental and autism spectrum disorder–related concerns. The parents expressed concerns that the EI services were not helping and questioned the validity of infant developmental screening in general and autism spectrum disorder (ASD) screening in particular.

Commentary

Environmental factors (socioeconomic status [SES] and social support, availability of language stimulation and learning experiences) begin to have a stronger influence on evaluation results (particularly cognitive and language abilities); in Jenny's case, environment would probably be a positive influence. Moreover, at this age cognitive and motor functions diverge, reasoning and language abilities are more readily assessed, and prediction to school-age function is better. Although evaluation moves from neuro-logic → motor → sensorimotor → cognitive function (Aylward, 2009b), prior to 18–24 months, many skills and functions are strongly *canalized*; these are essentially "prewired," self-righting, and fixed. These sensorimo-tor skills (e.g., midline behaviors, reaching, banging an object) are not highly complex, and the more strongly canalized the skill, the less it is affected by adverse biomedical circumstances. Conversely, the less cana-lized the behavior (i.e., greater complexity, such as producing two-word combinations or problem solving), the more susceptible the function is to adverse influences. Sensorimotor skills are strongly canalized, and these are typically prevalent in early screening and assessment (Aylward, 2009b). Therefore, the true magnitude of problems often cannot be identified early on. However, by 18–24 months, more complex, noncanalized behaviors are evaluated, and these provide insight into more complex, integrated functions.

Jenny was noted to display both cognitive and motor delays, these deficits being consistent over time (although they were becoming more obvious, perhaps as a function of the shift away from highly canalized skills). The fact that cognitive abilities were also affected, coupled with serial consistency and age at time of evaluation, tends to question the argu-ment that motor function primarily affects testing at this visit. In addi-tion, the toddler's medical–biological history, consistent developmental and neurodevelopmental concerns over the three serial assessments (despite the provision of EI services), and language and cognitive problems despite a supportive, nurturing environment all tend to underscore the fact that these deficits are potentially more long term. With regard to the ASD screening, it is estimated that 3.6–8% of children born EPT/ELBW have some type of ASD. This is a four- to twelvefold increase in prevalence in comparison with the general population. However, this issue is somewhat controversial, and specificity of diagnosis is compounded by the high rate of co-occurring developmental disabilities. That is to say, many symptoms resembling ASD could be attributable to behaviors that result from the developmental dis-ability and not from autism per se. Moreover, Asperger's disorder is rare, and social problems are more the result of inattention, distractibility, pro-cessing problems, and intellectual disability versus what is typical in true ASD. Jenny's parents were becoming increasingly overwhelmed and frus-trated with lack of improvement despite massive efforts on many fronts. This results in anger and questioning of information that is provided to them.

In addition to administering neurodevelopmental screening, the posi-tive M-CHAT results require that a follow-up M-CHAT interview be con-ducted by the pediatric psychologist, given the high rate of false-positive autism screening results and the likelihood that the findings could be attributable to developmental disabilities and not autism per se. The parents' frustration should be acknowledged and explored. Groundwork should be tactfully laid about the possibility of long-term deficits, still emphasizing that this is not certain and that the pediatric psychologist would be delighted to be proven wrong by Jenny.

Thirty-Six-Month Follow-Up

Jenny was seen at 3 years' chronological age for her last scheduled evaluation in the DCC. On the Bayley Scales of Infant and Toddler Development (Bayley-III; Bayley, 2006), she received a Cognitive Composite score of 80 (9th percentile), a Language Composite of 77 (6th percentile), and a Motor Composite of 73 (4th percentile). Jenny's cognitive abilities were grossly at a 27-month age level, receptive communication at 22 months, and expressive communication at 21 months. Fine motor skills were at a 25-month age equivalent, and gross motor abilities were at a 19-month age level. It was very difficult to keep Jenny focused on tasks, and there were numerous refusals, particularly with regard to language and motor items. Jenny displayed a distinct preference for using her left hand. She had aged out of EI and was in the process of being evaluated by the school system for placement in an early childhood education program with the anticipated eligibility designation of "developmental delay." Her parents expressed concerns regarding enrolling her in an out-of-home program, and they raised numerous questions regarding what to expect in terms of future cognitive and academic functioning. They had left Jenny with the grandparents on only a few occasions; when queried about the quality of their social life, they replied, "What social life?"

Commentary

"Intelligence" can be first tested at 3–4 years, although developmental indexes or quotients do not necessarily equate to intelligence quotients (Aylward, 2009b). At this point we had only developmental indexes available for Jenny. Nonetheless, concept development, precursors to academic skills, early indicators of executive function, and visual–motor integrative abilities can be assessed at this age. Verbal and nonverbal skills can be better differentiated now as well (Vohr et al., 2004). Prediction of later functioning is more accurate now than at earlier ages. Environmental influences are potent, but oftentimes in children born EPT/ELBW, medical–biological factors put a ceiling on malleability due to environmental factors. There also have been concerns raised in the literature that the Bayley–III may overestimate abilities (see Aylward & Aylward, 2011); however, this did not seem to be a major factor with Jenny because all her scores fell in the borderline range, with little variability.

With regard to predicting Jenny's intelligence, as a group, children born preterm score approximately 10 points lower than their full-term counterparts (.5–1.0 standard deviation below). The minority of children born at less than 25 weeks have average IQs, with most children born EPT having IQs in the low 80s. This does not occur in isolation but rather is in conjunction with other problems. Based on numerous studies, it is estimated that for each week of gestational age under 33 weeks, mean IQ scores decrease by 1.7–2.5 points per week (Aylward, 2005).

Jenny's parents also asked about future academic expectations. When predicting subsequent academic achievement, there was a high probability that Jenny would be at academic risk, with 60–70% of children born EPT/ELBW displaying learning disorders. There is a fivefold increase in learning problems when compared with full-term peers, and approximately one-third of these children will have multiple learning disabilities (LDs). LDs are most frequent with respect to math, followed by written output, spelling, and then reading. Those born at very low birthweight/very preterm (VLBW/VPT; < 1500 g, < 32 weeks) and younger have a greater incidence of nonverbal learning disabilities and a 20–40% rate of grade retention.

With regard to other areas of potential concern, most infants born at Jenny's gestational age manifest some type of visual–motor integrative/fine motor dysfunction (e.g., copying, spatial organization, visual memory, visual perception), with visual–motor integration scores typically being 1.5 standard deviations below average. This area of deficit has a particularly strong impact in early elementary grades because a high proportion of the day involves written activities and symbol manipulation (e.g., letters, numbers). Many basic language functions are intact in those born VPT and earlier; however, more complex components such as syntax, abstracting, and processing can be problematic. These issues are subtle but can have profound effects on learning and social interactions. Overall, there is a two- to threefold increase in language problems when compared with full-term counterparts.

Jenny is also at risk for executive function problems, particularly with the specific executive functions of initiating, working memory, shift/switching, planning/organizing, and monitoring. Children born ELBW/EPT have difficulty starting activities, display poor problem-solving flexibility, have working memory deficits, and cannot plan sequences of steps. At older ages they have difficulty extracting main points from lectures or written materials and cannot express themselves well when writing. Executive function problems are related to white matter damage, and this is a high probability, given Jenny's Grade III IVH. There is also the possibility of ADHD, which is 2.6–4 times more likely in preterm infants than in term peers. Some estimates are as high as 6 times greater, particularly in those born at less than 28 weeks' gestation. The manifestations of ADHD differ, with vigilance/alertness more affected than impulsivity. There is no male predominance or strong association with comorbidities, such as an oppositional defiant or conduct disorders, and a greater correlation with deficits in working memory or processing speed. This is sometimes considered a more "pure" form of ADHD. Many of these children have a "sluggish cognitive tempo," which is a combination of ADHD-inattentive subtype symptoms, executive dysfunction, and processing problems. Ventricular enlargement and parenchymal lesions (related to IVH) are found to be predictive of ADHD in those born prematurely.

There are also behavioral concerns that may evolve, with EPT/ELBW children displaying what has been termed a "preterm behavioral phenotype" (Johnson & Marlow, 2011). Components include inattention, anxiety, and social difficulties, with internalizing symptoms being more prominent than externalizing concerns. This behavioral tendency could be exacerbated further by parental behaviors that are in response to a vulnerable-child syndrome.

SUMMARY AND CONCLUSIONS

Many of the intervention functions and issues outlined in the previous encounters with Jenny and her family are still pertinent. Moreover, the process does not stop here. Periodic meetings with the family, encouragement and guidance through the education maze that begins with early childhood education, subsequent liaison activities with the school system, and periodic assessment to evaluate specific areas of concern could be provided by the pediatric psychologist. Throughout it should be emphasized that each child is unique and that Jenny is more like other children than not. In summary, the pediatric psychologist assumes many roles and functions in dealing with infants born at biological risk. Moreover, involvement should extend through school age and adolescence, due to the chronic nature of many issues faced by these children.

REFERENCES

Aylward, G. P. (1995). *Bayley Infant Neurodevelopmental Screener*. San Antonio TX: Psychological Corporation.

Aylward, G. P. (2005). Neurodevelopmental outcomes of infants born prematurely. *Journal of Developmental and Behavioral Pediatrics, 26*, 427–440.

Aylward, G. P. (2009a). Neonatology, prematurity, NICU, and developmental issues. In M. C. Roberts & R. Steele (Eds.), *Handbook of pediatric psychology* (4th ed., pp. 241–253). New York: Guilford Press.

Aylward, G. P. (2009b). Developmental screening and assessment: What are we thinking? *Journal of Developmental and Behavioral Pediatrics, 26,* 427–440.

Aylward, G. P., & Aylward, B. S. (2011). The changing yardstick in measurement of cognitive abilities in infancy. *Journal of Developmental and Behavioral Pediatrics, 32,* 465–468.

Bayley, N. (2006). *Bayley Scales of Infant and Toddler Development—Third edition.* San Antonio, TX: Psychological Corp.

Green, M. (1986). Vulnerable child syndrome and its variants. *Pediatrics in Review, 8,* 75–80.

Johnson, S., & Marlow, N. (2011). Preterm birth and childhood psychiatric disorders. *Pediatric Research, 69,* 11R–18R.

Robins, D. L., Fein, D., Barton, M. L., & Green, J. A. (2001). The Modified Checklist for Autism in Toddlers: An initial study investigating the early detection of autism and pervasive developmental disorders. *Journal of Autism and Developmental Disorders, 31,* 131–144.

Sherman, M. P., Aylward, G. P., & Shoemaker, F. (2011). Follow-up of the NICU patient. *Medscape.* Retrieved from *http://emedicine.medscape.com/ article/1833812-overview.* Updated October 27, 2011.

Vohr, B., Wright, L. L., Hack, M., Aylward, G., & Hirtz, D. (2004). Follow-up care of high-risk infants. *Pediatrics, 114*(5, Suppl.), 1377–1397.

CHAPTER 12

Pediatric Procedural Pain

ELIZABETH N. McLAUGHLIN
JOANNE M. GILLESPIE

Routine medical procedures, such as immunization and venipuncture, are typically experienced multiple times throughout childhood. Youth being assessed or treated for acute and chronic health conditions, accidents, or injuries may experience additional invasive procedures (e.g., lumbar puncture, port-a-cath access) as part of their medical care. A major stressor associated with acute and chronic illness, as reported by both parents and youth, is the pain and distress associated with needles and other medical procedures (Uman, Chambers, McGrath, & Kisely, 2006).

Fortunately, significant literature supports the efficacy of psychological interventions to help children and their families cope with medical procedures. The strongest evidence is for procedures involving needles in typically developing children (Blount et al., 2009; Taddio et al., 2010; Uman et al., 2006). There is additional evidence from research involving smaller samples or limited replication to support psychological interventions for children experiencing distress due to other types of procedures (e.g., magnetic resonance imaging [MRI]: Slifer, Koontz, & Cataldo, 2002; anesthesia induction: Kain et al., 2007).

Much is known about how parents and medical professionals (e.g., nurses, technicians, child life specialists) can help youth undergoing painful procedures. Children can benefit when adults provide timely and developmentally appropriate information about the procedure, engage them in coping-promoting behavior during the procedure, and make use of pharmacological options when indicated (see Blount et al., 2009). In routine cases, the pediatric psychologist may not play a direct role but instead may be involved in consultation and knowledge translation, in making relevant information accessible to caregivers and health care professionals, and in program development and evaluation. In more complicated situations, the existing literature can be used as a basis for tailoring individualized psychological treatment.

Given the vast array of medical procedures for which pediatric psychologists may be consulted, clinicians may be required to extrapolate effective psychological techniques from the available literature (e.g., on needles) to apply to less traditionally studied procedures that can cause distress for some youth (e.g., nasogastric tube insertion, dental extractions, tracheostomy changes, intraocular pressure testing). Furthermore, youth referred for psychological intervention often present for treatment following a history of traumatic medical experiences, with significant anticipatory anxiety, with individual differences (e.g., developmental challenges, disruptive behavior disorders), or with family variables (parent–child conflict, parental anxiety) that are underrepresented in typical research studies. Accordingly, pediatric psychologists may also need to draw upon the broader psychological literature (e.g., cognitive-behavioral therapy for anxiety disorders, behavioral interventions for youth with autism) to guide their interventions.

In this chapter, Ann, an 11-year-old girl with Down syndrome, is presented as a case example to illustrate how the pediatric psychologist can use a clinician-scientist approach to case conceptualization and the implementation of evidence-based intervention.

CASE EXAMPLE: ANN

Referral: "Please Assist Ann with Home Injections of MTX for JIA."

Ann was referred for assistance with weekly injections to be administered at home by her mother and stepfather. Medical chart review indicated that Ann, who has a mild intellectual disability, was diagnosed with juvenile idiopathic arthritis (JIA) 9 months prior, and a recent exacerbation in her disease did not respond to standard first-line treatment with oral nonsteroidal anti-inflammatory medication. As a result, her rheumatologist has recommended methotrexate (MTX) injections. MTX is a second-line disease-modifying antirheumatic drug given to reduce inflammation in children with JIA (refer to Rapoff, Lindsley, & Karlson, 2009, for a broader review of the medical and psychosocial aspects of JIA). There was no evidence of significant medical trauma from the hospital chart review, although it was noted that Ann did have regular blood work.

Consultation with the Referring Team and Treatment Planning

The referring clinic can be a valuable resource for relevant background information and behavioral observations. When contacted, the rheumatology clinic nurse indicated that Ann's parents seemed to be very committed to helping manage her arthritis and had been diligent about following treatment protocols. She reported that Ann was usually quite pleasant and cooperative during regular clinic visits but repeatedly asked whether she would be getting a needle. The clinic nurse indicated that Ann was known to have veins that were difficult to access, usually requiring more than one poke. She had observed the most recent blood draw, as it had taken place in the clinic instead of in the blood collection lab. Ann required restraint because she tried to hit and kick the adults present and would not sit still. Ann's mother reportedly cried while holding Ann, saying, "I'm sorry, it will be okay." After the blood test, Ann calmed down quickly, shortly after being given a small toy by her parents and a sticker by the phlebotomist.

The clinic nurse confirmed that Ann was to have her first MTX injection in the clinic in 6 weeks (at which point her parents would receive teaching about giving subsequent injections at home) and indicated that the family had a requisition for blood work to be completed at some point prior to the teaching session. During consultation with the referring team, the psychologist reviewed the steps involved in MTX injections and identified parts of the procedure about which Ann could make choices (e.g., which site would be used). She also confirmed that there would be no contraindication to Ann's using a topical anesthetic for the MTX injections or for her next blood test.

The nurse also shared her impression that presentation of MTX as a treatment option was met with some anxiety by the parents. Ann's mother reportedly stated that she felt Ann would never be able to get to the point of having injections at home, given how she responded to blood work. The family was aware that they would have the option of scheduling weekly appointments with Ann's primary care physician so that he could administer the MTX, but time from work and school made this a less-than-ideal alternative.

Several factors influence how an individual will cope with a medical procedure, including age, developmental level, temperament, culture, previous medical history, traumatic memories associated with medical events, and parental anxiety and behavior (Blount et al., 2009). Familiarity with this literature can help in developing an individualized assessment and treatment plan.

In Ann's case, it was hypothesized that the family's previous experience with blood collection would have a significant impact on home injections. The upcoming blood collection and first clinic-supported MTX injection, therefore, were seen as providing two important opportunities for intervention prior to the parent-administered injections at home. Because of the timeline for the upcoming MTX injection (and accompanying blood work), Ann's referral was triaged as a higher priority for intervention.

Initial Meeting with Ann and Her Parents

In the initial interview, Ann and her parents confirmed the rheumatology clinic nurse's report that her most recent blood test had been challenging and indicated that this was an accurate example of how Ann typically responds to venipuncture. They reported that Ann usually figures out that she is going to the hospital when she notices that her mother does not leave for work at the usual time. She will ask about the change of routine, and her parents will answer her truthfully. Her anxiety usually begins at that point, and it often takes significant coaxing just to get her into and out of the car. During her last visit, as they approached the doors of the hospital, Ann told her parents, "my heart is going too fast."

When reviewing Ann's experiences with other medical procedures, her parents were proud to report that 3 weeks prior Ann had had a successful trip to the dentist, during which she tolerated a cleaning with no difficulty. A visit to her family physician's office 2 months earlier for a flu shot was less successful. The flu shot was canceled because Ann refused to sit up on the examination table or allow her sleeve to be rolled up, and her physician and parents elected not to proceed with the injection.

Prior to embarking on a treatment plan, the psychologist collaborated with the family regarding the goals for treatment. Ann's parents were still contemplating whether they wanted Ann's injections to take place at home or in the family physician's office. As a first step, they were very interested in whatever strategies they could learn to assist with blood work. The pediatric psychologist considered discussing Ann's parents' ambivalence about completing injections at home. She hypothesized, however, that if Ann and her parents could experience success during blood work using cognitive-behavioral strategies, that accomplishment could increase their feelings of self-efficacy for administering injections at home. Ann clearly stated that she did not like blood tests but knew that her parents thought it was important. She described being held down as the worst part for her, and she wanted to find a way to avoid this.

Intervention

Psychoeducation was provided at a developmentally appropriate level to introduce the cognitive-behavioral model, including the physiological signs of arousal, the rationale for behavioral interventions, the effect of escape and avoidance, and the influence of cognitions. Examples were used from Ann's history to make this information more meaningful: "When you were trying to get out of the chair last time, that was your flight-or-fight response kicking in"; "When you left your doctor's office without having your flu shot, that probably made your fear stronger."

Replacing Unhelpful Thoughts

The cognitive-behavioral model posits that negative thoughts about the procedure or about one's perceived ability to cope with it will have an impact on behavior and mood. As such, another goal is to assess for the presence of maladaptive thoughts that may benefit from modification. Ann, for example, indicated that she had never looked at the syringe during blood work and believed that the needle was long enough to go right through her arm. Addressing the inaccuracy of this belief (including exposure to the needle typically used in the blood lab) was an important part of the psychological intervention for her needle fear.

When exploring her underlying belief about procedures, Ann reported thinking that she would "never be able to do it." Ann's recent successful dental appointment was used as evidence to argue against this thought and as an opportunity to build her self-efficacy. Ann's parents had prepared her for her dental exam by reading a number of children's books about going to the dentist. Her mother reported that during the exam, directing Ann's attention to the television on the ceiling was helpful. Ann and her family were praised for implementing these effective strategies.

After this exercise, Ann was assisted in coming up with the alternative thought, "I can do it," related to blood work, and she said that she agreed ("a little bit") with this statement. Although younger children, or those with developmental challenges, may not be able to engage in traditional cognitive therapy (i.e., identifying, challenging, and restructuring maladaptive cognitions), they can learn to repeat coping thoughts (e.g., "I am brave") or thoughts that focus on using coping strategies (e.g., "my job is to keep taking belly breaths"). Visual reminders (e.g., cue cards) or adult prompting may also be beneficial.

Distraction

A significant body of literature demonstrates the important role of distraction during medical procedures (e.g., Kleiber & Harper, 1999). We have had success in using and in coaching parents and other adults to use a variety of different types of distractors selected with the individual child in mind (e.g., bubbles, picture books, movies, smartphone and tablet applications). Some centers have access to virtual reality game systems and other multisensory distractors for use during more intense experiences, such as burn debridement (see Lange, Williams, & Fulton, 2006, for a review). Ann enjoyed her stepfather's portable computer, and he offered to download a new game for her to use at the hospital.

Relaxation

As with most children and youth, teaching Ann relaxation was an important step in helping her cope with painful procedures. She responded particularly well to diaphragmatic breathing. This strategy can be effective for children of all ages, and, because it does not require a lot of time or any special equipment, it can be implemented for most children as part of home practice and utilized during painful procedures. Progressive muscle relaxation is another active technique that many children enjoy and can practice at home (often with the assistance of a written script or digital recording). Ann's psychologist recommended that her parents coach her to practice her relaxation strategies daily at home. Helping caregivers to see themselves as supportive coaches who can encourage their children to use these coping strategies provides the opportunity for them to be actively involved in the procedure and to promote coping behavior in their children (Blount et al., 2009). Although not used with Ann, imagery can also be helpful during medical procedures. With appropriate training, clinicians may also consider introducing hypnosis.

Information Provision

Providing accurate, developmentally appropriate information is considered an important aspect of preparing a child for an upcoming painful procedure. Jaaniste, Hayes, and von Baeyer (2007) provide a thorough discussion of the factors to consider regarding the timing, type, and amount of information a child should be given in advance of a procedure. In Ann's case, she would become distressed after realizing on the morning of hospital visits that the family routine had changed. The psychologist recommended that Ann's parents remind her about the planned blood work 2 or

3 days in advance of the visit in order to give her an opportunity to manage her anxiety and participate more fully in preparation strategies.

Desensitization and Behavioral Rehearsal

When there is significant anticipatory anxiety, as with Ann, the additional steps of desensitization and behavioral rehearsal may also be indicated. For some individuals, a formal hierarchy can be generated, but for others, it may be sufficient for the pediatric psychologist to gradually expose the youth to different aspects of the procedure. Even talking about the procedure is a form of exposure to the feared event. For some children, this can elicit significant anxiety and may be an important early step in the desensitization process.

Other phases of exposure may involve imaginal exposure, role play in the psychologist's office with actual materials, and video modeling. Exposure to any stimuli that may serve as triggers for anxiety (e.g., an adult wearing a mask and gown, the smell of alcohol wipes) should be incorporated into rehearsal to give the youth an opportunity to habituate to them. Recognizing the limitations of generalizability and the fact that Ann was described by her parents as having difficulty adapting to unexpected changes, flexibility was built into Ann's exposure work (e.g., "This is a tourniquet. It may look like this one, it may look like this one, or it may even look like something else, but all of them have the same job . . . ").

Ann was able to use her diaphragmatic breathing as she moved through the steps of having a tourniquet put on her arm and pulled tight, having her arm washed with an alcohol swab, and being exposed to a butterfly needle. She responded well to praise for her efforts. Ann provided numerical ratings of anxiety for each step, as she had become familiar with rating her joint pain this way in rheumatology clinic. She was cued to take a breath and use her coping statement when her anxiety rose, and the step was repeated until her anxiety rating decreased. When Ann reported symptoms of arousal ("my heart is going fast"), or when symptoms of anxiety were observed, they were labeled as such and normalized (e.g., "That makes sense. It just means you are still a bit nervous about the needle") as per the anxiety sensitivity literature (McNally, 2002).

Although Ann very much wanted to complete the blood test without being held, given her history, the need for restraint remained a possibility. As such, restraint was incorporated into the rehearsal so that Ann would have an opportunity to habituate to the experience. Restraint was framed as a supportive aspect of the process that is sometimes necessary ("Your mom will hold your arm just in case your fight-or-flight response makes you start squirming"). The pediatric psychologist also planned for the unfortunate possibility of multiple pokes, given that Ann was known to have veins that were difficult to access ("If the needle doesn't go in the first time, your job is to take a belly breath and look at your game").

Once Ann was comfortable with each step in the pediatric psychologist's office, the rehearsal was moved to the blood collection lab. When working in the in vivo setting, it can be particularly helpful to have a new person (e.g., a phlebotomist) enter the room, as this can trigger anxiety. If time permits, the phlebotomist, nurse, or technician may even be able to participate in some of the behavioral rehearsal. For other types of referrals (e.g., computerized tomography [CT] scans), it may be more of a challenge to work in the in vivo setting due to the clinical demands on the environment. In these cases, it would still be valuable to rehearse outside of the psychology office (e.g., in a medical clinic with an examination table). Imaginal exposure may also be helpful. Ann was able to move through her hierarchy in an informal and flexible way, and she responded well to praise for each step. In other cases more strict application of behavior modification techniques, including removing attention from undesirable behavior, may be necessary (e.g., Mathews, Hodson, Crist, & LaRoche, 1992).

Interventions Focused on Adult Behavior

Parent behavior is known to have a significant impact on child coping during painful procedures (Blount et al., 2009). Caregivers should be educated about behaviors that promote child coping (e.g., distraction, coaching, humor) and those that promote distress (e.g., reassurance, criticism, apologies, empathy). Having caregivers distract a child during a procedure has been shown to reduce distress exhibited by the child. This intervention may also have the added benefits of helping caregivers to feel more self-efficacious because they are playing an active role in assisting the child with coping behavior, and reducing stress for both the caregiver and medical staff because the child is managing the procedure in a more positive way. During rehearsal, Ann's mother role-played directing Ann's attention to her computer game.

Ann's parents found it difficult to understand how intuitive behaviors such as reassurance and empathy could be distress-promoting. We find it especially helpful to describe specific research studies that support these claims (e.g., McMurtry, Chambers, McGrath, & Asp, 2010). During behavioral rehearsal and the procedure, Ann's psychologist modeled, prompted, and reinforced her parents' use of coping-promoting strategies and identified and provided constructive feedback regarding distress-promoting strategies.

Although most of the research has focused on parent behavior immediately before, during, and after the procedure, the psychologist should also assess for expressed feelings and thoughts in advance of the procedure that may influence the child's coping. For example, in the initial meeting with the psychologist, Ann's stepfather stated, "I don't know why they have to poke her so many times. She's just a kid. Needles are always so difficult." Ann's parents responded quite well to the suggestion that they try to convey a sense of confidence that Ann would be able to cope with the upcoming blood work.

Principles of Reinforcement

Adults also play an important role in the delivery of reinforcement (e.g., giving praise for coping). Important operant factors can also be in play, even if not specifically intended. For example, negative reinforcement may have a positive impact on coping if adults remove restraint when the child holds still. There is also the potential to inadvertently reinforce undesirable behavior. For example, tangible rewards (e.g., stickers, small toys) are often given to children by their parents and their medical team following painful procedures. These are often given just for completing the procedure and are not meant to be contingent on the child's behavior. Presumably this is done to help the child to view the experience as a positive one and to reduce the child's distress. We need to be mindful, however, that despite the intentions, these rewards could reinforce undesirable behavior. For example, when Ann received a sticker and toy after striking out during her last blood test, she may have inferred that her behavior was acceptable.

A formal reinforcement program may be deemed appropriate when intrinsic motivation to manage procedures differently is low, when refusal behavior has previously led to escape or avoidance of a procedure, or when it is important to extinguish maladaptive behaviors (e.g., physical aggression). Together with the parent and child, and taking into consideration the child's behavior during previous medical procedures, specific behavioral goals can be set in advance of the procedure. Rewards should be contingent on behaviors that increase the likelihood of a safe and successful procedure (e.g., getting on the exam table when directed, holding the arm still), rather than remaining stoic (e.g., not crying).

It can be difficult for parents and care providers alike to withhold tangible rewards for a child who has undergone a painful procedure, especially given other stressors that might be present (e.g., a new diagnosis, an acute illness). As such, psychologists may consider using a graded approach to contingent reward, with larger rewards reserved for behaviors that are particularly challenging for a given child and/or essential to the completion of the procedure.

Ann was intrinsically motivated to have her blood work completed without restraint, and she was encouraged by praise. It was suggested to her parents that they continue to offer a small toy or an activity-based reward but that they make it contingent on not hitting or kicking. With subsequent blood tests (or home injections), once physical aggression had been addressed, the target behavior to earn a reward could be then moved to other objective behaviors (e.g., remaining still).

Pharmacological Approaches

Much is known about the use of topical anesthetics and procedural sedation (see Blount et al., 2009), and the pediatric psychologist is often the first person to educate the family about combining pharmacological and psychological strategies. Ann had never used a topical anesthetic cream, and her parents were interested in trying it for her blood test. The psychologist suggested that her parents put it on both arms, given her history of being poked more than once per visit. For some, putting the cream on and taking the bandage off can be triggers for anxiety; this was not the case for Ann.

Planning the Procedure

Ann's pediatric psychologist also considered contextual factors in the scheduling of her blood work. Her mother described her as a "morning person" who was sometimes irritable at the end of a school day. The clinic was known to have longer waits early in the morning, so it was agreed to aim for a mid-morning visit. A plan for adults' roles was also established. Because Ann's parents had become effective participants in the rehearsal sessions, and given that there was a possibility of their administering needles at home, the psychologist decided to take a less active role in the blood work but remain present to observe and intervene if necessary. That is, Ann's mother would be the primary person to give instructions (e.g., "sit in the chair", "take a deep breath"), to direct Ann's attention to the computer game (e.g., "find the dog"), and to hold her arm still if necessary. Although her stepfather was also likely to be involved in future procedures, it was agreed that Ann would respond best to one person doing the coaching, as it was hypothesized that multiple individuals talking at once would increase her distress.

Ann's Blood Test

On the morning of the test, and with the Ann's parents' permission, the pediatric psychologist went to the blood collection lab to meet briefly with one of the phlebotomists and review the strategies the family had been practicing. Shortly before the procedure, the psychologist assessed Ann's anxiety and that of her parents, reviewed the plan for the procedure, and discussed Ann's reward (i.e., lunch in the hospital cafeteria with her parents) for not hitting or kicking. She also demonstrated the role of the topical anesthetic by touching areas with and without the cream. In the waiting room, Ann's parents and the psychologist engaged Ann in nonprocedural talk and were pleased to observe that Ann appeared calm and happy. Ann was praised when she completed early steps in the procedure (e.g., moving from the waiting room to the exam room).

Once in the lab, it was discovered that the computer had not been charged and could not be used. As such, less sophisticated distraction techniques (e.g., talking about a poster on the wall and engaging in nonprocedural talk) were introduced. When it was necessary to modify the previously determined plan, it was important for the pediatric psychologist to manage her own anxiety, to be flexible in problem solving concerning this difficulty, and to model coping and confidence. Ann's parents quickly responded to the psychologist's lead and talked with Ann about an upcoming desired event (a birthday party). Ann responded well to this improvisation and managed very well up to the moment of the needle. At that point, she could not be distracted, started to cry, and began moving her arm. Her mother held Ann's arm to ensure that the needle went in safely.

After the Procedure

It is important for pediatric psychologists to be cognizant of children's pain memory, as elevated recall of previous pain intensity has been positively correlated with increased distress during subsequent procedures (e.g., Chen, Zeltzer, Craske, & Katz, 2000). Positively reframing the painful event is an intervention that has been beneficial (Chen, Zeltzer, Craske, & Katz, 1999). The expressed thoughts and feelings of the parent after the procedure (e.g., "That was awful, I am so glad it is over" vs. "That was a tough procedure, but she did a great job staying still and practicing her breathing") should also be assessed for their potential impact on the child. Psychologists should consider meeting with a child and his or her caregivers (even briefly) following a procedure to discuss the event and to draw attention to what went well, with the purpose of influencing how the experience will be perceived, discussed, and remembered by the family.

Ann indicated that she felt bad that her mom had to hold her arm, but she was proud to have earned her special lunch for not hitting or kicking. She said she was surprised that the needle did not hurt. Ann's stepfather reported that he was proud of the improvement he saw in Ann's ability to cope before and during the blood test. Her mother agreed, and also stated, "that cream really works." The psychologist helped Ann and her parents to

focus on specific things that went well (e.g., Ann held still while the tourniquet was put on) and reviewed all of the strategies that they had used before
and during the procedure. Although the topical anesthetic did appear to
help, the psychologist helped them to conceptualize the cream as one of
several factors that seemed to make a difference. She recognized the value
of helping the family to identify their own behaviors as agents of change,
as a way of increasing their self-efficacy for coping with future procedures.

Home Injections

To this point, the intervention had not specifically targeted the original
reason for referral: parent-administered weekly intramuscular MTX injections. When examining treatment outcome in relation to the blood test,
it was clear that Ann and her parents had begun to learn and to see the
benefits of using cognitive-behavioral strategies. When debriefing about
the blood work, Ann's mother spontaneously stated, "I could really see
us learning how to give needles at home." The plan from this point was to
build on the skills learned in relation to blood work and to apply them to
the new goal. Behavioral rehearsal seemed to be an important component
of Ann's gains to date, and it was chosen as the main strategy for the next
phase of treatment.

SUMMARY

There is a significant amount of empirical literature supporting the efficacy
of cognitive-behavioral interventions to assist youth undergoing painful
medical procedures, especially those involving needles. Knowledge translation and consultation regarding effective strategies that can be implemented
by parents and health care providers should be viewed as important roles
for the pediatric psychologist in the multidisciplinary setting. For situations complicated by previous medical trauma, developmental differences,
or other individual-difference factors, the pediatric psychologist can com-
bine the available literature on procedural pain with knowledge regarding
these broader factors to design and implement an individualized treatment
plan that is evidence-based.

ACKNOWLEDGMENTS

The authors thank Christine Chambers, PhD, Jill Chorney, PhD, and Lindsay
Uman, PhD, for their helpful comments on an earlier draft of this chapter.

REFERENCES

Blount, R. L., Zempsky, W. T., Jaaniste, T., Evans, S., Cohen, L., Devine, K. A., et al. (2009). Management of pediatric pain and distress due to medical procedures. In M. C. Roberts & R. G. Steele (Eds.), *Handbook of pediatric psychology* (4th ed., pp. 171–188). New York: Guilford Press.

Chen, E., Zeltzer, L. K., Craske, M. G., & Katz, E. R. (1999). Alteration of memory in the reduction of children's distress during repeated aversive medical procedures. *Journal of Consulting and Clinical Psychology, 67,* 481–490.

Chen, E., Zeltzer, L. K., Craske, M. G., & Katz, E. R. (2000). Children's memories for painful cancer treatment procedures: Implications for distress. *Child Development, 71,* 933–947.

Jaaniste, T., Hayes, B., & von Baeyer, C. L. (2007). Providing children with information about forthcoming medical procedures: A review and synthesis. *Clinical Psychology: Science and Practice, 14,* 124–143.

Kain, Z. N., Caldwell-Andrews, A., Mayes, L., Weinburg, M. E., Wang, S. M., MacLaren, J., et al. (2007). Family-centered preparation for surgery improves perioperative outcomes in children: A randomized controlled trial. *Anesthesiology, 106,* 65–74.

Kleiber, C., & Harper, D. C. (1999). Effects of distraction on children's pain and distress during medical procedures: A meta-analysis. *Nursing Research, 48,* 44–49.

Lange, B., Williams, M., & Fulton, I. (2006). Virtual reality distraction during pediatric medical procedures. *Pediatric Pain Letter, 8*(1), 6–10.

Mathews, J. R., Hodson, G. D., Crist, W. B., & LaRoche, G. R. (1992). Teaching young children to use contact lenses. *Journal of Applied Behavior Analysis, 25,* 229–235.

McMurtry, C. M., Chambers, C. T., McGrath, P. J., & Asp, E. (2010). When "don't worry" communicates fear: Children's perceptions of parental reassurance and distraction during a painful medical procedure. *Pain, 150,* 52–58.

McNally, R. J. (2002). Anxiety sensitivity and panic disorder. *Biological Psychiatry, 52,* 938–946.

Rapoff, M. A., Lindsley, C. B., & Karlson, C. (2009). Medical and psychosocial aspects of juvenile rheumatoid arthritis. In M. C. Roberts & R. G. Steele (Eds.), *Handbook of pediatric psychology* (4th ed., pp. 366–380). New York: Guilford Press.

Slifer, K. J., Koontz, K. L., & Cataldo, M. F. (2002). Operant-contingency-based preparation of children for functional magnetic resonance imaging. *Journal of Applied Behavior Analysis, 35,* 191–194.

Taddio, A., Appleton, M., Bortolussi, R., Chambers, C. T., Dubey, V., Halperin, S., et al. (2010). Reducing the pain of childhood vaccination: An evidence-based clinical practice guideline. *Canadian Medical Association Journal, 182,* E843–E855.

Uman, L. S., Chambers, C. T., McGrath, P. J., & Kisely, S. (2006). Psychological interventions for needle-related procedural pain and distress in children and adolescents [Review]. *Cochrane Database of Systematic Reviews, Issue 4.*

CHAPTER 13

Pediatric Chronic and Episodic Pain

ANNE M. LYNCH-JORDAN

Chronic abdominal pain (CAP) is a prominent feature of many functional gastrointestinal disorders (Rasquin et al., 2006) and a common pediatric chronic pain condition (Dahlquist & Nagel, 2009). CAP arises from the interplay of genetic and environmental factors, psychosocial stressors, and mood and coping responses (Banez & Cunningham, 2009; Dahlquist & Nagel, 2009). Interdisciplinary treatment is advocated, and psychologists are often in the best position to address pain-related impairment. Empirical evidence supports the application of psychological interventions, namely, cognitive-behavioral therapy (CBT), to treat a wide range of pediatric acute (Uman, Chambers, McGrath, & Kisely, 2008) and chronic pain conditions (Palermo, Eccleston, Lewandowski, Williams, & Morley, 2010), including CAP (Huertas-Ceballos, Logan, Bennett, & Macarthur, 2008). This chapter illustrates how CBT interventions for chronic pain are implemented using a prototypical example of an adolescent with CAP and the clinical considerations for intervention delivery.

CASE EXAMPLE: LUCY

Presenting Information

Lucy was a 16-year-old Caucasian female referred to a behavioral medicine clinic at a large children's hospital from the Division of Gastroenterology

177

for problems coping with chronic pain. Lucy described having chronic abdominal pain in the periumbilic region of her abdomen. Pain duration was 6 months, with onset following a 1-week viral illness accompanied by fatigue, nausea, and vomiting. Lucy reported that pain and nausea had persisted following the illness, although vomiting had abated. Pain was constant and described as sharp and stabbing, with daily flare-ups lasting varying amounts of time. Pain was worse at bedtime, whereas nausea peaked in the morning. Exacerbating factors included certain foods (greasy), eating large quantities of food, physical activity, and stress. Pain was moderately alleviated by rest and distracting activities, such as listening to music and watching TV. Lucy was initially treated by her pediatrician without symptom relief and subsequently referred to a pediatric gastroenterology clinic. Diagnostic tests revealed no organic disease or inflammatory processes contributing to her symptoms, and her pain was characterized as "functional." Lucy felt that this diagnosis implied that she was faking or magnifying her symptoms. Medication management (Elavil) had only slightly reduced her symptoms and improved her sleep.

Assessment

Lucy and her mother participated in an initial assessment with a pediatric psychologist, the focus of which included pain-related functional impairment, mood changes, and current coping attempts, both successful and unsuccessful. Pain characteristics, such as location, onset, duration, frequency, and quality (e.g., sharp, burning), were obtained. Alleviating and exacerbating factors were determined, with attention to those that might be amenable to behavioral interventions (e.g., stress, sleep problems, physical overexertion).

The use of objective measures to monitor clinical outcomes is strongly recommended as a basis for evaluating patient progress and the efficacy of interventions. The Functional Disability Inventory (FDI; Walker & Greene, 1991) was developed to measure impairment in youth with chronic pain; clinical cutoffs have been established to aid interpretation (Kashikar-Zuck et al., 2011). The FDI was administered during the evaluation to establish a baseline level of functional disability and at all subsequent sessions to mark treatment progress. Lucy's initial FDI score was 30 (range 0–60), suggesting severe pain-related functional disability.

No known clinical measure exists to assess pain coping efficacy in children; however, quantifying coping is necessary given the focus of psychological treatment. We have used the Pain Coping Questionnaire's (PCQ) three pain coping efficacy questions to derive a coping score to evaluate treatment progress (range: 3–15; Reid, Gilbert, & McGrath, 1998). Although this brief measure was not explicitly developed for clinical purposes, our anecdotal evidence suggests that it adequately captures coping, is responsive to treatment, and appropriately varies as a function of disability. Pain coping efficacy was assessed at baseline and at every subsequent session to mark treatment progress. Lucy's initial coping score was quite low (6), reflecting poor pain coping.

Finally, pain intensity ratings were collected via a 0–10 numeric rating scale (NRS). Although not a primary treatment focus, pain reduction is a result of CBT interventions (Eccleston, Palermo, Williams, Lewandowski, & Morley, 2009) and thus worth measuring. Lucy's average pain was rated at the evaluation (8/10) and subsequent sessions.

Based on her interview and data, Lucy experienced significant pain-related functional disability across multiple domains. At home, Lucy engaged in sedentary activities, using rest and TV as her primary (and passive) coping strategies. She had stopped meeting family expectations, including running errands, attending church and family functions, and completing chores. When she did leave the house, outings were brief due to low endurance and cautiousness about being away from home too long while in pain.

Academic functioning had been significantly affected by her health. Lucy had many absences, went home early when pain intensity flared, or was tardy due to nausea and fatigue. Normally an A student in honors classes, Lucy was far behind, with several "Incompletes" and no specific plan for how best to prioritize her growing amount of makeup work. Lucy's teachers knew about her health issues; their responses varied from encouraging to indifferent to frustrated. Lucy experienced similar reactions from peers, with close friends providing support but other peers questioning the veracity of her medical issues. In terms of hobbies, Lucy was the manager of the basketball team, but she had stopped attending practices or participating in conditioning with the team due to pain and fatigue. She frequently opted out of social events, feeling unable to push herself through anything more than required activities such as school and homework.

Lucy's eating habits had changed dramatically since pain onset. Due to nausea, she avoided eating breakfast in the morning. Depending on her school schedule (e.g., a test), she occasionally skipped lunch to prevent a disabling pain flare-up that might impair her concentration. After school, Lucy was so hungry that she ate a large snack despite the consequence of having a pain flare-up.

Finally, Lucy's mood had suffered from the chronicity of health problems and change in functioning. Lucy and her family described her as irritable, withdrawn, tired, and easily frustrated. She reported sadness that worsened with greater pain intensity but denied severe depression or suicidal ideation. Lucy stated that she had always been a "worrier" or "thinker"—particularly conscientious about her grades and performance.

She liked to excel academically but had difficulty disengaging from her busy schedule and "to do" list, which created considerable stress. Lucy regularly worried about the pain, its etiology, duration, and how best to cope with it. Current family stressors contributed to her anxiety, including her parents' disagreements about how to handle Lucy's health problems. Lucy described her father as too strict in his expectations that pain should not interfere with daily life and her mother as overly concerned about her, resulting in frequent health-related questions and monitoring. Both anxiety and pain routinely disrupted sleep onset and maintenance, which contributed to ongoing fatigue.

Initial Case Conceptualization

A biopsychosocial approach to case conceptualization is suggested. Lucy's chronic abdominal pain was likely initiated by viral illness but maintained by a host of factors. Biologically, sensory inputs from the gut to the brain were intensified secondary to visceral hyperalgesia (increased sensitivity in the visceral lining of organs, such as the stomach) and Lucy's chronic physiological arousal due to anxiety. Behaviorally, Lucy had stopped engaging in many daily routines and normal activities that would have provided pleasant distractions from her symptoms. Excessive sedentary activities contributed to deconditioning, poor endurance for physical activities of even modest intensity, and mood changes by providing more time to ruminate about her health. Dysregulated mood and sleep likely made it quite difficult to engage in adaptive coping techniques and normal functioning despite pain. Additionally, eating habits alternated between under- and overeating, the former potentially exacerbating ongoing nausea and the latter related to distention of the stomach and gastrointestinal (GI) tract, promoting flare-ups of already sensitized nerves.

Clinical Decision Making

Several factors were considered prior to recommending CBT. Intrapersonal factors (age, development level, and cognitive functioning) can affect the ability to learn and implement CBT. Lucy was sufficiently old enough (generally over 8 years) to acquire the skills and had no significant impairments in attention or cognitive functioning that might affect skill application. Additionally, her comorbid mood changes were not severe, life threatening (e.g., active suicidal ideation), or likely to prevent treatment progress (as with, e.g., intrusive flashbacks from PTSD, frequent panic attacks). Thus she was deemed a good candidate for pain-focused CBT. In other cases, a referral for psychiatric medication or general mental health services would preempt pain coping skills training.

Cognitive-Behavioral Therapy

Gate-Control Theory of Pain

Treatment began with psychoeducation to teach Lucy why and how behavioral interventions for pain were effective. Given her history of inconclusive diagnostic findings and perceived physician skepticism about her symptoms, Lucy needed validation that her pain was real and that physiological changes in the nervous system likely contributed to symptom maintenance. A developmentally appropriate explanation using nontechnical language was delivered via the Gate Control Theory of Pain. Education provided a framework for her ongoing pain and helped Lucy understand why her symptoms wax and wane due to attention or distraction, mood changes, and her degree of tension and arousal related to anxiety. Lucy expressed relief in learning that there were logical, physiological triggers for flare-ups. By the next session, disability and coping efficacy scores began improving solely with this information.

Clinical Outcome Measures

Education about the clinical outcome measures was also provided to define treatment success, which was based on a rehabilitative approach with expected improvements in functioning and coping and not primarily pain reduction. This was an important conversation in order for Lucy to understand that pain intensity was not purposefully being ignored but would also not be the focus of evaluating her treatment progress. Lucy was informed that disability ratings should decrease and coping response improve following CBT.

Family Behavioral Guidelines

Family guidelines for behavioral pain management were reviewed with both Lucy and her mother to instruct her parents on how to provide the most adaptive environment to enhance functioning and coping. The emphasis was a transition away from a medical crisis-oriented mind-set toward wellness behaviors despite chronic pain symptoms. Specifically, her parents were to foster Lucy's independent coping by encouraging her to rely on her new coping techniques rather than seeking refuge at home in her bed. Praising positive functioning, ignoring pain behaviors, and reducing pain-focused conversations were advised so that Lucy's health was not her identity or the sole focus of family attention. Lucy was instructed to resume normal activities despite pain, with reassurance that modifications would be made to address her fatigue, poor endurance, and flare-ups. She was reminded that school attendance and socialization with friends were powerful distractions and also provided a consistent routine at a time when her health seemed unpredictable. Finally, her mother was advised to stop health-related worry in front of Lucy and special treatment on "bad days" that unintentionally reinforced disability. Lucy's mother admitted that she asked too frequently about Lucy's pain, had many medical conversations in Lucy's presence, and had become overly cautious about allowing Lucy to try activities that seemed too taxing. Adherence to these behavioral guidelines was reassessed throughout treatment and ongoing support provided to Lucy's mother to reduce her own anxiety and improve her comfort with Lucy's independent management of pain.

Pain Diaries

Self-monitoring via daily diaries was introduced during the first treatment session. Part of Lucy's pain-related anxiety was the unpredictability of her flare-ups. A daily diary was provided to record pain intensity, stressors, and therapeutic homework assignments. Completion of daily self-monitoring allowed Lucy to track flare-ups, which increased awareness of triggering factors and identifications of symptom patterns.

Biofeedback-Assisted Relaxation Training

Relaxation techniques were taught first to improve parasympathetic responses and also to provide ample time for problem solving about their implementation throughout treatment. Diaphragmatic breathing was presented as a portable technique that assists in reducing physiological and emotional arousal. Lucy practiced the technique in session with the psychologist and reported feeling calmer but also having a slight increase in abdominal pain. The technique was modified to reduce expansion of the abdominal area (which aggravated sensitized nerves) and emphasize slow, deep breaths. A practice schedule was developed for Lucy with twice-daily practices of 5–10 minutes in a quiet location. Small stickers were also provided as cues for "mini relaxation." Lucy was instructed to place the stickers in familiar locations (e.g., locker, iPod) and to take 1–2 deep breaths whenever she saw one to enhance her memory for and application of this technique throughout the day.

Guided imagery was personalized for Lucy related to her favorite vacation to the mountains. The imagery exercise was recorded digitally and given to Lucy to listen to on her portable device at home with a daily practice schedule. In a similar fashion, progressive muscle relaxation (PMR) was taught in session and recorded, with an emphasis on PMR being another method of initiating a parasympathetic response to pain. To increase compliance with home practice without overburdening her time, Lucy was instructed to practice breathing daily and to alternate the practice of imagery and PMR daily until she discerned which techniques maximized her relaxation response, at which time she could elect to focus on those. Consistent practice was required even on "good days" to maintain her skills and serve as prevention tools.

Biofeedback technology was used as a teaching tool to highlight the body's physiological responses in a state of relaxation; there is some support for its use with abdominal pain (Dahlquist & Nagel, 2009). Electromyography (EMG) and thermal modalities were utilized to explore muscular and peripheral temperature changes during relaxation. Lucy liked this scientific aspect of body awareness training, which gave further credibility to behavioral strategies. Given her perfectionistic tendencies, Lucy was cautioned that it might take several weeks before appreciable physiological changes in EMG or thermal ratings were noted, as she was still learning relaxation training.

Behavioral Activation and Activity Pacing

Once Lucy had begun to experience efficacy mastering her physiological reactions to pain and anxiety, she was less resistant to coping with pain outside of her comfort zone (home). Lucy identified a number of enjoyable distraction activities that had been limited due to her health, such as going to friends' houses or resuming her basketball team manager position. These activities were prioritized, and Lucy chose to tackle her team commitments first. Due to her sedentary lifestyle and deconditioning, Lucy was not capable of fully completing these duties without a subsequent flare-up that would compromise school attendance. Thus activity pacing was introduced.

It was explained to Lucy that underexertion and fear of pain flare-ups had led to avoidance of normal activity, which consequently increased muscle weakness and deconditioning and resulted in a cycle of further increased pain and avoidance. Then she was shown how overexertion without breaks on "good days" typically resulted in frequent, debilitating flare-ups requiring excessive rest and recuperation. Instead of either of these approaches, it was emphasized that dividing activity into smaller episodes with brief (5–10 minutes) breaks would proactively reduce flare-ups, promote comfort, and build endurance. This concept was applied to school, to her eating habits, and to physical activity in the following manner. A detailed review of her daily school schedule revealed that Lucy's pain progressively worsened throughout the day, often resulting in early departures from school to manage flare-ups. Together with Lucy, a pacing plan was established whereby she routinely took a 5- to 10-minute break in a quiet location to practice relaxation techniques mid-morning and mid-afternoon. These breaks were described as opportunities to improve coping, reduce distress, and prevent pain levels from elevating. Because school staff members showed varying levels of awareness of her symptoms, the psychologist wrote a letter to the school describing (1) the purpose of planned pacing and (2) the fact that breaks should be routinely scheduled and not "as needed." The latter was done to reduce the burden on Lucy of having to interrupt class and request special treatment. Additionally, it prevented teachers from subtly pressuring her to ignore symptoms or to push through them so as not to miss class. Finally, it was emphasized that this preventive technique would facilitate better attendance, performance, and effort, which were the goals of Lucy, her parents, and the teachers.

A pacing plan was developed related to her team manager duties. Because of the intense practice schedule, Lucy received approval from her coach to attend one practice and one game per week. During practices, Lucy took 5-minute rest breaks on the bleachers to engage in her breathing exercises. The frequency of breaks varied, but Lucy reported that she generally needed to proactively rest every 20–25 minutes to prevent a flare-up from excessive standing or physical activity. Having team commitments only 2 days per week left other days free for medical appointments, makeup work, and recuperation.

Finally, Lucy's eating habits had unintentionally suffered from her behaviors aimed to reduce flare-ups. Lucy had difficulty differentiating the physiological sensations of hunger, need for a bowel movement, and pain. One of her responses to pain was to target a known trigger—eating. Thus Lucy engaged in food avoidance (breakfast and/or lunch) to prevent symptom magnification at school, a strategy that resulted in hunger by mid-afternoon and frequent overeating (too fast and too large a quantity), leading to a flare-up. To address these issues, Lucy first provided a recall of food (type and quantity) consumed the previous day. A plan was developed to normalize food consumption with modest portions, including the use of relaxation techniques to address anticipatory anxiety about eating. Lucy agreed to engage in diaphragmatic breathing 3–5 minutes prior to food consumption to reduce physiological arousal. At breakfast, Lucy chose to eat a small portion of protein (cheese) with her preferred food (crackers), feeling that this combination would not aggravate her nausea excessively. In her letter to the school, the psychologist requested permission for Lucy to consume a snack during her mid-morning break. For lunch, Lucy chose to make her lunch at home with regular-sized portions; she then divided the meal in half, eating one half during her lunch period and the other half after school for a mid-afternoon snack. In this way, Lucy consumed a wide array of foods but in appropriate portions that would not distend her stomach and flare up sensitized nerves. A similar approach to dinner portions was encouraged. An evening snack was optional but suggested to prevent morning nausea that might be due to excessive hunger.

Lucy agreed to practice this plan for 1 week; she was asked to make no adjustments to it in order to fully adapt to the new eating schedule. At the next session, review of the plan revealed the need for additional intervention, such as finding practical snack options for school and in vivo food consumption so the psychologist could coach Lucy on the application of relaxation during meals and monitor the speed of eating. Over time, with problem solving and this systematic approach, Lucy felt efficacious in preventing flare-ups. (It should be noted that a thorough assessment of Lucy's eating behaviors was completed, which revealed a primary goal of food restriction to avoid pain flare-ups and nausea, not due to body image concerns suggestive of an eating disorder.)

Cognitive Restructuring

Formal training in cognitive restructuring occurred later in the treatment for several reasons. Sharing personal thoughts and feelings is often threatening to patients (particularly adolescents) if done early in the intervention. For adolescents with negative therapy experiences or who have "trust issues," these conversations are often more productive once a relationship has been established. Over time, the psychologist also collects evidence of maladaptive thinking and can offer his or her own observations if the patient is less insightful about thoughts and emotions. Negative cognitions are not ignored in early treatment sessions, but the psychologist may selectively choose which thoughts to address at any given time. If extremely rigid, inflexible, and negative cognitions impair treatment progress, then addressing cognitive restructuring becomes paramount and supersedes all other skills. In such cases, the patient may require treatment for more prominent concerns (e.g., depression or obsessive–compulsive disorder) or a referral to psychiatry for medication management if untreated symptoms prevent the acquisition and utilization of pain coping skills (e.g., attention-deficit/hyperactivity disorder).

Throughout treatment, Lucy was able to vocalize worries related to her pain and appeared relatively insightful about the impact of stress on her symptoms. She was less adept at modifying her thinking to neutralize negative cognitions. Thus Lucy was educated about the connection between thoughts, emotions, physiological reactions, and behaviors using salient examples from her life. Lucy also introduced to common cognitive errors (e.g., black-and-white thinking, fortune telling) related to pain and health that frequently result in anxiety. She articulated several worries, including the etiology of her pain (e.g., "What if I really need surgery to fix this problem?"), the duration of the pain (e.g., "I'm afraid I will always have pain"), and whether or not planned activities would have to be aborted due to her symptoms (e.g., "The team is going to hate me if I miss one more game"). Lucy tended to scan her body each morning, evaluating her symptoms to determine whether or not it would be a "good day." With an unfavorable impression, she often had significant anticipatory anxiety related to how bad she would feel and how she would cope.

Lucy was taught several methods to modify this thinking style. First, she created a list of positive self-statements that she could review under increased symptom intensity. This list focused on reasonable statements to neutralize her worries, such as "This flare-up won't last forever"; "I have many techniques to help me cope"; or "I've made it through the school day before with pain." Second, Lucy was coached to investigate her thinking by asking herself such questions as "Do I know for sure the pain will get worse?" or "Will it matter in 5 years that I got a bad grade on this quiz because of my pain?" When thoughts were framed in this manner, Lucy recognized how her pain-related catastrophizing frequently made the situation worse and resulted in producing the outcome that she feared. However, Lucy endorsed difficulty using cognitive modification techniques "in the moment" and was provided with a thought diary to track her negative thoughts and to cue her to engage in more adaptive, flexible thinking.

End of Active Treatment and Maintenance Considerations

In total, Lucy's treatment comprised one session for evaluation, one session for psychoeducation, three sessions for relaxation training, two sessions for activity pacing and school reentry plans, and one session for cognitive restructuring. At times, topics were revisited across multiple sessions (e.g., school reentry plan). A typical session included a status update, a review of clinical outcome data and therapy homework, problem solving related to flare-ups and homework barriers, skill introduction and rehearsal, homework assignment, and review of session content with parents. At the end of active treatment, outcome data reflected improvements in functioning, coping, and pain. Her FDI score decreased by 50% (from 30, "severe disability," to 15, "moderate disability"). Her PCQ coping efficacy score increased from 6 to 13, suggesting that Lucy felt successful in managing her pain and emotions. Although it was not a primary outcome, Lucy's average pain intensity also decreased by 50% (8/10 to 4/10), with some pain-free episodes throughout the day. She attributed these outcomes to use of coping techniques, a better understanding of her body, and resuming a more normal lifestyle. Lucy also was scheduled to return to her gastroenterologist for follow-up to monitor the lingering symptoms that had not improved despite pain coping skills training.

It was important to prepare Lucy for effective coping without regular attendance in therapy. Thus issues concerning maintenance were addressed.

During review, Lucy was able to label and describe each coping skill, when she used it, and what barriers might affect implementation in the future (e.g., eating habits changing over summer vacation, less motivation to use techniques on the weekends when symptoms are less intense). A 1-month follow-up was scheduled to evaluate Lucy's independent self-management and to solve problems that had arisen. Lucy was told to expect that brief flare-ups would likely happen in the future, and she prepared positive self-statements in anticipation to prevent catastrophizing. Finally, Lucy was coached to recognize when she might need a therapy "tune-up" in the future (e.g., stressful times such as exam week) and encouraged to schedule appointments accordingly on an as-needed basis. In this way, sustained positive coping was expected, but Lucy did not feel abandoned or unable to seek professional support if pain-related functioning or disability became problematic.

SUMMARY AND CONCLUSIONS

Lucy's case illustrates how CBT for behavioral pain management is brief and skills-focused yet comprehensively addresses important domains affected by health. Her psychologist helped Lucy to improve her functional disability by developing concrete behavioral plans to facilitate change and teaching coping tools to promote physical and emotional comfort. Tailoring these techniques to the developmental level of the patient is critical, and the inclusion of parents in this intervention is more prominent with younger children. Thus CBT provides an effective complement to the medical management of pediatric chronic pain.

REFERENCES

Banez, G., & Cunningham, C. L. (2009). Abdominal pain-related gastrointestinal disorders: Irritable bowel syndrome and inflammatory bowel disease. In M. C. Roberts & R. G. Steele (Eds.), *Handbook of pediatric psychology* (4th ed., pp. 403–419). New York: Guilford Press.

Dahlquist, L. M., & Nagel, M. S. (2009). Chronic and recurrent pain. In M. C. Roberts & R. G. Steele (Eds.), *Handbook of pediatric psychology* (4th ed., pp. 153–170). New York: Guilford Press.

Eccleston, C., Palermo, T. M., Williams, A. C., Lewandowski, A., & Morley, S. (2009). Psychological therapies for the management of chronic and recurrent pain in children and adolescents. *Cochrane Database of Systematic Reviews*, CD003968.

Huertas-Ceballos, A., Logan, S., Bennett, C., & Macarthur, C. (2008). Psychosocial interventions for recurrent abdominal pain (RAP) and irritable bowel syndrome (IBS) in childhood. *Cochrane Database of Systematic Reviews,* CD003014.

Kashikar-Zuck, S., Flowers, S. R., Claar, R. L., Guite, J. W., Logan, D. E., Lynch-Jordan, A. M., et al. (2011). Clinical utility and validity of the Functional Disability Inventory among a multicenter sample of youth with chronic pain. *Pain, 152,* 1600–1607.

Palermo, T. M., Eccleston, C., Lewandowski, A. S., Williams, A. C., & Morley, S. (2010). Randomized controlled trials of psychological therapies for management of chronic pain in children and adolescents: An updated meta-analytic review. *Pain, 148,* 387–397.

Rasquin, A., Di Lorenzo, C., Forbes, D., Guiraldes, E., Hyams, J. S., Staiano, A., et al. (2006). Childhood functional gastrointestinal disorders: Child/adolescent. *Gastroenterology, 130,* 1527–1537.

Reid, G. J., Gilbert, C. A., & McGrath, P. J. (1998). The Pain Coping Questionnaire: Preliminary validation. *Pain, 76,* 83–96.

Uman, L. S., Chambers, C. T., McGrath, P. J., & Kisely, S. (2008). A systematic review of randomized controlled trials examining psychological interventions for needle-related procedural pain and distress in children and adolescents: An abbreviated Cochrane review. *Journal of Pediatric Psychology, 33,* 842–854.

Walker, L. S., & Greene, J. W. (1991). The Functional Disability Inventory: Measuring a neglected dimension of child health status. *Journal of Pediatric Psychology, 16,* 39–58.

CHAPTER 14

Pediatric Sleep Disorders

JODI A. MINDELL
LISA J. MELTZER

Sleep problems are highly common, occurring in 25–40% of typically developing children (Meltzer & Mindell, 2009). When children and adolescents do not obtain sufficient sleep, there are numerous consequences, affecting growth, development, cognitive functioning, performance, health, mood, and family functioning (Mindell & Owens, 2009). Further, disrupted sleep can often be associated with concomitant physical or psychiatric illness.

Psychologists play a primary role in the treatment of pediatric sleep disorders, with many pediatric sleep centers including psychologists as part of their teams. One study (Meltzer, Moore, & Mindell, 2008) of 265 consecutive patients evaluated in an interdisciplinary sleep center that included attendings in pulmonary medicine, neurology, and psychology found that over half of the patients seen had comorbid medical diagnoses and that 31% had comorbid psychiatric diagnoses. Over one-third of patients received at least one behavioral recommendation.

As with most areas of pediatric psychology, a thorough evaluation of a wide array of underlying medical and psychiatric contributors to sleep disturbances is essential, especially as the same symptom can be related to physiological or behavioral causes. In an exemplary situation, the patient is evaluated by an interdisciplinary team that has a wide array of expertise, but a thorough assessment within a psychological practice that incorporates an understanding of the plethora of factors that can contribute to sleep disturbances can be done (for complete information on assessment, see Mindell & Owens, 2009). This chapter provides an overview of three cases that exemplify treatment of behaviorally based interventions for a broad spectrum of sleep disturbances.

CASE EXAMPLE 1: OSCAR

Oscar was an 8-month-old boy who presented with his mother with difficulties falling asleep at bedtime and naptime without nursing, as well as frequent night wakings.

Assessment and Further Evaluation

Clinical Interview

Sleep History. Oscar had an evening routine that included a bath at approximately 8:30 P.M., followed by reading stories with his 3-year-old sister, and then being nursed to sleep around 9:15–9:30 P.M. Oscar was then placed in his crib asleep, which was in his parents' bedroom. Once put down at bedtime, he would often wake and begin crying. His mother would then have to pick him back up and nurse him until he returned to sleep. Once asleep, Oscar woke 2–4 times per night. His mother would again nurse him to help him return to sleep. By the second waking, she would bring him to her bed, where he would continue to wake, crying, at least another two times during the night. Nap times were also difficult, with Oscar's mother again nursing him to sleep, but she would then need to hold him throughout nap time so that he would remain asleep.

Other Relevant History. Oscar was born full term with no complications. He had a significant history of reflux-related symptoms, which had not been treated. His mother was highly tearful throughout the appointment. She had been assessed for depression at 6 weeks postpartum but had not pursued treatment, as she was "overwhelmed." She did have an appointment scheduled for the following week to see a therapist. Her husband was a full-time MBA student, and the family lived in a one-bedroom apartment with a den, where the older daughter slept. The family had moved to the area 1 year prior, and the mother had no local support system. She did attend a play group, but it only met once every 2 weeks.

2-Week Sleep Diary

Oscar's mother completed a daily sleep diary for 2 weeks prior to the appointment (Figure 14.1). Highly fragmented sleep was indicated throughout the night, with highly variable nap times.

Differential Diagnosis

Reflux is highly common in infants and often contributes to sleep difficulties. Reflux could be contributing to Oscar's nighttime awakenings but would not account for his difficulties in falling asleep independently. Oscar clearly met diagnostic criteria for behavioral insomnia of childhood—sleep onset association type (American Academy of Sleep Medicine, 2005), given his association of nursing with sleep onset at bedtime, following naturally occurring night wakings, and at nap times.

Intervention and Outcomes

Oscar was referred to a gastroenterologist for evaluation for reflux. His symptoms had been progressively getting better, so no medical intervention was implemented.

Behavioral interventions are highly successful in the treatment of bedtime problems and night wakings in infants and toddlers (Mindell, Kuhn, Lewin, Meltzer, & Sadeh, 2006). First, an earlier bedtime of 7:00 was established, as late bedtimes are noted to be associated with increased difficulties falling asleep and maintaining sleep in young children (Mindell, Meltzer, Carskadon, & Chervin, 2009). Second, nursing was moved to the start of the bedtime routine and occurred in the living room rather than in the bedroom. During the first week, his mother continued to rock him to sleep at bedtime. Once nursing was no longer associated with falling asleep at bedtime, a graduated extinction approach was recommended, with Oscar to be put down awake at bedtime and his parents to institute a checking method every 5–10 minutes until he fell asleep. It was recommended that Oscar's father manage the bedtime sleep training, as his mother was unsure whether she could be consistent if Oscar became upset. While helping Oscar to fall asleep independently, his mother was to respond consistently to night wakings, nursing him back to sleep. After 5 days, Oscar was falling asleep easily on his own at bedtime, and he began to sleep for significantly longer stretches at night. At week 3, his mother stopped all nighttime nursing, and at 1-month follow-up Oscar was sleeping well at night. His mother was starting to work on putting him down awake at nap times.

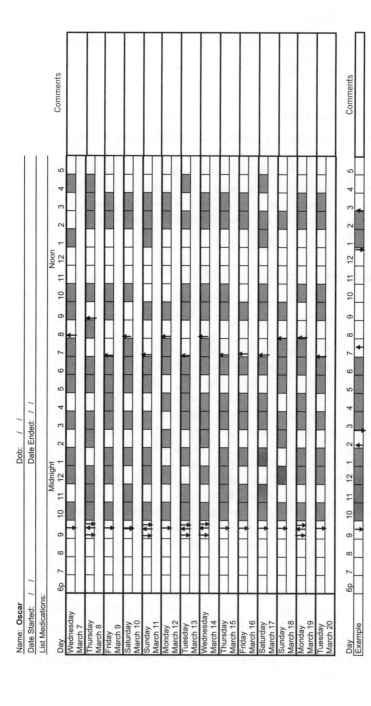

FIGURE 14.1. Sleep diary for Oscar.

192

Issues and Challenges

Postpartum depression was a significant concern in this case, and it is known to be associated with sleep disruption (Dorheim, Bondevik, Eberhard-Gran, & Bjorvatn, 2009). Oscar's mother was encouraged to keep her upcoming appointment with a therapist. A thorough evaluation at the sleep clinic appointment was conducted to ensure that Oscar's mother was not at risk of harming herself or either of her children, and recommendations were made as to what she should do if she began having such thoughts. A plan was developed to have Oscar's father manage more of the child care over the upcoming weeks, while the sleep intervention was being implemented. Oscar's mother was also encouraged to initiate contact with other mothers from her play group on a more frequent basis. Initially, daily calls were made with the mother to provide support and continually assess her functioning.

CASE EXAMPLE 2: TONY

Tony was a 9-year-old boy with high-functioning autism spectrum disorder (ASD), eczema, and allergic rhinitis who presented, with his parents, with complaints of a lifetime history of prolonged sleep onset latency, as well as frequent and prolonged night wakings.

Assessment and Further Evaluation

Clinical Interview

Sleep History. Tony's sleep routine included a "bedtime goal" of between 8:00 and 8:30 P.M. on weekdays and 9:00 P.M. on weekends. However, he would often "dawdle" at bedtime and not want to get ready for bed. Once he was finally in bed it would take about 60 minutes for him to fall asleep. Most nights his mother would return to the room and rub Tony's back until he was "pretty close to asleep." His mother thought that on some nights he was asleep prior to her leaving the room.

While asleep, Tony had frequent congestion at night but no symptoms of sleep-disordered breathing. He would wake once each night and come into his parents' room. Sometimes he would complain of itching or a bad dream, but most often he would complain that he could not sleep. His parents would attempt to return him to his bed, but most nights he would return to the parents' bed. These night wakings would last up to 2 hours. Tony did not nap during the day.

Other Relevant History. Tony was diagnosed with high-functioning ASD and was taking hydroxyzine twice a day for his eczema. He was also taking "half a dropper" of melatonin, although his parents did not know the dosing of the melatonin.

2-Week Sleep Diary

Prior to his appointment, Tony's parents completed a daily sleep diary for 2 weeks (Figure 14.2). A prolonged sleep onset latency was recorded for only one night; however, prolonged night awakenings were clearly visible every night.

Differential Diagnosis

A number of factors likely contributed to Tony's sleep difficulties. First, 44–83% of children with ASD have difficulties with sleep initiation, sleep maintenance, early morning sleep termination, and/or shorter total sleep duration (Richdale & Schreck, 2009). This would suggest a possible diagnosis of insomnia due to a psychiatric condition. Second, 60–83% of children with eczema have difficulties with sleep initiation and/or sleep maintenance due to itching (Camfferman, Kennedy, Gold, Martin, & Lushington, 2010), suggesting a possible diagnosis of insomnia due to a medical condition. Third, Tony's bedtime resistance, followed by an inability to fall asleep or return to sleep without a parent present, is suggestive of behavioral insomnia of childhood, combined type. Any one of these diagnoses would have been appropriate in this case.

Intervention

Tony's parents were encouraged to follow up with his allergist to better manage Tony's eczema. The following plan was designed to target the behavioral aspects of Tony's sleep problems. First, a bedtime chart was recommended to prevent bedtime stalling and resistance. A bedtime chart includes a picture of each step of the bedtime routine (e.g., snack, bath, toilet, toothbrush, book, bed). In general, children with ASD respond well to consistent routines and visual cues. Thus this chart provides a constant reminder and a predictable routine every night. Second, to help teach Tony to fall asleep independently, his mother began taking a short break at bedtime, returning to help Tony fall asleep. Each night this break was progressively longer, with the goal of Tony falling asleep while his mother was not in the room. Once he fell asleep, Tony earned an immediate reward of a sticker under his pillow. Finally, as melatonin has been shown to improve sleep onset in youth with ASD (Doyen et al., 2011; Malow et al., 2011; Rossignol & Frye, 2011), Tony began taking a full dropper of melatonin (which was the equivalent of 1 mg of melatonin) 30 minutes before bed.

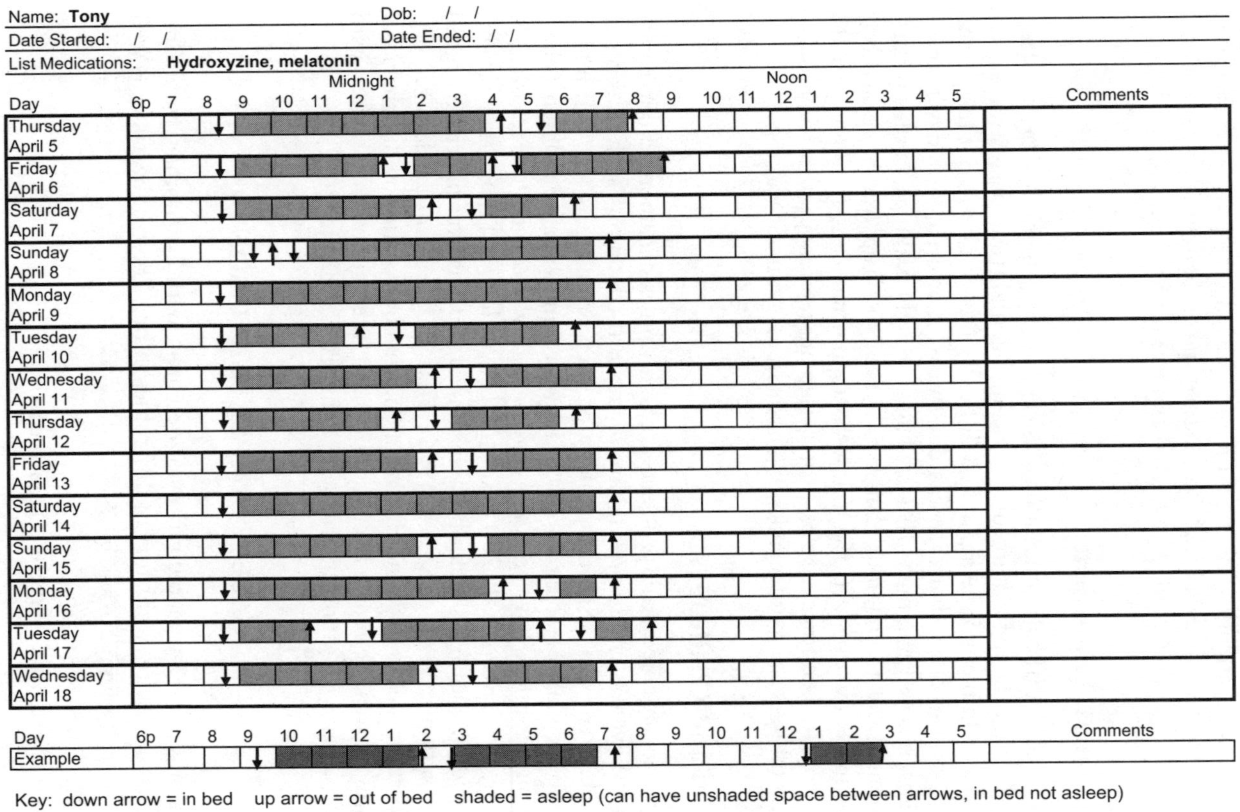

Name: **Tony**   Dob: / /

Date Started: / /   Date Ended: / /

List Medications: **Hydroxyzine, melatonin**

FIGURE 14.2. Sleep diary for Tony.

Key: down arrow = in bed   up arrow = out of bed   shaded = asleep (can have unshaded space between arrows, in bed not asleep)

195

For his night wakings, Tony was given a "nighttime pass" each night (Moore, Friman, Fruzzetti, & MacAleese, 2007). If he came into his parents' room seeking attention, he would have to give up the pass. However, if he chose to stay in his own bed, he could save and exchange the passes for small rewards (e.g., a bike ride with his father, an extra 5 minutes of television).

Outcomes Assessment

Tony had a difficult time falling asleep the first night but began sleeping through the night immediately, using his nighttime passes for desired rewards. On night 5, he again had difficulty falling asleep, but his parents noted on the diary that this was due to a special event that day that got him overexcited. On night 10 Tony had two night wakings, but his parents attributed this to coughing that required cough syrup, and he returned to sleep in his own bed. At the follow-up appointment the family reported a less stressful bedtime routine, shorter sleep onset latency (with Tony consistently falling asleep independently), and almost no night wakings.

Issues and Challenges

As previously noted, sleep problems are highly prevalent among children with ASD, as well as children with chronic medical conditions such as eczema. For children with ASD, the etiology of sleep problems is not well understood (Richdale & Schreck, 2009). However, individually tailored behavioral interventions have been shown to be highly effective (Piazza, Fisher, & Sherer, 1997; Reed et al., 2009; Reynolds & Malow, 2011). Further, parents of children with ASD prefer behavioral interventions over pharmacological interventions (Wiggs & Stores, 1996). That said, a recent randomized placebo-controlled trial found that melatonin in combination with behavioral treatment was the most effective short-term intervention for children with ASD (Cortesi, Giannotti, Sebastiani, Panunzi, & Valente, 2012).

CASE EXAMPLE 3: ALLISON

Allison was a 15-year-old girl who presented, with her mother, with complaints of a multiyear history of difficulties falling asleep at bedtime, as well as infrequent night awakenings.

Assessment and Further Evaluation

Clinical Interview

Sleep History. Allison's sleep routine included taking a shower at 10:00 P.M., after doing homework, followed by texting her friends and being on the computer while in bed. Between 11:00 and 11:30 P.M. she would turn out the lights and "toss and turn," finally falling asleep between 1:00 and 2:00 A.M. If she felt frustrated that she was not asleep, she would turn her computer back on or text. Most nights, Allison reported waking between 3:00 and 4:00 A.M. and would not return to sleep for another 30–45 minutes. Her wake time on school days was 6:00 A.M. On weekends, lights-out was usually between midnight and 1:00 A.M., and it would also take her 1–3 hours to fall asleep. She would usually "sleep in" until 11:00 A.M. on weekends. Allison reported having sleep problems for the past few years, although it had gotten worse in the past year.

Allison had no symptoms of sleep-disordered breathing. She did not report any uncomfortable sensations in her legs at bedtime, and she was not described as a restless sleeper. Allison reported feeling tired during the day, especially after a poor night's sleep, but she did not report any significant daytime sleepiness, and she did not take any planned or spontaneous naps. Allison stated that she often worried throughout the day about how well she was going to sleep that night and "dreaded" bedtime.

Other Relevant History. Allison reported that she thought that she was more anxious than her peers. She excelled in school, although her poor sleep had begun to interfere with her school performance over the past year. Family history was significant for insomnia in her mother.

2-Week Sleep Diary

Prior to her appointment, Allison completed a daily sleep diary for 2 weeks (Figure 14.3). Allison consistently reported a sleep onset latency of 1–3 hours, and night wakings were indicated on 10 of the 14 nights recorded.

Differential Diagnosis

Poor sleep hygiene is a common reason that adolescents have difficulty falling asleep. Although Allison did engage in electronic use prior to bed and sometimes after lights-out, she did have a consistent bedtime and bedtime routine, she did not take daily naps that interfered with sleep onset, and she did not drink any caffeinated beverages. Other sleep disorders, primarily restless legs syndrome (RLS) and delayed sleep phase disorder (DSPD), can also result in difficulties falling asleep. RLS involves uncomfortable sensations in the legs, primarily at bedtime, and an uncontrollable urge to move the legs, which relieves the sensations (American Academy of Sleep Medicine, 2005). Allison denied symptoms of RLS. DSPD is highly common during adolescence, with a prevalence rate of approximately 7% (Mindell & Owens, 2009). However, in DSPD there is typically no difficulty falling asleep when lights-out is at the adolescent's naturally occurring sleep

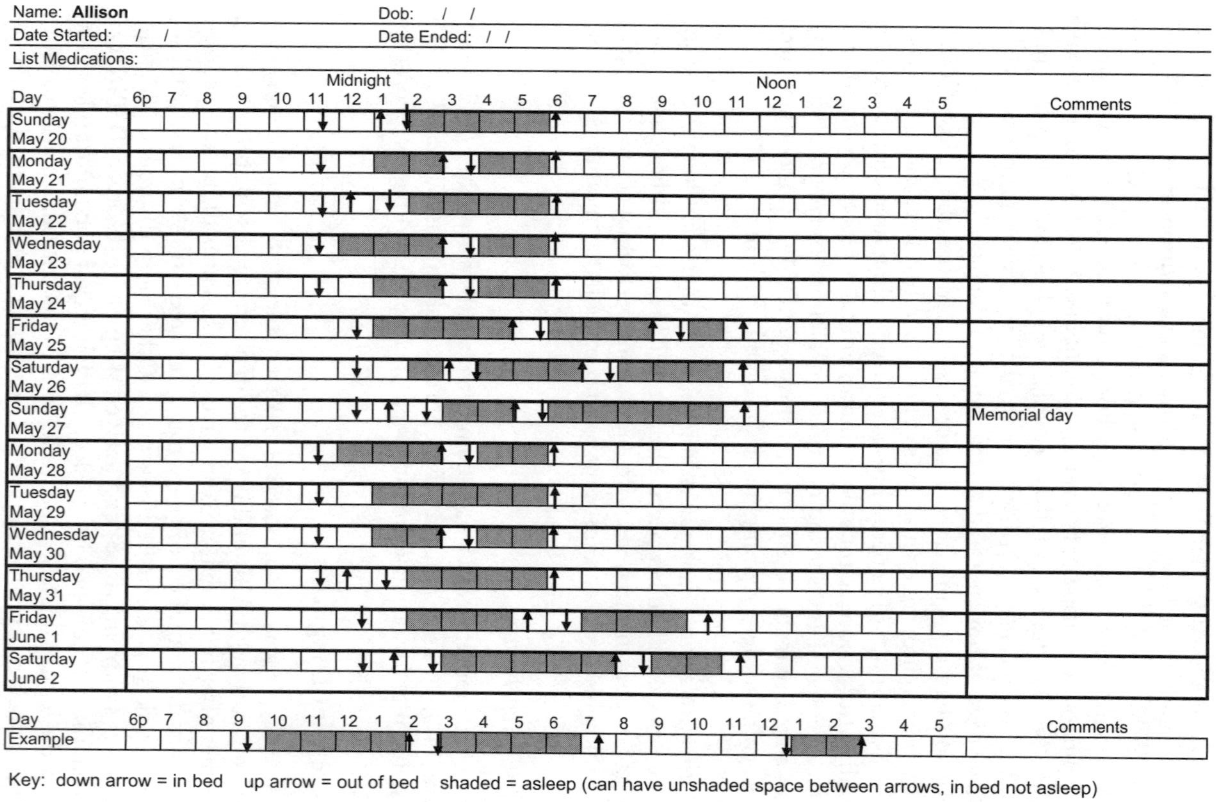

FIGURE 14.3. Sleep diary for Allison.

198

onset time, and rarely are night awakenings present. Allison had a prolonged sleep onset latency regardless of bedtime, as well as frequent night awakenings. Allison clearly met diagnostic criteria for psychophysiological insomnia (American Academy of Sleep Medicine, 2005), as indicated by (1) complaint of difficulties initiating and maintaining sleep for at least 1 month, (2) heightened arousal about sleep, including excessive focus on anxiety about sleep, (3) adequate opportunity and circumstances for sleep, and (4) daytime impairment. Approximately 9–13% of adolescents experience chronic insomnia, with up to 35% experiencing frequent insomnia symptoms (Dohnt, Gradisar, & Short, 2012). Insomnia is more common in girls postpuberty.

Intervention

A behavioral intervention plan was developed in conjunction with Allison and her mother, starting with stimulus control. This included (1) no activities in bed that were not conducive with sleep (e.g., electronics use), (2) moving her alarm clock across the room so that she was not watching the clock throughout the night, (3) moving lights-out closer to her naturally occurring sleep onset time, (4) getting in bed only when she was sleepy (in this case, 1:00 A.M.), and (5) getting out of bed if she was not asleep after 15–20 minutes and engaging in a nonstimulating activity (e.g., reading a book that she had read many times), only returning to bed when she felt sleepy. Once she began falling asleep more quickly, Allison was instructed to begin moving her bedtime earlier by 15 minutes every few nights.

Outcomes Assessment

Although resistant at first to the idea of getting out of bed when she was not asleep, Allison found that she had to get out of bed only one time per night for the first week or so. She found that going to bed much later was quite helpful, as this initially restricted her sleep duration, with the increased sleepiness reducing her cognitive arousal at bedtime. After 2 weeks, Allison was falling asleep within 20–30 minutes most nights.

Issues and Challenges

Behavioral interventions are highly effective for insomnia (Morin, Hauri, et al., 1999), although there is limited research on its use with adolescents. As expected, the recommendation to limit electronics use in bed was met by resistance, as well as the instruction to get out of bed after 20 minutes of wakefulness. Furthermore, families may expect pharmacological management with immediate results and can be frustrated by behavioral recommendations that require significant effort and diligence. However, there are no Food and Drug Administration–approved medications for insomnia in children and adolescents. Furthermore, research indicates that behavioral interventions are as effective as medications in the short term and have better outcomes long term (Morin, Colecchi, Stone, Sood, & Brink, 1999).

SUMMARY

As exemplified by the preceding cases, the key to successful treatment is the inclusion of a thorough evaluation, as well as tailoring evidence-based interventions to meet the needs of individual patients. Referral to a medical sleep specialist should occur in situations in which a child or adolescent has symptoms of other underlying sleep disrupters (e.g., obstructive sleep apnea) or excessive daytime sleepiness despite sufficient sleep duration. For patients who fail to respond to common behavioral interventions, a referral to a behavioral medicine specialist with expertise in treating sleep problems may be warranted.

REFERENCES

American Academy of Sleep Medicine. (2005). *International classification of sleep disorders: Diagnostic and coding manual* (2nd ed.). Westchester, IL: Author.

Camfferman, D., Kennedy, J. D., Gold, M., Martin, A. J., & Lushington, K. (2010). Eczema and sleep and its relationship to daytime functioning in children. *Sleep Medicine Reviews, 14*(6), 359–369.

Cortesi, F., Giannotti, F., Sebastiani, T., Panunzi, S., & Valente, D. (2012). Controlled-release melatonin, singly and combined with cognitive behavioural therapy, for persistent insomnia in children with autism spectrum disorders: A randomized placebo-controlled trial. *Journal of Sleep Research, 21*(6), 700–709.

Dohnt, H., Gradisar, M., & Short, M. A. (2012). Insomnia and its symptoms in adolescents: Comparing DSM-IV and ICSD-II diagnostic criteria. *Journal of Clinical Sleep Medicine, 8*(3), 295–299.

Dorheim, S. K., Bondevik, G. T., Eberhard-Gran, M., & Bjorvatn, B. (2009). Sleep and depression in postpartum women: A population-based study. *Sleep, 32*(7), 847–855.

Doyen, C., Mighiu, D., Kaye, K., Colineaux, C., Beaumanoir, C., Mouraeff, Y., et al. (2011). Melatonin in children with autistic spectrum disorders: Recent and practical data. *European Child and Adolescent Psychiatry, 20*(5), 231–239.

Malow, B., Adkins, K., McGrew, S., Wang, L., Goldman, S., Fawkes, D., et al. (2011). Melatonin for sleep in children with autism: A controlled trial examining dose, tolerability, and outcomes. *Journal of Autism and Developmental Disorders, 42,* 1729–1737.

Meltzer, L. J., & Mindell, J. A. (2009). Pediatric sleep. In M. C. Roberts & R. G. Steele (Eds.), *Handbook of pediatric psychology* (4th ed.). New York: Guilford Press.

Meltzer, L. J., Moore, M., & Mindell, J. A. (2008). The need for interdisciplinary pediatric sleep clinics. *Behavioral Sleep Medicine, 6*(4), 268–282.

Mindell, J. A., Kuhn, B., Lewin, D. S., Meltzer, L. J., & Sadeh, A. (2006). Behavioral treatment of bedtime problems and night wakings in infants and young children. *Sleep, 29*(10), 1263–1276.

Mindell, J. A., Meltzer, L. J., Carskadon, M. A., & Chervin, R. D. (2009). Developmental aspects of sleep hygiene: Findings from the 2004 National Sleep Foundation Sleep in America Poll. *Sleep Medicine, 10*(7), 771–779.

Mindell, J. A., & Owens, J. A. (2009). *A clinical guide to pediatric sleep: Diagnosis and management of sleep problems* (2nd ed.). Philadelphia: Lippincott Williams & Wilkins.

Moore, B. A., Friman, P. C., Fruzzetti, A. E., & MacAleese, K. (2007). Brief report: Evaluating the Bedtime Pass Program for child resistance to bedtime—a randomized, controlled trial. *Journal of Pediatric Psychology, 32*(3), 283–287.

Morin, C. M., Colecchi, C., Stone, J., Sood, R., & Brink, D. (1999). Behavioral and pharmacological therapies for late-life insomnia: A randomized controlled trial. *Journal of the American Medical Association, 281*(11), 991–999.

Morin, C. M., Hauri, P. J., Espie, C. A., Spielman, A. J., Buysse, D. J., & Bootzin, R. R. (1999). Nonpharmacologic treatment of chronic insomnia: An American Academy of Sleep Medicine review. *Sleep, 22*(8), 1134–1156.

Piazza, C. C., Fisher, W. W., & Sherer, M. (1997). Treatment of multiple sleep problems in children with developmental disabilities: Faded bedtime with response cost versus bedtime scheduling. *Developmental Medicine and Child Neurology, 39*(6), 414–418.

Reed, H. E., McGrew, S. G., Artibee, K., Surdkya, K., Goldman, S. E., Frank, K., et al. (2009). Parent-based sleep education workshops in autism. *Journal of Child Neurology, 24*(8), 936–945.

Reynolds, A. M., & Malow, B. A. (2011). Sleep and autism spectrum disorders. *Pediatric Clinics of North America, 58*(3), 685–698.

Richdale, A. L., & Schreck, K. A. (2009). Sleep problems in autism spectrum disorders: Prevalence, nature, and possible biopsychosocial aetiologie. *Sleep Medicine Reviews, 13*(6), 403–411.

Rossignol, D. A., & Frye, R. E. (2011). Melatonin in autism spectrum disorders: A systematic review and meta-analysis. *Developmental Medicine and Child Neurology, 53*(9), 783–792.

Wiggs, L., & Stores, G. (1996). Severe sleep disturbance and daytime challenging behaviour in children with severe learning disabilities. *Journal of Intellectual Disability Research, 40,* 518–528.

CHAPTER 15

Juvenile Idiopathic Arthritis

CATHERINE BUTZ
KATHLEEN LEMANEK
CYNTHIA A. GERHARDT

Juvenile idiopathic arthritis (JIA) comprises a variety of rheumatic diseases and affects an estimated 294,000 children in the United States (Helmick et al., 2008). Although other tissue and organ systems may be affected, it is primarily marked by unpredictable flares or acute inflammation of musculoskeletal tissue. (For a recent review of medical and psychosocial aspects of the disease, see Rapoff, Lindsley, & Karlson, 2009). In brief, symptoms and prognosis vary widely depending on disease type and severity, and many children have recurrent disease or functional limitations into adulthood (Foster, Marshall, Myers, Dunkley, & Griffiths, 2003; Oen et al., 2002). Treatment to reduce common symptoms, such as pain and inflammation, is multifaceted and often includes nonsteroidal anti-inflammatory drugs (NSAIDs), disease-modifying antirheumatic drugs (DMARDs), corticosteroid injections in the muscle or joints, and physical therapy to maintain functioning and prevent deformities.

Given the symptoms, treatment demands, and potential for long-term functional limitations due to JIA, there has been concern for the psychosocial well-being of affected children and their families. Most youth with arthritis do not have severe or lasting psychological difficulties, but there may be some risk for internalizing problems (Adam et al., 2005; LeBovidge, Lavigne, Donenberg, & Miller, 2003), reduced social activities

(Aasland, Flato, & Vandvik, 1997; Feldmann, Weglage, Roth, Foell, & Frosch, 2005), school absences (Billings, Moos, Miller, & Gottlieb, 1987; Lovell et al., 1990), and difficulty achieving developmental milestones, particularly regarding employment, as they mature (Foster et al., 2003; Packham & Hall, 2002). Children with more severe forms of arthritis, longer disease duration, or greater pain tend to have more psychosocial difficulties (Billings et al., 1987; Sandstrom & Schanberg, 2004; Sawyer et al., 2005). However, a more complex, reciprocal association between disease and psychosocial factors also has been suggested (Schanberg, Gil, Anthony, Yow, & Rochon, 2005).

CASE EXAMPLE: JULIE

The complexities of the foregoing associations are exemplified in the case of Julie M, an 11-year-old white female with juvenile polyarticular rheumatoid arthritis, who was referred for psychological treatment by her rheumatologist. The rheumatologist reported that Julie's pain and disease process were relatively stable with initial use of corticosteroids and maintenance therapy with NSAIDs and steroid injections. However, there was concern that Julie was not coping adequately with her diagnosis, as evidenced by school absences, poor sleep hygiene, and suspected depressive symptoms. This chapter discusses the psychologist's assessment of these concerns, case conceptualization, selection and implementation of evidence-based treatments, and the various roles the psychologist served to facilitate a positive outcome for Julie.

An initial assessment and clinical interview were scheduled with Julie and her parents to assess mood, school functioning, and sleep problems. Julie lived with her mother, father, and two older brothers. Her parents had been together for 18 years but had recently separated. Although they reconciled, Mr. and Mrs. M acknowledged ongoing marital conflict and significant financial stress. Julie's father worked in a factory, but he feared losing his job. Julie's mother was unemployed. The family history was significant for depression in Julie's mother, anxiety in Julie's father, and behavioral problems for her brother, but the family had never sought treatment for any of these issues. These family factors are discussed later in more detail and in terms of their relevance to Julie's presenting problem and treatment.

Julie was described as a good student with a normal course of development and no significant history of psychosocial difficulties or treatment. She was in the sixth grade, had a history of numerous absences, and had not attended school for 2 months prior to meeting with the psychologist. As a result, her grades significantly declined. Some educational accommodations were in place at school, such as a decrease in writing assignments and a scribe for tests, but her parents noted that the implementation of these interventions was inconsistent. Although it appeared that Julie's poor attendance could be related to the timing of her diagnosis, other individual and familial factors were discovered as contributing factors.

During the initial meeting, Julie reported symptoms suggesting an anxiety disorder (e.g., worry, school avoidance), but she did not meet diagnostic criteria. In addition, symptoms consistent with depression (e.g., poor sleep patterns, disordered eating, irritability) were seen, more so as a result of poor lifestyle habits and routine. She was compliant with medical treatment, and there was also no evidence of a behavior problem outside of school attendance. However, her sleep patterns resembled a delayed sleep phase disorder, in which sleep onset was significantly shifted to a time of day that was maladaptive. Although she was in bed for an adequate amount of time, she slept every night with her mother from 3 A.M. to 11 A.M., which interfered with school attendance. There was an initial concern that corticosteroids, which can affect mood and sleep (Reddy & Subramanian, 2009), may have contributed to Julie's poor sleep patterns. However, Julie denied nightmares and fragmented sleep, and her sleep patterns reportedly developed prior to her diagnosis due to nighttime fears and a growing dependence on her mother as a co-sleeper. Her mother's own history of depression and disrupted sleep interfered with implementation of an age-appropriate routine for Julie. Thus Julie's exacerbated pain and school absences seemed rooted in her poor sleep patterns and not her diagnosis or treatment (Bromberg, Gil, & Schanberg, 2012). Given the obvious detriment this sleep pattern had on Julie's school attendance, improvement of sleep hygiene was a necessary first step in therapy.

Evidence-based approaches to the treatment of psychosocial issues among families of children with JIA or similar rheumatic diseases have primarily relied on psychoeducational and cognitive-behavioral strategies to address adherence or self-management (Rapoff et al., 2002; Rapoff & Lindsley, 2007; Stark et al., 2005), pain (Lavigne, Ross, Berry, Hayford, & Pachman, 1992; Walco, Varni, & Ilowite, 1992), and coping (Degotardi et al., 2006; Kashikar-Zuck, Swain, Jones, & Graham, 2005). Because the number of intervention studies focused specifically on JIA is small, clinicians often reference the broader literature on successful interventions for children with other health conditions. Julie was deemed a good candidate for several of these interventions: (1) a general behavioral approach to improve sleep hygiene, (2) cognitive-behavioral therapy (CBT) to improve emotional functioning, and (3) a modified JIA-specific intervention (Lavigne et al., 1992; Walco et al., 1992) involving relaxation training with biofeedback for pain control.

Julie's family was willing to engage in treatment to improve her sleep once the physiological effects of sleep deprivation on pain were thoroughly discussed. It was first recommended that the family create a regular sleep schedule and start bedtime 30 minutes earlier every few nights (see Table 15.1). In addition, the importance of a routine was emphasized, such that Julie was encouraged to take the same steps every night, beginning 1 hour before an identified bedtime, to facilitate sleep onset. These steps included a light snack, bathing, watching television, and/or reading outside of the bedroom.

In addition, Julie's mother was coached on behavioral fading, whereby Julie would become better able to fall asleep on her own and in her own bed. Julie's mother was encouraged to approach fading in steps. This involved first having Julie sleep in her own bed with her mom, then having her mother leave during the night to return to her own room, and finally having her mother help Julie during her routine but leave her room before Julie fell asleep. Co-sleeping was strongly discouraged, and Julie's parents were instructed to return Julie to her bed if she awoke during the night. Moreover, Julie was instructed on breathing techniques that she could practice during her nightly routine to help her relax, manage nighttime fears, and return to sleep. After 5 weeks, Julie reported significant improvement in her sleep, mood, and pain. In addition, although she continued to express hesitancy about school, she began attending sporadically.

CBT was applied throughout treatment to help Julie better identify triggers for her symptoms of anxiety. The association between her mood and pain was discussed. For instance, Julie began to recognize that an irregular sleep schedule led to pain and school absences. Missing school and other age-appropriate activities subsequently contributed to a decline in mood and an increase in anxiety about returning to school. Moreover, Julie was able to recognize her resentment over her diagnosis and that

TABLE 15.1. Julie's Sleep Schedule and School Attendance for the First Five Sessions of Treatment

Week	Approximate sleep (hours)	Average pain score (0–10)[a]	School attendance (days)
1	2:00 A.M.–10:00 A.M.	8	0
2	1:00 A.M.–9:00 A.M.	6	0.5
3	11:30 P.M.–8:00 A.M.	7	1
4	11:00 P.M.–7:00 A.M.	3	2
5	10:00 P.M.–6:30 A.M.	3	3.5

[a] Higher scores indicate worse pain.

she actively distracted herself from her own self-care by aligning with her mother's poor functioning and lifestyle. Her mood would become more despondent as she had more contact with her mother, and her avoidance of school would increase. As such, her negative cognitions about her health, school functioning, peer relations, and family conflict were identified and addressed.

Common in CBT, treatment focused on identifying how the link between cognition and behavior related to poor functioning. Over time, Julie began to recognize distortions that she had about her condition and her perceived limitations. Although she felt debilitated at times, she felt accomplished when she attended school. In addition, she was able to reframe her physical limitations by identifying more aspects of life that had remained stable and/or positive. Julie admitted that her school attendance was poor not because of pain and poor mobility but because of worry about her mother, as well as a fear of judgment from peers. To address her worry about her mother, Julie arranged times when she could contact her father during the day to inquire about her mother, thereby creating some healthy distance from her mother that allowed for age-appropriate independence. In addition, she wrote about her worries in a journal and was encouraged to use scheduled 5- to 10-minute worry periods to help compartmentalize this tendency. To reframe concerns regarding peers, Julie created a letter for her classmates that explained her diagnosis and the reasons why she had been absent. To explain her need for accommodations, Julie also demonstrated how she used a writing device. Answering questions from classmates allowed her to feel knowledgeable and eliminated the misconception that her classmates were judging her. As a result, her school attendance and peer interactions improved.

The benefits of relaxation training and biofeedback were discussed early in treatment as an important tool for proactive coping among patients with chronic pain (Lavigne et al., 1992; Walco et al., 1992). Although Julie used breathing techniques to manage nighttime anxiety and promote sleep, she did not understand how these techniques could be applied to pain. Therefore, treatment shifted to psychoeducation on the physiological impact of pain and stress as a rationale for relaxation. As such, Julie became more open to this approach, and instruction on specific relaxation techniques were resumed as the last step of treatment.

Care was taken in deciding what relaxation technique to employ for Julie, as she had limited mobility in key joints. Although progressive muscle relaxation (PMR) might have been helpful to relieve tension in some areas, coordination with Julie's physical therapist was needed to determine in which areas this technique could be applied. Julie was introduced to PMR, but more time was spent teaching her passive relaxation techniques. She reported great benefit from imagery and began regular practice in the evening and when receiving steroid injections. Biofeedback was instrumental in illustrating the control Julie could gain in her physiological response to pain and anxiety, and this control contributed to more consistent practice of PMR at home.

As noted, members of Julie's family were also having difficulties. Several studies have examined functioning among parents and siblings of children with JIA that suggest that the majority do well relative to controls or measurement norms (Gerhardt et al., 2003; Reid, McGrath, & Lang, 2005; Weiss, Schiaffino, & Ilowite, 2001). However, parents who experience the illness as more intrusive and who have older children may have a greater risk for distress (Andrews et al., 2009). Furthermore, the extent to which families, particularly parents, have premorbid risk factors or difficulty adapting to the stress of JIA may predict outcomes for affected children (Drotar, 1997; Palermo & Eccleston, 2009). Specifically, parental stress has been related to child reports of pain and anxiety among families of children with JIA (Anthony, Bromberg, Gil, & Schanberg, 2011), and parent distress may be linked to child depressive symptoms, particularly when the illness is more intrusive for the child (Wagner et al., 2003). The impact of parental distress, particularly on the part of Julie's mom, was important during Julie's therapy.

It is notable that several intervention studies in JIA have included family members in the child's treatment (Hagglund et al., 1996; Lavigne et al., 1992; Rapoff et al., 2002; Stark et al., 2005; Walco et al., 1992), but only one has specifically targeted outcomes for mothers (Ireys, Sills, Kolodner, & Walsh, 1996). Although CBT was generally helpful for Julie, interventions had to be discussed within a broader family systems context, as there was significant conflict and instability in Julie's family during treatment. Six months into treatment, Julie's mother reported a history of substance abuse and was admitted to an inpatient drug treatment program. This admission forced Julie, her brother, and her father to move multiple times, cohabitating with different family members. Thus treatment goals shifted to a family approach to address this instability. For example, the focus of one dyadic session was on Mrs. M's own emotional problems, and in this session Julie was able to process her anxiety about her mother and create realistic expectations for their relationship. In a subsequent session with Julie's brother, his anger issues and their impact on the home environment were discussed, prompting a referral for his treatment. Julie's father was unable to attend sessions consistently, so he was kept abreast of her therapeutic goals via phone contact, as he was most adept at maintaining some structure in the household. Other family members (e.g., paternal aunt, grandmother) also took part in sessions to optimize generalization of skills. Ultimately, facilitating stability within the family had an overall positive impact on Julie's mood, sleep, and school attendance.

SUMMARY AND CONCLUSIONS

In this case example, the psychologist filled several roles to ensure that a patient with JIA and a complicated psychosocial history could have a positive outcome. It was important to establish rapport and a good relationship with the patient, as well as other family members, to ensure that critical issues were identified and that a plan was established to address the family factors contributing to Julie's problem. Meeting with other caregivers was necessary to maintain progress during times of instability in living arrangements. In addition, the role of advocate was essential to coordinating services in school, as well as in-home counseling for the family. The psychologist was a liaison, often communicating with other medical personnel (e.g., rheumatologist, physical therapist), as well as other treatment facilities, to coordinate care.

This case also highlighted the importance of flexibility in approach, not only in dealing with psychosocial complexities and inconsistent attendance at therapy but also in acknowledging Julie's acceptance of the treatment approach. Fortunately, the family had public insurance, which did not limit the number of sessions. If a finite number of sessions was allotted, a skilled therapist would need to determine treatment plans earlier and identify the focus of treatment based on patient engagement and preference. In this case, delaying relaxation training until a good understanding of CBT was established proved to be beneficial to optimize therapeutic gains. In conclusion, empirically based interventions, thoughtfully implemented in the context of the unique characteristics of the illness and family, are fundamental to the successful treatment of children affected by JIA.

REFERENCES

Aasland, A., Flato, B., & Vandvik, I. H. (1997). Psychosocial outcome in juvenile chronic arthritis: A nine-year follow-up. *Clinical and Experimental Rheumatology, 15,* 561–568.

Adam, V., St. Pierre, Y., Fautrel, B., Clarke, A. E., Duffy, C. M., & Penrod, J. R. (2005). What is the impact of adolescent arthritis and rheumatism? Evidence from a national sample of Canadians. *Journal of Rheumatology, 32,* 354–361.

Andrews, N. R., Chaney, J. M., Mullins, L. L., Wagner, J. L., Hommel, K. A., & Jarvis, J. N. (2009). The differential effects of child age on illness intrusiveness:

Parent distress relationship in juvenile rheumatic disease. *Rehabilitation Psychology*, *54*, 45–50.

Anthony, K. K., Bromberg, M. H., Gil, K. M., & Schanberg, L. E. (2011). Parental perceptions of child vulnerability and parent stress as predictors of pain and adjustment in children with chronic arthritis. *Children's Health Care*, *40*, 53–69.

Billings, A. G., Moos, R. H., Miller, J. J., & Gottlieb, J. E. (1987). Psychosocial adaptation in juvenile rheumatic disease: A controlled evaluation. *Health Psychology*, *6*(4), 343–359.

Bromberg, M. H., Gil, K. M., & Schanberg, L. E. (2012). Daily sleep quality and mood as predictors of pain in children with juvenile polyarticular arthritis. *Health Psychology*, *31*, 202–209.

Degotardi, P. J., Klass, E. S., Rosenberg, B. S., Fox, D. G., Gallelli, K. A., & Gottlieb, B. S. (2006). Development and evaluation of a cognitive-behavioral intervention for juvenile fibromyalgia. *Journal of Pediatric Psychology*, *31*, 714–723.

Drotar, D. (1997). Relating parent and family functioning to the psychological adjustment of children with chronic health conditions: What have we learned? What do we need to know? *Journal of Pediatric Psychology*, *22*(2), 149–165.

Feldmann, R., Weglage, J., Roth, J., Foell, D., & Frosch, M. (2005). Systemic juvenile rheumatoid arthritis: Cognitive function and social adjustment. *Annals of Neurology*, *58*(4), 605–609.

Foster, H. E., Marshall, N., Myers, A., Dunkley, P., & Griffiths, I. D. (2003). Outcome in adults with juvenile idiopathic arthritis: A quality of life study. *Arthritis and Rheumatism*, *48*(3), 767–775.

Gerhardt, C. A., Vannatta, K., McKellop, J. M., Zeller, M., Taylor, J., Passo, M., et al. (2003). Comparing parental distress, family functioning, and the role of social support for caregivers with and without a child with juvenile rheumatoid arthritis. *Journal of Pediatric Psychology*, *28*(1), 5–15.

Hagglund, K. J., Doyle, N. M., Clay, D. L., Frank, R. G., Johnson, J. C., & Pressly, T. A. (1996). A family retreat as a comprehensive intervention for children with arthritis and their families. *Arthritis and Rheumatism*, *9*, 35–41.

Helmick, C. G., Felson, D. T., Lawrence, R. C., Gabriel, S., Hirsch, R., Kwoh, C. K., et al. (2008). Estimates of the prevalence of arthritis and other rheumatic conditions in the United States. *Arthritis and Rheumatism*, *58*, 15–25.

Ireys, H. T., Sills, E. M., Kolodner, K. B., & Walsh, B. B. (1996). A social support intervention for parents of children with juvenile rheumatoid arthritis: Results of a randomized trial. *Journal of Pediatric Psychology*, *21*(5), 633–641.

Kashikar-Zuck, S., Swain, N. F., Jones, B. A., & Graham, T. B. (2005). Efficacy of a cognitive-behavioral intervention for juvenile primary fibromyalgia. *Journal of Rheumatology*, *32*, 1594–1602.

Lavigne, J. V., Ross, C. K., Berry, S. L., Hayford, J. R., & Pachman, L. M. (1992). Evaluation of a psychological treatment package for treating pain in juvenile rheumatoid arthritis. *Arthritis Care and Research*, *5*, 101–110.

LeBovidge, J. S., Lavigne, J. V., Donenberg, G. R., & Miller, M. L. (2003).

Psychological adjustment of children and adolescents with chronic arthritis: A meta-analytic review and comparison with existing models. *Journal of Developmental and Behavioral Pediatrics, 28,* 29–39.

Lovell, D. J., Athreya, B., Emery, H. M., Gibbas, D. L., Levinson, J. E., Lindsley, C. B., et al. (1990). School attendance and patterns, special services and special needs in pediatric patients with rheumatic diseases: Results of a multicenter study. *Arthritis Care and Research, 3,* 196–203.

Oen, K., Malleson, P. N., Cabral, D. A., Rosenberg, A. M., Petty, R. E., & Cheang, M. (2002). Disease course and outcome of juvenile rheumatoid arthritis in a multicenter cohort. *Journal of Rheumatology, 29,* 1989–1999.

Packham, J. C., & Hall, M. A. (2002). Long-term follow-up of 246 adults with juvenile idiopathic arthritis: Social function, relationships, and sexual activity. *Rheumatology, 41,* 1440–1443.

Palermo, T. M., & Eccleston, C. (2009). Parents of children and adolescents with chronic pain. *Pain, 146,* 15–17.

Rapoff, M. A., Belmont, J., Lindsley, C., Olson, N., Morris, J., & Padur, J. (2002). Prevention of non-adherence to nonsteroidal anti-inflammatory medications for newly diagnosed patients with juvenile rheumatoid arthritis. *Health Psychology, 21,* 620–623.

Rapoff, M. A., & Lindsley, C. B. (2007). Improving adherence to medical regimens for juvenile rheumatoid arthritis. *Pediatric Rheumatology, 5.* Retrieved from *www.ped-rheum.com/content/5/1/10.*

Rapoff, M. A., Lindsley, C. B., & Karlson, C. (2009). Medical and psychosocial aspects of juvenile rheumatoid arthritis. In M. C. Roberts & R. G. Steele (Eds.), *Handbook of pediatric psychology* (4th ed., pp. 366–380). New York: Guilford Press.

Reddy, R. M., & Subramanian, S. (2009). Sleep disturbances due to pulmonary medications. *Current Respiratory Medicine Reviews 5,* 225–229.

Reid, G. J., McGrath, P. J., & Lang, B. A. (2005). Parent–child interactions among children with juvenile fibromyalgia, arthritis, and healthy controls. *Pain, 113,* 201–210.

Sandstrom, M. J., & Schanberg, L. E. (2004). Brief report: Peer rejection, social behavior, and psychological adjustment in children with juvenile rheumatic disease. *Journal of Pediatric Psychology, 29,* 29–34.

Sawyer, M. G., Carbone, J. A., Whitman, J. N., Roberton, D. M., Taplin, J. E., Varni, J. W., et al. (2005). The relationship between health-related quality of life, pain, and coping strategies in juvenile arthritis: A one-year prospective study. *Quality of Life Research, 14,* 1585–1598.

Schanberg, L. E., Gil, K. M., Anthony, K. K., Yow, E., & Rochon, J. (2005). Pain, stiffness, and fatigue in juvenile polyarticular arthritis. *Arthritis and Rheumatism, 52,* 1196–1204.

Stark, L. J., Janicke, D. M., McGrath, A. M., Mackner, L. M., Hommel, K. A., & Lovell, D. (2005). Prevention of osteoporosis: A randomized clinical trial to increase calcium intake in children with juvenile rheumatoid arthritis. *Journal of Pediatric Psychology, 30,* 377–386.

Wagner, J. L., Chaney, J. M., Hommel, K. A., Page, M. C., Mullins, L. L., White, M. M., et al. (2003). The influence of parental distress on child depressive symptoms in juvenile rheumatic diseases: The moderating effect of illness intrusiveness. *Journal of Pediatric Psychology, 28,* 453–462.

Walco, G. A., Varni, J. W., & Ilowite, N. T. (1992). Cognitive-behavioral pain management in children with juvenile rheumatoid arthritis. *Pediatrics, 89,* 1075–1079.

Weiss, K. A., Schiaffino, K. M., & Ilowite, N. (2001). Predictors of sibling relationship characteristics in youth with juvenile chronic arthritis. *Children's Health Care, 30,* 67–77.

CHAPTER 16

Pediatric Human Immunodeficiency Virus

JERILYNN RADCLIFFE
LINDA A. HAWKINS
CINDY L. BUCHANAN

HIV (human immunodeficiency virus) and its progression to AIDS (acquired immune deficiency syndrome) have affected children and adolescents since shortly after the condition was recognized in 1981 (Armstrong, Willen, & Sorgen, 2003). At first viewed as a fatal disease of infants and young children born to mothers with HIV, understanding of HIV illness has changed dramatically over the past decades to its current status as a chronic health condition. This shift in perspective has been gradual, attributable to many causes, although two notable catalysts have been the earlier diagnosis of asymptomatic individuals and improved medications.

HIV is transmitted when the virus enters the bloodstream of an individual. Once within the bloodstream, the viral cells attach and then enter vital cells within the human immune system. There, the virus alters the cell's reproductive capabilities in such a way that instead of reproducing identical healthy cells, the cell generates HIV cells. These newly formed HIV cells then attach to additional cells within the immune system, overcome their reproductive systems, and transform these cells into those that reproduce even more HIV cells. In this way, HIV spreads throughout the individual, damaging the immune system so that the individual is left vulnerable to a host of other infectious agents, known as "opportunistic infections." Left untreated, most individuals infected with HIV become progressively weakened by the spreading virus, as well as by other infections, and die prematurely (Kalichman, 1998).

In the United States, more than 1 million people live with HIV, including approximately 6,000 children under 13 years old (Centers for Disease Control and Prevention, 2012a). Mother-to-child transmission has become relatively rare in the United States, now estimated at 100–200 infants annually, as compared with 27% transmission rate before the implementation of prenatal or perinatal HIV preventive medications (Connor et al., 1994). In 2009, an estimated 8,000 youth ages 13–24 years were diagnosed with HIV (Centers for Disease Control and Prevention, 2011). The spread of HIV among youth in the United States occurs predominantly through sexual contact, though not all sexual contact that results in transmission is consensual. In 2008, fully 78% of youth ages 13–24 with HIV diagnoses had become infected through sexual activity without barrier protection, whereas 22% of infected youth acquired HIV through hemophilia, blood transfusion, birth, or other modes of transmissions. HIV has a disproportionate impact on ethnic minority children and youth, particularly sexual minority males and those of color. In 2009, young men who have sex with men (YMSM) accounted for 69% of all new HIV diagnoses among persons ages 13–29. New HIV diagnoses in YMSM of color increased 48% from 2006 through 2009 (Centers for Disease Control and Prevention, 2011). However, estimates of HIV prevalence are limited because there is no uniform system of reporting HIV diagnoses within the United States and because field reports have shown that approximately 20% of youth infected with HIV are unaware of their status (Centers for Disease Control and Prevention, 2012b).

In the United States, youth with HIV are largely ethnic minority adolescents, many living in poverty. Those infected at birth have typically had medical care throughout their lives, have learned of their diagnoses years after they were given, and have frequently lost other family members to HIV/AIDS. Their upbringing often included members of their extended families or adoptive and foster families who assumed parenting roles when birth parents became unable to continue this role due to illness or death. HIV, even for those children and youth, remains a stigmatized disease. There is variation in terms of when, how, and by whom children with HIV are informed of their diagnoses, given the implications for the HIV status of their parents. These youth are often cautioned not to share their diagnoses with others outside a trusted small circle of medical care providers, family, and possibly friends. Although the diagnosis of HIV is medically the same for individuals diagnosed at birth as it is for those who acquire HIV through behavioral means later in life, the psychosocial impacts are very different. So different are the needs and resources that some hospitals maintain separate clinics for the two groups of patients. Because of these important differences, this chapter does not presume to cover both areas comprehensively and instead focuses on those youth who acquire HIV behaviorally, as these are the patients most likely to be served currently by pediatric psychologists.

The large majority of youth living with HIV are diagnosed in adolescence. Unlike nearly all other pediatric diseases, a diagnosis of HIV may not be communicated directly to parents or families until the youth chooses to make this disclosure. Due to federal and state reporting laws that restrict sharing of information regarding HIV, youth are often able to decide who is given access to their diagnosis, including their own parents and, in some states, their partners. Stigma surrounding HIV may be heightened for these youth because contracting HIV is perceived as avoidable and because HIV stigma is combined with the equally significant stigma that is attached to same-gender sexual activity (Radcliffe, Doty, et al., 2010). This makes sharing an HIV diagnosis with loved ones even more challenging because of the potential "coming out" regarding sexual orientation that may challenge cultural and religious beliefs within the family and the community. Youth may choose to avoid this confrontation altogether by simply not sharing their diagnosis with others. As a result, these youth often begin medical treatment on their own, without the support of family or friends. They may also choose to forgo access to housing or medical resources (e.g., family health insurance) and, as a result, experience increased stressors and even more compromised health.

Treatment for HIV requires close surveillance of physical health, through at least quarterly visits to health care providers. These medical appointments are focused on addressing typical health issues for adolescents, as well as on the specialized needs of immuno-compromised individuals. Medical care may include health and wellness vaccinations, such as for influenza and human papillomavirus (HPV). These visits are also used to closely monitor the progression of the virus in the youth's immune system by tracking CD4 count and viral load. Highly active anti-retroviral treatment (HAART) medication is initiated only after careful planning to select the optimal regimen for the youth, a regimen that is based on the youth's physical indices and lifestyle preferences. HAART regimens can include taking medications once to twice a day, within a specified time frame, sometimes with or without food, and most medications have side effects including fatigue and gastrointestinal distress (cramping and diarrhea). Another layer of adherence to HIV treatment is preventing any additional sexually transmitted infections (STIs) from others to them, as well as from them to others. Youth living with HIV receive counseling and instruction about how to reduce the risk of acquiring additional STIs or potentially exposing a sexual partner to HIV. However, balancing an age-appropriate need for social connection with the need to avoid being stigmatized, rejected, or punished through disclosure of their HIV diagnosis can be extremely difficult for youth living with HIV.

Although adjusting to any chronic disease is challenging, the psychosocial, sociopolitical, and racial/ethnic stigma still attached to HIV as a sexually transmitted illness results in a more demanding process of adaptation for youth diagnosed with HIV, even today. This is particularly so for youth whose sexual orientation is other than heterosexual and for those youth who are part of cultural/ethnic groups historically intolerant of diversity in sexual orientation. These youth, who are doubly or triply stigmatized for reasons of HIV, race/ethnicity, and sexual orientation, are often marginalized as far as essential family and community support that would have otherwise helped them to manage their illness and maintain a healthy lifestyle. As a result, the medical treatment team may become a major source of support and, sadly, for some youth their only support for living with HIV.

CASE EXAMPLE: KEVIN

Kevin, 16, was tested for HIV at his primary care clinic as part of routine screening for all sexually transmitted infections. He identified himself to his medical provider as a gay male and reported having had unprotected sex in the past year. When the test results were known, Kevin's doctor told him that the HIV test was positive. Kevin sat quietly as he heard this information. The doctor let Kevin know that he would begin working with a multidisciplinary team who specialize in working with youth who live with HIV and that one of the team members was available in the primary care office to answer any questions and help Kevin get connected to the HIV specialty care clinic.

Individual reactions to this diagnosis can range from fear and shock to stoic acceptance. Pediatric psychologists are well advised to assess reaction to diagnosis as part of the initial assessment. Examining other parameters of reaction to diagnosis may include such questions as: Was finding out that you had HIV a surprise? Do you know other people who are living with HIV? What have you heard about living with HIV? Who is currently in your life that can be supportive? Appreciating how a youth contextualizes the diagnosis will assist the psychologist in providing initial emotional support and in beginning to consider the use of other therapeutic approaches, especially if the reaction includes suicidal or homicidal ideation.

When asked, Kevin said that he was not completely surprised that he had HIV. Since identifying as gay starting at around 10 years of age, and later becoming familiar with the local gay community, he had heard a lot about HIV. He also had heard in the neighborhood that one of the young men with whom he had had sex might have HIV. Although Kevin was not happy about his diagnosis, he described feeling that it was inevitable as a young gay black male. Kevin was anxious to find out about how having HIV would affect his health, his life, his future relationships, and his potential to become a parent. When asked if Kevin wanted to share his diagnosis with his parents, with whom he lives, he stated that he did not. He said that his mother had kicked him out of the house for 2 weeks when, at age 14, he informed her that he was gay. He did not believe that this new health information would go over well and needed some time to adjust to the information himself first before informing his family. He stated that, for now, he would rely on friends for emotional support over the diagnosis.

HIV remains an extremely stigmatized and stigmatizing diagnosis in society (Kalichman, 1998). Unlike with other chronic conditions, a youth's HIV diagnosis does not ensure that the family will be supportive, helpful, and/or comforting. Many youth report fearing they will be kicked out of their homes after sharing their HIV diagnosis with their parents (Futterman, Chabon, & Hoffman, 2000). As a result, youth may seek out friends, other community members who act as "chosen family," and even clinic staff to fill their needs for support, help, and comfort (Valenzuela et al., 2011). Pediatric psychologists can help the youth to identify sources of support; these individuals are vital resources for the youth's journey from diagnosis to adjustment and then treatment. These supportive resources may be found in schools, community centers and organizations, churches, and diagnosis-based groups within hospitals and clinics.

Besides identifying external resources available to the youth, psychologists can help the youth identify internal resources that help support coping. This is important early in building the therapeutic relationship between the psychologist and the youth (Naar-King et al., 2006). Many youth diagnosed with HIV have already experienced multiple traumas in their lives (Radcliffe, Beidas, Hawkins, & Doty, 2010). Utilizing a motivational interviewing style of inquiry with a youth to understand how he or she successfully navigated other challenging experiences in his or her life can add to the resilience repertoire of behaviors in future work with the youth (Naar-King et al., 2006). Living successfully with HIV requires the ability to understand and process a huge amount of information. Medical appointments will be filled with terms and concepts that are very specific to this diagnosis and its treatment. Additionally, making the physical and behavioral modifications that are necessary for a long and healthy life with HIV requires a depth and breadth of strong communication strategies and coping skills, as with any chronic illness (Safren, Gonzalez, & Soroudi,

2008). Pediatric psychologists can help to empower youth to utilize these skills during medical visits (e.g., taking notes, asking questions), while they are completing lifestyle changes (e.g., adherence logs), or while seeking out support (e.g., asking a friend to attend an appointment with them, using online programs for medication reminders).

Overall comprehensive assessment of youth should include cognitive screening; family mental health history; historic and current support resources, including experiences with mental health providers; substance use/abuse; history of suicidal ideation and attempts; and multiply stigmatized identities (race, ethnicity, gender identity, sexual orientation, physical disability). A thorough assessment of traumatic life events is crucial in both appreciating what events have influenced the life and development of the patient and assisting in placing the diagnosis of HIV within the context of the youth's life. A multilayered assessment should also include exploration of personal strengths and strategies that the youth has utilized to make it through past life challenges. Future goals are important to explore as well. Understanding the youth's strengths, challenges, and life goals from a broad-based assessment is fundamental to developing an appropriate mental health treatment plan. Additionally, pediatric psychologists can help advocate for the patient and help the multidisciplinary team understand the patient based on the broad-based assessment.

> Kevin was a sophomore at a local public high school and had repeated ninth grade. He did not attend special classes or have an individualized education plan, but while he was in the specialty care clinic he showed difficulties retaining information from one visit to the next. A cognitive screening conducted as part of his initial assessment within the clinic found that although his overall IQ was in the low-average range, his verbal abilities were deficient, whereas his nonverbal performance skills were average range or higher.
>
> The cognitive limitations identified through the cognitive screen alerted the team to provide Kevin with simple verbal explanations of his disease and its treatment and to incorporate illustrations, diagrams, and charts as much as possible. The pediatric psychologist advised the treatment team to ask Kevin to summarize key information shared with him to evaluate his understanding and recall for important information related to his care.
>
> When asked if he had ever been in counseling before, Kevin replied that he had talked with one counselor at school when a teacher found out that he was being bullied for being gay. He reported that he had had only a few short sessions with the counselor, and he felt that it had just touched the surface of what was going on in his life (school, home, and relationships). He added that at around age 15 he had started drinking alcohol, which he says was fun and helped him "stress less" about everything going on in his life.

Addressing mental health needs within a multidisciplinary medical team can be challenging, because there may be many issues of concern, as indicated in Kevin's case. Kevin's alcohol use was of some concern but not considered alcohol dependence, and so a plan was formulated to follow his alcohol use over time and make a referral for substance abuse treatment if this became a greater clinical concern. Further discussions with Kevin brought to light many symptoms of depression (e.g., diminished appetite, interruptions in sleep, depressed and irritable mood). Depressive symptoms are common among youth with HIV; depressive symptoms in individuals with HIV are known to lead to difficulties with treatment adherence and decreases in quality of life (Reisner et al., 2009). Because of the extent of Kevin's depressive symptoms, concern about how these would potentially affect his HIV care, and the other information from the comprehensive diagnostic evaluation, a plan was made to offer treatment for depression. Cognitive-behavioral therapy (CBT) has been found effective for adolescents with depressive symptoms (Compton et al., 2004; Spirito, Esposito-Smythers, Wolff, & Uhl, 2011). Treatment trials for adults with HIV support the use of several psychotherapies, including CBT, educational programs, and stress management programs (Antoni, 2003; Blanch et al., 2002; Weiss et al., 2003).

> As Kevin processed his alcohol use with the team psychologist through weekly CBT sessions, he was able to identify the reasons for initiating his use (to reduce stress). He began to build new resources to reduce stress through journaling, guided imagery, music, and systematic relaxation. However, HIV progression required that Kevin prepare to begin HAART in the coming months. The pediatric psychologist worked with the team to develop a plan for teaching the complicated medication information that was based on Kevin's cognitive strengths and challenges. When Kevin was informed that he must begin HAART medications, his mood deteriorated significantly. He stopped leaving the house, missed several therapy sessions, and stated that he stopped eating. When asked, he said that the food restriction was a form of self-harm.

Preparing for optimal medication adherence to HAART is a multifaceted process. Due to the highly adaptable nature of HIV, even a brief period of nonadherence to the precise guidelines of the medication regimen (requiring that medications be taken at certain times of day, with or without food) can cause the virus to adapt to the medications and eventually resist the medication benefit. As a result, great time and attention is given to the adherence preparation process. The role of the pediatric psychologist on the medical team is important in addressing the cognitive, mental health, and support issues that may impede optimal HAART adherence.

For Kevin, cognitive challenges, lack of support at home (where the medications would be taken and any side effects would be noticed), and depression were all essential to address before the plan for him to start HAART could begin.

> Continuing CBT, Kevin and his psychologist determined that two additional supports would be necessary for his success with beginning and adhering to his medications. In addition to his weekly CBT sessions, Kevin expressed willingness to consider adding a psychotropic medication to assist with alleviating his depression symptoms. He also stated that he would like to tell his mother about his diagnosis so that she could support him generally, allow him to store medications at home, and reduce potential challenges that could arise if he experienced medication side effects.

Pairing psychotropic medications with CBT has been found highly effective in promoting adherence to HAART (Safren et al., 2004). Thus, partnering with a psychiatrist who is knowledgeable about the intricate nature of HIV, as well as aware of the challenges of multiply stigmatized adolescents, can be helpful. HIV medications may be accompanied by psychological side effects (e.g., depression, anxiety, nightmares) that may intensify preexisting mood disorders. Although psychotropic medications may be taken safely in conjunction with HAART, selecting the most appropriate psychotropic medication for an individual youth requires special expertise and close monitoring. In Kevin's case, his monthly meetings with the psychologist and the psychiatrist resulted in close monitoring of his response to medications designed to reduce his depressive symptoms and promote continued adherence to his care plan.

Initial side effects of HAART can resemble flu-like symptoms, including fatigue, nausea, and diarrhea. Additionally, when individuals are hiding their diagnosis and medications from others, experiencing these side effects can raise challenging questions and concerns from family members and thus increase anxiety for the youth. Preparing a youth for how he or she would manage these situations if they were to arise is important to maintaining adherence. In this case, Kevin decided that it would be too hard to hide the potential side effects from his mother. Considering how he would work around those issues caused significant anxiety in sessions. Through weekly work on a pro–con decision-making paradigm, Kevin was able to identify that disclosing the diagnosis to his mother was far less challenging than it would be to manage the side effects alone and to deal with any questions that would possibly arise.

> Kevin was successful in taking his antidepressant medication for a month while he and his therapist role-played the scenario of disclosing

to his mother. They considered the multiple potential outcomes to this disclosure and how he would respond to each one. The worst case, being kicked out of his house, was considered as well. The solution that Kevin developed was to move in with his aunt, to whom he disclosed his HIV status as part of the rehearsal for disclosing his status to his mother. His aunt was supportive, to his relief, and offered to house Kevin if necessary. Kevin decided to ask his mother to come with him to a clinic visit so that he could disclose his status to her within this supportive setting. He wanted his mother to see how hard he had been working to care for his health, and he wanted the medical team to be on hand to answer any questions she had.

The role of liaison between the patient and the medical team is an important role for the pediatric psychologist in helping to develop and implement an optimal mental health, wellness, and medication plan for the youth. For Kevin, having the support of another person to assist him with daily medication adherence was important in light of his cognitive challenges, as has been empirically demonstrated (Reynolds et al., 2004). Kevin's realization of this was facilitated by the use of the guided pro–con decision-making paradigm and developing the plan to have his mother informed of his diagnosis in the clinic setting. This required that the team be prepared to field questions about why his mother had not been previously informed about her son's diagnosis. Their explanations to Kevin's mother included education about the rules of confidentiality, as well as praise for Kevin in being able to manage his medical care independently.

Kevin's mother had many questions about the diagnosis, the medications, and the prognosis for her son. The medical team was able to address those questions and concerns immediately and offered to meet with her as needed to provide information and support. Kevin began his HAART regimen with his mother's support and experienced some of the initial side effects, which subsided after a few weeks. He continued with monthly therapy, which serves to support his ongoing success with medication adherence, and began to address new issues that arose, such as new relationships, additional diagnosis disclosures, and working toward future goals.

SUMMARY AND CONCLUSIONS

This case illustrates only some of the many complex issues concerning youth living with HIV for which the input of the pediatric psychologist can be essential to the success of the multidisciplinary team in providing optimal care. Broader issues, such as racial and ethnic health disparities and how these affect access to psychology services, management of pain, empirically supported treatments (or lack thereof), palliative care, transition to adult care, and advocacy, all play important, interconnecting roles in affecting the care of children and youth living with HIV (Roberts & Steele, 2009).

REFERENCES

Antoni, M. (2003). Stress management and psychoneuroimmunology in HIV infection. *CNS Spectrum, 8*(1), 40–51.

Armstrong, F. D., Willen, E. J., & Sorgen, K. (2003). HIV and AIDS in children and adolescents. In M. C. Roberts (Ed.), *Handbook of pediatric psychology* (3rd ed., pp. 358–374). New York: Guilford Press.

Blanch, J., Rousand, A., Hautzinger, M., Martinez, E., Peri, J. M., Andres, S., et al. (2002). Assessment of the efficacy of a cognitive-behavioral group psychotherapy programme for HIV-infected patients referred to a consultation-liaison psychiatry department. *Psychotherapy and Psychosomatics, 71*(2), 77–84.

Centers for Disease Control and Prevention. (2011). *HIV among youth*. Retrieved December 20, 2011, from *www.cdc.gov/hiv/youth/pdf/youth.pdf*.

Centers for Disease Control and Prevention. (2012a). *Mother-to-child HIV transmission and prevention*. Retrieved May 1, 2012, from *www.cdc.gov/hiv/topics/perinatal/resources/factsheets/perinatal.htm*.

Centers for Disease Control and Prevention. (2012b). *HIV among gay and bisexual men*. Retrieved June 21, 2012, from *www.cdc.gov/hiv/topics/msm/pdf/msm.pdf*.

Compton, S. N., March, J. S., Brent, D., Albano, A. M., Weersing, V. R., & Curry, J. (2004). Cognitive-behavioral psychotherapy for anxiety and depressive disorders in children and adolescents: An evidence-based medicine review. *Journal of American Academy of Child and Adolescent Psychiatry, 43*, 930–959.

Connor, E. M., Sperling, R. S., Gelber, R., Kiselev, P., Scott, G., O'Sullivan, M. J., et al. (1994). Reduction of maternal-infant transmission of human immunodeficiency virus type 1 with zidovudine treatment. *New England Journal of Medicine, 331*, 1173–1180.

Futterman, D., Chabon, B., & Hoffman, N. (2000). HIV and AIDS in adolescents. *Pediatric Clinics in North America, 47*(1), 171–188.

Kalichman, S. C. (1998). *Understanding AIDS: Advances in research and treatment* (2nd ed.). Washington, DC: American Psychological Association.

Naar-King, S., Wright, K., Parsons, J., Frey, M., Templin, T., Lam, P., et al. (2006). Healthy choices: Motivational enhancement therapy for health risk behaviors in HIV-positive youth. *AIDS Education and Prevention, 18*, 1–11.

Radcliffe, J., Beidas, R., Hawkins, L., & Doty, N. (2011). Trauma and sexual health risk among sexual minority African American HIV+ adults. *Traumatology, 17*, 24–33.

Radcliffe, J., Doty, N., Hawkins, L., Gaskins, C. S., Beidas, R., & Rudy, B. (2010). Stigma and sexual health risk among HIV+ African American sexual minority youth. *AIDS Patient Care and STDs, 23*(8), 493–499.

Reisner, S., Mimiaga, M., Skeer, M., Perkovich, B., Johnson, C., & Safren, S. (2009). A review of HIV antiretroviral adherence and intervention studies among HIV-infected youth. *Topics in HIV Medicine, 17*(1), 14–25.

Reynolds, N. R., Testa, M. A., Marc, L. G., Chesney, M. A., Neidig, J. L., Smith, S. R., et al. (2004). Factors influencing medication adherence beliefs and self-efficacy in persons naïve to antiretroviral therapy: A multicenter, cross-sectional study. *AIDS Behavior, 8,* 141–150.

Roberts, M. C., & Steele, R. G. (2009). *Handbook of pediatric psychology* (4th ed.) New York: Guilford Press.

Safren, S. A., Gonzalez, J. S., & Soroudi, N. (2008). *Coping with chronic illness: A cognitive-behavioral therapy approach for adherence and depression.* Oxford, UK: Oxford University Press.

Safren, S. A., Hendriksen, E. S., Mayar, K. H., Mimiaga, M. J., Pickard, R., & Otto, M. W. (2004). Cognitive-behavioral therapy for HIV medication adherence and depression. *Cognitive and Behavioral Practice, 11,* 415–423.

Spirito, A., Esposito-Smythers, C., Wolff, J., & Uhl, K. (2011). Cognitive-behavioral therapy for adolescent depression and suicidality. *Child and Adolescent Psychiatric Clinics of North America, 20*(2), 191–204.

Valenzuela, J., Buchanan, C., Radcliffe, J., Ambrose, C., Hawkins, L., Tanney, M., et al. (2011). Transition to adult services among behaviorally infected adolescents with HIV: A qualitative study. *Journal of Pediatric Psychology, 36,* 134–140.

Weiss, J. J., Mulder, C. L., Antoni, M. H., de Vroome, E. M., Garssen, B., & Goodkin, K. (2003). Effects of a supportive-expressive group intervention on long-term psychosocial adjustment in HIV-infected gay men. *Psychotherapy and Psychosomatics, 72*(3), 132–140.

CHAPTER 17

Pediatric Asthma

BARBARA JANDASEK
DAVID A. FEDELE

Jose was an 8-year-old Hispanic male with asthma who had had two recent ER visits. He was prescribed quick relief and controller medications. Jose lived with his mother, who often worked late at a local restaurant, and a 17-year-old sister. Jose was described as nervous; he often complained of difficulty breathing at bedtime and wanted to take his asthma medicine. His school nurse stated that he frequently complained of stomachaches and trouble breathing. Jose's mother had concerns about medication side effects and was confused about medication administration.

Maggie was a 16-year-old Caucasian female living with her biological parents. She had a history of severe persistent asthma and multiple hospitalizations. Her asthma had been relatively stable for the past few years but had recently worsened. Maggie reported increased asthma symptoms and decided to forgo soccer tryouts this fall. During a recent visit with her pediatrician, it was clear that Maggie was not taking her controller medicine regularly. When asked about school and friends, she said, "I'm stressed right now and can't think about my asthma!" Maggie's mother was concerned about her declining school grades, her moodiness, and her not wanting to spend time with the family and said that Maggie often came home smelling of smoke.

Pediatric psychologists offer a variety of valuable services when working with families with asthma. Referrals may occur in the context of outpatient therapy, inpatient consultation, or informal consultation with medical- and school-based colleagues. Psychologists may serve as an educational resource, utilizing psychological intervention techniques to promote effective family-based asthma management and helping to identify and address psychosocial barriers to effective asthma management (McQuaid & Abramson, 2009). Information regarding each of these roles is highlighted in what follows and is linked to the cases for illustrative purposes. Given the high prevalence rates of asthma, pediatric psychologists commonly encounter children presenting with primary psychological concerns who also happen to have asthma. Information relevant to assessment and treatment of youth with asthma also is presented according to co-occurring psychological disorders.

THE PEDIATRIC PSYCHOLOGIST AS AN EDUCATIONAL RESOURCE

Depending on the psychologist's expertise in asthma, he or she may be able to provide education directly or facilitate access to local educational resources to promote asthma management. If the psychologist is not familiar with local educational programming, he or she should work with the client's medical team to identify appropriate resources. A variety of online resources and games are also available (e.g., *http://asthma.starlight.org*). With regard to Maggie, an educational approach would focus on the different mechanisms of quick relief and controller medicines and the impact of smoking on asthma. For Jose, appropriate medication use and knowledge also should be emphasized, in addition to medication beliefs, potential side effects, and strategies used to minimize side effects.

THE ROLE OF PSYCHOLOGICAL INTERVENTIONS IN MEDICAL MANAGEMENT OF ASTHMA

A large role for psychologists is to promote asthma management, such as adherence to daily medications to control exacerbations in individuals with persistent asthma. Behavioral and multicomponent interventions have demonstrated stronger effects on adherence and health outcomes than interventions utilizing educational approaches alone (Graves, Roberts, Rapoff, & Boyer, 2010). Organizational interventions also have been described as "probably efficacious" for asthma (Lemanek, Kamps, & Chung, 2001).

The psychologist should be aware that the burden of asthma is greater for ethnic minority and socioeconomically disadvantaged youth (Akinbami et al., 2012) and that these factors may affect asthma management. Some addressable contributing factors in the context of treatment include misperception of respiratory symptoms, medication beliefs, adherence, and health care access and utilization (e.g., Fritz et al., 2010; Jandasek et al., 2011; McQuaid et al., 2009; Warman, Silver, & Stein, 2001).

Asthma knowledge and self-monitoring of symptoms provide essential foundations for effective asthma management but are not necessarily sufficient; addition of developmentally tailored behavioral strategies may further enhance adherence behavior and health outcomes (Graves et al., 2010). For 8-year-old Jose, treatment would heavily emphasize supervision and training of family members in behavioral principles (e.g., token reinforcement; daCosta, Rapoff, Lemanek, & Goldstein, 1997).

Although adolescents display a greater capacity for involvement in management and higher levels of knowledge than children, they continue to benefit from continued parental assistance and supervision (Bender, Milgrom, Rand, & Ackerson, 1998; McQuaid, Kopel, Klein, & Fritz, 2003). These efforts should be balanced with strategies targeting individual motivation, problem solving, and independent self-management (e.g., Seid et al., 2012). Adolescents, such as Maggie, may benefit from motivational interviewing to clarify personal motivations and perceived disadvantages related to self-management (Rollnick, Miller, & Butler, 2008). Use of problem solving would help Maggie identify specific situations in which adherence is challenging and teach her to generate, evaluate, and choose between alternative actions. Integration of technology-based strategies used to provide individualized feedback may also be highly acceptable to youth and promote self-management (Seid et al., 2012).

Recommendations for asthma management also emphasize close collaboration between the family, patient, and health care providers (National Heart, Lung, and Blood Institute [NHLBI], 2007). Organizational strategies include interventions designed to improve this collaboration, increase physician supervision, and tailor the treatment regimen. Use of an asthma action plan that outlines individualized instructions for prevention and treatment of asthma exacerbations is encouraged. The psychologist may help families identify barriers to asthma management and teach effective communication strategies for health care visits and with school personnel. Jose's family also could be coached to use a color-coded system to differentiate between types of medications. Finally, use of a calendar to record asthma exacerbations and medication use could improve collaboration within the family, as well as accuracy of symptom reports to the physician.

PROMOTING EFFECTIVE
FAMILY-BASED ASTHMA MANAGEMENT

The impact of the family system on asthma can be significant (see Kaugars, Klinnert, & Bender, 2004). Family factors (e.g., caregiver distress, health beliefs) are associated with negative asthma management practices and increased morbidity (Bartlett et al., 2001; Chen, Bloomberg, Fisher, & Strunk, 2003; McQuaid et al., 2009). Incorporating family-based strategies into treatment may help to minimize burden and distress related to asthma management and improve asthma outcomes (e.g., Ng et al., 2008).

Validated measures assessing family-based asthma management include the Family Ritual Questionnaire (Fiese, Wamboldt, O'Connor, & Markson, 1998) and the Family Asthma Management System Scale (FAMSS; Klinnert, McQuaid, & Gavin, 1997; McQuaid, Walders, Kopel, Fritz, & Klinnert, 2005). Attention to family routines and rituals is key in promoting effective asthma management; specific recommendations based upon the work of Fiese and Wamboldt (2000) are outlined in Figure 17.1.

In the case of Jose, integrating both his mother and sister into treatment may provide perspective on the distribution of responsibility for asthma management across family members and offer insight into family stressors that affect Jose's adjustment and asthma management. The psychologist should work with the family to identify areas of misunderstanding among family members about how to manage asthma and negotiate specific, developmentally appropriate roles in asthma management for each member.

ASSESSING ASTHMA OUTCOMES

If treated effectively, asthma symptoms should be well controlled with minimal functional impact (NHLBI, 2007). Psychological interventions targeting asthma management should assess changes in asthma control using well-established measures (e.g., the Asthma Control Test; Nathan et al., 2004). The psychologist should also collaborate with the treating physician to gain information pertaining to objective measures of lung function. Other measures, such as the Pediatric Asthma Quality of Life Questionnaire (Juniper et al., 1996) and the Asthma Self-Efficacy Questionnaire (Tobin, Wigal, Winder, Holroyd, & Creer, 1987) are also informative. Depending on clinical presentation, addressing other potential psychological issues that may influence adherence and adjustment to illness is crucial. In the next sections, we outline potential psychological issues, including anxiety, depression, behavior problems, and tobacco use.

---

1. Assess currently existing organization and routinization within the family (e.g., dinnertime, weekend activities).

2. Assess the degree to which asthma management disrupts family routines and how these situations are handled.

3. Identify established family routines and roles specific to asthma management.

4. Facilitate adaptation and planning relevant to asthma management strategies into the family system.

FIGURE 17.1. Family-based strategies to increase treatment adherence (Fiese & Wamboldt, 2000).

COMMONLY CO-OCCURRING
PSYCHOLOGICAL CONDITIONS

Anxiety

Children such as Jose, who present with nervousness, somatic complaints, and potential overuse of their asthma medications, are likely to be among the most common referrals to pediatric psychologists. Anxiety is a common comorbid psychological condition (Vila, Nollet-Clemencon, de Blic, Mouren-Simeoni, & Scheinmann, 2000), especially for youth with elevated asthma severity (e.g., Wamboldt, Fritz, Mansell, McQuaid, & Klein, 1998).

Anxiety is related to overperception of asthma symptoms (Steptoe & Vogele, 1992), potentially leading to misuse of quick relief medications (Mawhinney et al., 1993). Panic symptoms may promote or escalate asthma symptoms via the inflammatory bodily responses to stress following periods of panic or other panic symptoms such as hyperventilation (Lehrer, Feldman, Giardino, Song, & Schmaling, 2002). Asthma symptoms such as chest tightening and breathing difficulties may also lead to panic symptoms (Lehrer et al., 2002). Children and adolescents with asthma who have experienced asthma-related trauma (e.g., intubation) may also experience posttraumatic stress or even develop posttraumatic stress disorder (PTSD; Kean, Kelsay, Wamboldt, & Wamboldt, 2006).

Assessment of anxiety symptomatology is a crucial first step in determining the treatment course. Several non-asthma-specific measures are used to assess anxiety (see Holmbeck et al., 2008; Mash & Barkley, 2007); however, endorsement of respiratory-based symptoms of anxiety should be interpreted with caution. The Youth Asthma-Related Anxiety Scales (Bruzzese, Unikel, Shrout, & Klein, 2011), a recently developed tool, is designed to measure children's anxiety in relation to asthma management.

Conducting a clinical interview with the child and caregiver may further explicate the nature of the child's anxiety surrounding asthma. For Jose, contextual factors related to medication use, somatic complaints,

panic symptoms, and his subjective experience during periods of hyperventilation and dyspnea should be gathered prior to initiating psychological
treatment. Consultation with Jose's physician should be conducted to place
individual and familial concerns and perceptions in the context of clinical
history and objective medical information.

Empirically supported treatments to reduce anxiety in this population
are scant. Cognitive-behavioral treatment should incorporate differentia-
tion and connections between asthma and anxiety symptoms and appropriate course of self-management. Identification of anxious cognitions and
subsequent modification and use of relaxation electromyography (EMG)
biofeedback techniques can also be beneficial (see Kazdin & Weisz, 2003),
particularly for children whose asthma symptoms are emotionally triggered
(McQuaid & Nassau, 1999). Additional clinical intervention is indicated
if children and adolescents are evidencing symptoms of panic. Treatment
could include additional components, such as breathing training and expo-
sures (Lehrer et al., 2008).

Depression

Depression is significantly more likely to occur among adolescents with
asthma than among healthy peers (Bender, 2007). Adolescents with depression, such as Maggie, are at risk for poor medication adherence (Smith et
al., 2006), increased symptom frequency and missed school days (Bender &
Zhang, 2008), and risky behavior (Bender, 2006). As depressive symptoms
affect several areas of functioning beyond asthma management, referrals
to psychologists may stem from the patient him- or herself, from concerned
family members, or from school personnel.

Given the lack of empirically supported treatments specific to adolescents with asthma and co-occurring depressive symptoms, the role of the psychologist is to operate within existing treatments (see Kazdin & Weisz, 2003)
to incorporate asthma-related information. It is important to consider how
asthma may be linked to depressive symptoms, for example, how Maggie's
mood is related to the daily demands of asthma management and activity
restrictions. Exploring Maggie's attitudes toward her illness and treatment
expectations, providing education surrounding asthma medications and
effects of nonadherence, and focusing on the deleterious effects of smoking
on asthma symptoms are important treatment targets. Treatment for youth
with depression and asthma also should directly address feelings of hopelessness and low self-efficacy in an effort to boost health-promoting behavior.

Behavior Problems

Children with asthma appear less likely to manifest externalizing than
internalizing symptoms (Blackman & Gurka, 2007). However, children

with asthma, particularly those whose illness is more severe, are at greater risk for behavioral difficulties compared with healthy children (McQuaid, Kopel, & Nassau, 2001). Asthma-specific factors directly contributing to symptom presentation should be considered. For instance, symptoms of hyperactivity and behavioral dysregulation may be related to medication side effects. Children from families who do not have a history of asthma and who may be less comfortable with asthma management may experience even greater risk for behavioral difficulties (Calam et al., 2005).

Objective assessments and parent report of executive functioning also may be helpful in identifying children whose attentional difficulties may affect asthma morbidity (see Koinis Mitchell et al., 2009; McQuaid et al., 2008). The psychologist should also assess and help to address contextual and familial factors potentially affecting both behavioral adjustment and asthma management (e.g., poverty, family stress, family routines). Treatment should incorporate education regarding the child's individual asthma symptom presentation and triggers and emphasize behavioral strategies targeting recognition of asthma symptoms and awareness of triggers (e.g., exercise), problem solving in the face of symptoms, and reinforcement of appropriate self-management behaviors.

Tobacco Use

Adolescents with asthma are *more* likely to smoke than adolescents without asthma (Hublet et al., 2007). These youth are also more likely to engage in other risk behavior and poorer health practices and to belong to a "risky" peer group (Bender, 2007; Hublet et al., 2007). Thus, psychologists working with youth such as Maggie should conduct a detailed assessment of risk behavior (e.g., alcohol use) and health practices (medication adherence; Bender, 2006). Effective smoking interventions should include cognitive-behavioral aspects, motivational components, and attention to peer influences (Sussman, Sun, & Dent, 2006). Asthma-specific components, such as the increased likelihood of exacerbations and their impact on the youth's preferred activities, should be incorporated to build motivation for change. Treatment should also attend to other potential maintaining factors, such as the use of smoking in an attempt to control weight (Tomeo, Field, Berkey, Colditz, & Frazier, 1999).

CONCLUSIONS AND FUTURE DIRECTIONS

Considerable research within pediatric psychology has been devoted to pediatric asthma; however, much work remains, particularly in the field of intervention research. Existing research has focused primarily on determining psychosocial correlates of asthma and evaluating interventions that target adherence and, to a lesser extent, anxiety. Continued work in this area should focus on "unpacking" of adherence interventions to determine the relative impact of each intervention component, as well as continued integration of innovative strategies, such as technology. In addition, further development and evaluation of intervention and prevention programs designed to address specific co-occurring psychological conditions (e.g., depression, tobacco use) are needed. Finally, there is a need for more tailored interventions targeting youth at highest risk for poor health outcomes.

REFERENCES

Akinbami, L. J., Moorman, J. E., Bailey, C., Zahran, H. S., King, M., Jonson, C. A., et al. (2012, May). Trends in asthma prevalence, health care use, and mortality in the United States, 2001-2010. *NCHS Data Brief, no 94.*

Bartlett, S. J., Kolodner, K., Butz, A. M., Eggleston, P., Malveaux, F. J., & Rand, C. S. (2001). Maternal depressive symptoms and emergency department use among inner-city children with asthma. *Archives of Pediatric and Adolescent Medicine, 155,* 347–353.

Bender, B. G. (2006). Risk taking, depression, adherence, and symptom control in adolescents and young adults with asthma. *American Journal of Respiratory and Critical Care Medicine, 173,* 953–957.

Bender, B. G. (2007). Depression symptoms and substance abuse in adolescents with asthma. *Annals of Allergy, Asthma, and Immunology, 99,* 319–324.

Bender, B., Milgrom, H., Rand, C., & Ackerson, L. (1998). Psychological factors associated with medication nonadherence in asthmatic children. *Journal of Asthma, 35,* 347–353.

Bender, B., & Zhang, L. (2008). Negative affect, medication adherence, and asthma control in children. *Journal of Allergy and Clinical Immunology, 122(3),* 490–495.

Blackman, J. A., & Gurka, M. J. (2007). Developmental and behavioral comorbidities of asthma in children. *Journal of Developmental and Behavioral Pediatrics, 28,* 92–99.

Bruzzese, J. M., Unikel, L. H., Shrout, P. E., & Klein, R. G. (2011). Youth and parent versions of the Asthma-Related Anxiety Scale: Development and initial testing. *Pediatric Allergy, Immunology, and Pulmonology, 24,* 95–105.

Calam, R., Gregg, L., Simpson, A., Simpson, B., Woodcock, A., & Custovic, A. (2005). Behavior problems antecede the development of wheeze in childhood: A birth cohort study. *American Journal of Respiratory and Critical Care Medicine, 171,* 323–327.

Chen, E., Bloomberg, G. R., Fisher, E. G., Jr., & Strunk, R. C. (2003). Predictors of repeat hospitalizations in children with asthma: The role of psychosocial and socio-environmental factors. *Health Psychology, 22,* 12–18.

daCosta, I. G., Rapoff, M. A., Lemanek, K., & Goldstein, G. L. (1997). Improving adherence to medication regimens for children with asthma and its effect on clinical outcome. *Journal of Applied Behavior Analysis, 30,* 687–691.

Fiese, B., & Wamboldt, F. (2000). Family routines, rituals, and asthma management: A proposal for family-based strategies to increase treatment adherence. *Families, Systems, and Health: Journal of Collaborative Family Healthcare, 18*, 405–418.

Fiese, B. H., Wamboldt, F. S., O'Connor, S., & Markson, S. (1998). *Family Routines Questionnaire: Asthma Version.* Syracuse, NY: Department of Psychology, Syracuse University.

Fritz, G. K., McQuaid, E. L., Kopel, S. J., Seifer, R., Klein, R. B., Mitchell, D. K., et al. (2010). Ethnic differences in perception of lung function: A factor in pediatric asthma disparities? *American Journal of Respiratory and Critical Care Medicine, 182*, 12–18.

Graves, M. M., Roberts, M. C., Rapoff, M., & Boyer, A. (2010). The efficacy of adherence interventions for chronically ill children: A meta-analytic review. *Journal of Pediatric Psychology, 35*, 368–382.

Holmbeck, G. N., Thill, A. W., Bachanas, P., Garber, J., Miller, K. B., Abad, M., et al. (2008). Evidence-based assessment in pediatric psychology: Measures of psychosocial adjustment and psychopathology. *Journal of Pediatric Psychology, 33*, 958–980; discussion 981–982.

Hublet, A., De Bacquer, D., Boyce, W., Godeau, E., Schmid, H., Vereecken, C., et al. (2007). Smoking in young people with asthma. *Journal of Public Health (Oxford), 29*, 343–349.

Jandasek, B., Ortega, A. N., McQuaid, E. L., Koinis Mitchell, D., Fritz, G. K., Kopel, S. J., et al. (2011). Access to and use of asthma health services among Latino children: The Rhode Island–Puerto Rico Asthma Center Study. *Medical Care Research and Review, 68*, 683–698.

Juniper, E., Guyatt, G., Feeny, D., Griffith, L., Ferrie, P., & Townsend, M. (1996). Measuring quality of life in children with asthma. *Quality of Life Research, 5*, 35–46.

Kaugars, A. S., Klinnert, M. D., & Bender, B. G. (2004). Family influences on pediatric asthma. *Journal of Pediatric Psychology, 29*, 475–491.

Kazdin, A. E., & Weisz, J. R. (2003). *Evidence-based psychotherapies for children and adolescents.* New York: Guilford Press.

Kean, E. M., Kelsay, K., Wamboldt, F., & Wamboldt, M. Z. (2006). Posttraumatic stress in adolescents with asthma and their parents. *Journal of the American Academy of Child and Adolescent Psychiatry, 45*, 78–86.

Klinnert, M., McQuaid, E., & Gavin, L. (1997). Assessing the family asthma management system. *Journal of Asthma, 34*, 77–88.

Koinis Mitchell, D., McQuaid, E., Seifer, R., Kopel, S., Nassau, J., Klein, R., et al. (2009). Symptom perception in children with asthma: Cognitive and psychological factors. *Health Psychology, 28*, 226–237.

Lehrer, P., Feldman, J., Giardino, N., Song, H. S., & Schmaling, K. (2002). Psychological aspects of asthma. *Journal of Consulting and Clinical Psychology, 70*, 691–711.

Lehrer, P. M., Karavidas, M. K., Lu, S. E., Feldman, J., Kranitz, L., Abraham, S., et al. (2008). Psychological treatment of comorbid asthma and panic disorder: A pilot study. *Journal of Anxiety Disorders, 22*, 671–683.

Lemanek, K. L., Kamps, J., & Chung, N. B. (2001). Empirically supported treatments in pediatric psychology: Regimen adherence. *Journal of Pediatric Psychology, 26*, 279–282.

Mash, E. J., & Barkley, R. A. (2007). *Assessment of childhood disorders.* New York: Guilford Press.

Mawhinney, H., Spector, S. L., Heitjan, D., Kinsman, R. A., Dirks, J. F., & Pines, I. (1993). As-needed medication use in asthma usage patterns and patient characteristics. *Journal of Asthma, 30*, 61–71.

McQuaid, E. L., & Abramson, N. W. (2009). Pediatric asthma. In M. C. Roberts & R. G. Steele (Eds.), *Handbook of pediatric psychology* (4th ed., pp. 254–270). New York: Guilford Press.

McQuaid, E., Kopel, S., Klein, R., & Fritz, G. (2003). Medication adherence in pediatric asthma: Reasoning, responsibility, and behavior. *Journal of Pediatric Psychology, 28*, 323–333.

McQuaid, E. L., Kopel, S. J., & Nassau, J. H. (2001). Behavioral adjustment in children with asthma: A meta-analysis. *Journal of Developmental and Behavioral Pediatrics, 22*, 430–439.

McQuaid, E. L., & Nassau, J. H. (1999). Empirically supported treatments of disease-related symptoms in pediatric psychology: Asthma, diabetes, and cancer. *Journal of Pediatric Psychology, 24*, 306–328.

McQuaid, E. L., Vasquez, J., Canino, G., Fritz, G. K., Ortega, A. N., Colon, A., et al. (2009). Beliefs and barriers to medication use in parents of Latino children with asthma. *Pediatric Pulmonology, 44*, 892–898.

McQuaid, E., Walders, N., Kopel, S., Fritz, G., & Klinnert, M. (2005). Pediatric asthma management in the family context: The Family Asthma Management System Scale. *Journal of Pediatric Psychology, 30*, 492–502.

McQuaid, E. L., Weiss-Laxer, N., Kopel, S. J., Koinis-Mitchell, D., Nassau, J. H., Wamboldt, M. Z., et al. (2008). Pediatric asthma and problems in attention, concentration, and impulsivity: Disruption of the family management system. *Families, Systems, and Health, 26*, 16–29.

Nathan, R. A., Sorkness, C. A., Kosinski, M., Schatz, M., Li, J. T., Marcus, P., et al. (2004). Development of the Asthma Control Test: A survey for assessing asthma control. *Journal of Allergy and Clinical Immunology, 113*, 59–65.

National Heart, Lung, and Blood Institute. (2007). *Guidelines for the diagnosis and management of asthma.* Retrieved from *www.nhlbi.nih.gov/guidelines/asthma/asthsumm.pdf.*

Ng, S. M., Li, A. M., Lou, V. W., Tso, I. F., Wan, P. Y., & Chan, D. F. (2008). Incorporating family therapy into asthma group intervention: A randomized waitlist-controlled trial. *Family Process, 47*, 115–130.

Rollnick, S., Miller, W. R., & Butler, C. C. (2008). *Motivational interviewing in health care: Helping patients change behavior.* New York: Guilford Press.

Seid, M., D'Amico, E. J., Varni, J. W., Munafo, J. K., Britto, M. T., Kercsmar, C. M., et al. (2012). The in vivo adherence intervention for at risk adolescents with asthma: Report of a randomized pilot trial. *Journal of Pediatric Psychology, 37*, 390–403.

Smith, A., Krishnan, J. A., Bilderback, A., Riekert, K. A., Rand, C. S., & Bartlett, S. J. (2006). Depressive symptoms and adherence to asthma therapy after hospital discharge. *Chest, 130*, 1034–1038.

Steptoe, A., & Vogele, C. (1992). Individual differences in the perception of bodily sensations: The role of trait anxiety and coping style. *Behaviour Research and Therapy, 30,* 597–607.

Sussman, S., Sun, P., & Dent, C. W. (2006). A meta-analysis of teen cigarette smoking cessation. *Health Psychology, 25,* 549–557.

Tobin, D. L., Wigal, J. K., Winder, J. A., Holroyd, K. A., & Creer, T. L. (1987). The "Asthma Self-Efficacy Scale." *Annals of Allergy, 59,* 273–277.

Tomeo, C. A., Field, A. E., Berkey, C. S., Colditz, G. A., & Frazier, A. L. (1999). Weight concerns, weight control behaviors, and smoking initiation. *Pediatrics, 104,* 918–924.

Vila, G., Nollet-Clemencon, C., de Blic, J., Mouren-Simeoni, M. C., & Scheinmann, P. (2000). Prevalence of DSM-IV anxiety and affective disorders in a pediatric population of asthmatic children and adolescents. *Journal of Affective Disorders, 58,* 223–231.

Wamboldt, M., Fritz, G. K., Mansell, A., McQuaid, E. L., & Klein, R. B. (1998). Relationship of asthma severity and psychological problems in children. *Journal of the American Academy of Child and Adolescent Psychiatry, 37,* 943–950.

Warman, K. L., Silver, E. J., & Stein, R. E. (2001). Asthma symptoms, morbidity, and anti-inflammatory use in inner-city children. *Pediatrics, 108,* 277–282.

CHAPTER 18

Pediatric Diabetes

LISA M. BUCKLOH

There are several variants of diabetes mellitus, including type 1 (DM1), type 2 (DM2), maturity-onset diabetes of youth (MODY), and cystic-fibrosis-related diabetes (CFRD). Diabetes mellitus is characterized by impaired glucose metabolism due to either insulin deficiency (DM1 and MODY) or insulin resistance (DM2 and CFRD). The treatment of DM1 and MODY consists of self-monitoring of blood glucose (SMBG) typically 4–6 times daily, multiple daily insulin injections or use of an insulin pump, daily exercise, and regulation of carbohydrate intake (Chase, 2006). Youth with DM2 with insulin resistance typically are treated with daily oral medications that enhance insulin action and sensitivity (e.g., Metformin). If DM2 progresses to insulin deficiency, youth usually will be managed with daily insulin injections and a regimen similar to that for DM1. Diabetes mellitus is associated with potential long-term risks of kidney, heart, eye, and nerve disease. Maintaining near normal hemoglobin A_{1c} (HbA_{1c}; e.g., < 7.5) has been found to reduce these risks greatly (Diabetes Control and Complications Trial Research Group, 1994; U.K. Prospective Diabetes Study Group, 1998).

The demands of diabetes affect and are affected by many psychological processes, and family and other social spheres (e.g., school, peers, health care settings) are important in the management of this complex disease. Most of the literature has focused on youth with DM1, but there are ongoing studies of psychological components for children with DM2. Interventions targeting family management of diabetes have empirical support in improving glycemic control and psychological outcomes in youth with DM1. For example, behavioral modification (e.g., Carney, Schechter, & Davis, 1983) and behavioral contracting (e.g., Epstein et al., 1981) have been found to improve treatment adherence. Behavioral family systems therapy (BFST) is a family-based intervention targeting problem-solving skills, family communication, and cognitive restructuring using an ecological–family systems perspective and has been found to improve treatment adherence and glycemic control (Wysocki et al., 2007), as well as family communication (Wysocki, Harris, et al., 2008). Multisystemic therapy (MST), an intensive, home-based, problem-focused therapy involving multiple systems (family, school, peers, health care) also has yielded effects on adherence (Ellis et al., 2005; Ellis, Templin, et al., 2007).

Interventions targeting individual coping and adjustment also have been effective with youth with DM1. For example, coping skills training has been related to improved glycemic control, better diabetes self-efficacy and coping, and less negative impact on quality of life in teens with DM1 (Grey, Boland, Davidson, Li, & Tamborlane, 2000). Other cognitive-behavioral interventions, including those involving self-monitoring, stress management, and cognitive restructuring, have had positive effects on psychological outcomes (e.g., Mendez & Belendez, 1997). See Gage and colleagues (2004) and Wysocki (2006) for reviews and Winkley, Landau, Eisler, and Ismail (2006) for a meta-analysis of psychological interventions to improve glycemic control in patients with DM1.

Social support interventions involving peers have shown positive effects for youth with DM1 (e.g., Greco, Pendley, McDonell, & Reeves, 2001; Pendley et al., 2002). These interventions may be especially important for adolescents with diabetes, because managing peer impressions is a key interest for this age group (Thomas, Peterson, & Goldstein, 1997). Finally, community involvement at the school and health care system levels also is very important in the successful management of diabetes. See Wysocki, Buckloh, and Greco (2009) for a comprehensive review of empirically validated measures and treatments within the domains of family management, individual coping and psychological adjustment, and the greater social context of diabetes.

The following case example illustrates how a pediatric psychologist's expertise can be applied to a family of a teen with type 1 diabetes who is having problems with poor adherence and problematic adjustment to her disease. As is illustrated, many factors affected this teen's adjustment and treatment outcome, including psychosocial stresses and inconsistent psychotherapy attendance. A number of interventions were utilized, including BFST, cognitive-behavioral interventions targeting coping and adjustment, and educational and social support interventions. Psychological treatment occurred within multidisciplinary care for this teen.

CASE EXAMPLE: ASHLEY

History of Presenting Illness

Ashley, a 15-year-old Caucasian female with DM1, was referred by her endocrinologist for concerns about her poor diabetes management and glycemic control. She had been struggling with her diabetes management for the past year and was dealing with numerous psychosocial stresses. The family reported that Ashley was checking her blood glucose (BG) only about once a week and fabricating BG values. She was on an insulin pump, was bolusing (injecting a dosage of) her insulin without checking her BG, and was snacking and eating lunch at school without bolusing insulin. Moreover, Ashley was not changing her pump site and insulin cartridges regularly. She and her mother reported some family communication problems related to her diabetes care, and her mother was not monitoring her diabetes care closely. Ashley's father had moved to another state to take a new job several months before, which has been stressful for the family. Ashley's school grades declined recently, from B's and C's to F's. Ashley reported having some anxiety but denied significant symptoms of depression or any current or past suicidal ideation. Her mother reported that Ashley acted sad and tired and that she tended to be a shy, quiet teenager who had trouble advocating for herself. Ashley had friends and a boyfriend and was her volleyball team captain.

Psychosocial History

Ashley was living with her mother and 19-year-old sister. Ashley was in the ninth grade and had never repeated a grade nor had special education services. Her mother denied any family history of psychiatric, learning, or attentional problems, alcohol or drug abuse, seizures, or tics. Ashley had not received any previous psychiatric or psychological assessment or treatment.

Developmental/Medical History

Ashley was born full term with no complications during her mother's pregnancy, labor, or delivery. Her developmental milestones were normal for her age. Ashley's medical history was significant for DM1, diagnosed when she was 7 years old. Her most recent HbA_{1c} was 14% (3 weeks prior), up from 8.5% (7 months prior; see Figure 18.1). She had no known allergies.

Diagnosis

Ashley was diagnosed as having adjustment disorder with anxiety (309.24); rule out depressive symptoms.

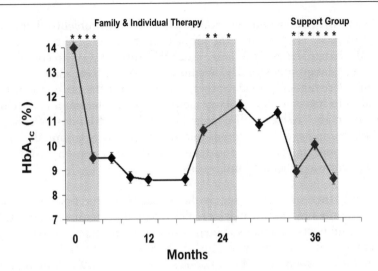

FIGURE 18.1. Changes in Ashley's HbA_{1C} over the course of treatment. * = intervention sessions.

Treatment Plan

Individual and family therapy were recommended on a weekly to biweekly basis. Ashley's treatment goals included improving her diabetes management/compliance, coping and anxiety/stress management skills, and family communication and relationships.

Because Ashley was experiencing significant diabetes management problems, elements of BFST (Wysocki, Harris, Greco, Mertlich, & Buckloh, 2001) were considered as a means to improve her diabetes compliance, glycemic control, and family communication. BFST is a manualized therapy targeting problem solving, family communication, and cognitive restructuring skills from an ecological family systems perspective. In addition, individual therapy using cognitive-behavioral interventions was indicated to help Ashley to manage her anxiety and depressive symptoms and to develop better coping skills.

Therapy Session 1

Session 1, a 50-minute family therapy session with Ashley and her mother, took place 2 weeks later. The family reported that Ashley had improved in checking her BG more regularly. Ashley and her mother were taught problem-solving skills, using materials from BFST (Wysocki et al., 2001). Because changing her pump site regularly was identified as a main concern for the family, Ashley and her mother practiced the problem-solving skills using this goal. They defined the problem (not changing site on time), set the goal (change site every 3 days), and brainstormed ways to complete the goal (e.g., change site Monday, Wednesday, Friday; have materials in the kitchen as a reminder; provide a reward for changing the site on time; set up reminders in Ashley's phone). They then agreed on solutions and developed an action plan ("Ashley will change her site every Monday, Wednesday, and Friday and have the materials out in the kitchen as a reminder."). The contract would be reviewed and revised at the next session. A follow-up appointment was scheduled in 2 weeks.

Family therapy was chosen as the modality for the first two sessions because family functioning plays a major role in diabetes management. The literature supports problem solving (Wysocki, Iannotti, et al., 2008), family communication (Bobrow, AvRuskin, & Siller, 1985), and parental support and involvement (e.g., Ellis, Podolski, et al., 2007; Wiebe et al., 2005) as important family variables affecting DM1 care. It was important to get Ashley's mother more involved in monitoring her diabetes care. A common mistake that parents make is to back off from monitoring because they think their teen has the diabetes knowledge and skills to manage his or her diabetes. However, although diabetes knowledge and skills increase with age, children and parents are still prone to errors (e.g., Delamater et al., 1988), and diabetes knowledge is weakly related to treatment adherence and glycemic control (Heidgerken et al., 2007).

Therapy Session 2

Session 2, a 50-minute family therapy session with Ashley and her mother, took place 2 weeks later. The family reported success with Ashley's behavioral goals, including changing her pump site regularly. Ashley indicated improvements in her mood and coping, as well as her academics. Ashley and her mother talked about how to increase the frequency of her checking her BG to every 2 hours. They went through the structured problem-solving steps and generated several goals, including Ashley's mother agreeing to check Ashley's BG in the middle of the night and to discuss with teachers when and where Ashley could check her BG. Ashley agreed to check her BG at lunch and to use a log book to record her BG numbers.

Because Ashley had been successful using some of the solutions from the previous session, the family tackled a new problem using the same format and developed an action plan. Getting the school involved in a student's diabetes care is important but can be a challenge, as there often is limited support and monitoring at school. Pediatric psychologists often need to work with families to remove barriers to diabetes management at school. For example, students may not be allowed to carry their diabetes supplies with them, so they must go to the office or nurse to manage their diabetes. Teenagers often do not want to take extra time to do this or do not want to be singled out to leave class early to manage their diabetes. Sometimes creative ways to get around these barriers must be sought. The American Diabetes Association (2002) has recommendations for school accommodations, including training school personnel in diabetes care.

Therapy Session 3

Session 3, a 50-minute individual psychotherapy session with Ashley and her maternal grandmother, took place 2 weeks later. Ashley's HbA_{1c} decreased to 9.5%, showing good improvement in her glycemic control. She reported having some trouble with meeting the new diabetes goal (checking BG more frequently). She continued to change her pump site regularly. Ashley worked individually with the provider on problem-solving additional ways to accomplish her diabetes management goals by removing potential barriers. Ashley explored her feelings about psychosocial issues. She learned basic coping skills from a cognitive-behavioral approach to manage her anxiety and stress. At the next session, the plan was to introduce behavioral contracting and effective family communication skills, both elements of BFST. The family did not make a follow-up appointment.

Psychological stress can affect adolescents' ability to manage their diabetes by decreasing both glycemic control and adherence (Wysocki et al., 2009). Anxiety and depression appear to play significant roles in individual adaption to DM1, although their relationship to glycemic control is not clear (Dantzer, Swendsen, Maurice-Tison, & Salamon, 2003). Moreover, coping style may affect glycemic control, with certain styles, such as avoidance coping (e.g., Grey, Lipman, Cameron, & Thurber, 1997), possibly being related to poorer DM1 outcomes. Ashley was taught cognitive-behavioral strategies to manage her stress and mood, such as positive thinking skills (cognitive restructuring), distraction techniques, and relaxation techniques (deep breathing, visualization). Unfortunately, there are many practical barriers to keeping families with a child with DM1 engaged in the therapy process. DM1 is a burdensome disease with a complex regimen, requiring frequent medical appointments (with, e.g., an endocrinologist, a dietician, a diabetes educator). In addition, many families travel from a distance away, as major medical centers with endocrinology and other subspecialties are usually not available in more rural areas. Ashley was lost to psychology follow-up but was seen regularly by an endocrinologist. At each endocrinology appointment, Ashley and her mother were encouraged to return to psychotherapy. However, it took another year for the family to return for psychological services.

Therapy Session 4

Session 4, a 50-minute family therapy session with Ashley and her mother, took place 1 year later. The family returned to therapy with concerns that Ashley was not checking her BG frequently enough, was sometimes taking insulin without checking her BG, was eating without taking insulin, and was not keeping up with her diabetes supplies. She also was not communicating about diabetes to her mother well enough when she was out with friends. Behavioral contracting was introduced to the family. Ashley and her mother developed a behavioral contract for Ashley to check her BG 5–6 times a day and to download her BG meter every 7 days. She would earn an incentive (to go out with friends) if she fulfilled this over the next 2 weeks and a bonus (an additional privilege) if she needed no reminders from her mother.

Ashley's return to psychotherapy was prompted by concerns again about her poor diabetes management and lack of independence with her diabetes regimen. The family was given a step-by-step guide to creating a behavioral contract and written examples. They were encouraged to choose a problem behavior that can be reliably measured. They defined the problem behavior in concrete terms. They then problem-solved ways to improve that behavior and identified rewards that would provide motivation for Ashley to succeed. The desired behavior was specified (quantified) in a way that could be accurately observed and counted. The contract was negotiated by Ashley and her mother, was written on paper, and was signed by both family members. Behavioral contracting helps parents and teens to have reasonable, achievable goals, with realistic ways of monitoring progress, and incentives to motivate youth. Incentives that often work with teenagers are social in nature, such as time with friends and driving privileges. Bonuses for additional positive behavior, such as teens taking more initiative (not needing to be reminded), can be built into the contract.

Therapy Session 5

Session 5, a 50-minute family therapy session with Ashley and her mother took place 2 weeks later. Ashley's mother reported privately that there had been significant family stress: The house was in foreclosure, the parents were divorcing (which Ashley was not yet aware of), and her father was not as involved with Ashley. Her mother reported that Ashley often seemed quiet and unmotivated. The behavior contract was reviewed. The family thought it had been successful and wanted to continue it. The family problem-solved how to remove barriers to get Ashley to check her BG mid-morning and during lunch at school. The provider spoke with Ashley's mother privately about how to talk with her daughters about and help them adjust to the divorce. Ashley's affect was flat, and she was less engaged in the session. The next session was scheduled in 3 weeks.

It became clear in this session that family stresses were likely contributing heavily to Ashley's decline in treatment adherence. It was important to address these issues and to assist in Ashley's adjustment. It also was important to get Ashley more motivated and to address ways to remove the barriers to her diabetes care. Motivational interviewing (MI) techniques could have been a good approach to use here. MI involves building awareness, generating alternatives, solving problems, making choices, setting goals, and avoiding confrontation and has been found to have positive effects on glycemic control in teens with DM1 (Channon et al., 2007). Informal reassessment of her mood was made (observations by her mother and her own self-report), but this also could have been a good time to assess more formally with standardized measures such as the Behavior Assessment System for Children-2 (BASC-2; Reynolds & Kamphaus, 2004).

Therapy Session 6

Session 6, a 50-minute individual psychotherapy session with Ashley and her mother, took place 2 months later. Two psychology appointments had been canceled in the interim. The family returned indicating many recent stresses, including the divorce, their home in foreclosure, and Ashley, her mother, and her sister moving in with maternal grandparents. Ashley had been anxious, and her diabetes management slipped. Ashley discussed her feelings about psychosocial stresses and strained family relationships within the context of supportive therapy. She problem-solved how to improve her diabetes management once she settled in at her grandparents' home. For example, ideas to get her grandmother involved in helping her remember to check her BG were generated. Ashley was taught additional coping strategies, and ways to improve communication with her father were brainstormed. The provider recommended cognitive-behavioral and supportive therapy to help Ashley adjust to her parents' divorce and loss of her home. It was planned to work on diabetes self-management (improving BG testing and bolusing insulin at mealtimes) at the next session. An appointment was scheduled in 1 month.

Extended family often is important to involve in diabetes management and support, as in this case involving Ashley's grandmother. Although Ashley's father was not present to benefit from communication skills training, working with the teenager alone on communication skills can also be beneficial. Communication skills training is a component of BFST and involves identifying positive communication skills (roles of the speaker and the listener), as well as negative communication patterns and alternatives to those patterns (e.g., lecturing, reminding/nagging, silent treatment, yelling). Ashley's mother canceled the next scheduled appointment, and the family did not return to psychotherapy. Ashley's HbA_{1c} increased over time (see Figure 18.1). At all of her endocrinology appointments, she was advised to return to psychotherapy to address treatment adherence and psychosocial issues. The family did not seem interested and reported that they did not have enough time to follow up with psychotherapy. They eventually were referred to the endocrinology social worker for follow-up. Six months later, they saw the social worker as part of their multidisciplinary team.

Social Work Initial Assessment

Ashley's mother indicated that she wanted Ashley to be more independent with her diabetes care now that she was 18 years old. Ashley continued to have problems involving not checking her BG or bolusing insulin at school or when socializing with friends. Ashley denied anxiety or depressive symptoms but admitted to feeling frustrated and angry at times. She no longer had contact with her father. She was a senior and getting average grades.

Ashley was enrolled in the Individualized Diabetes Education and Support Clinic (IDEAS), a multidisciplinary education and support group for teens with DM1 in poor control ($HbA_{1c} > 9.0\%$). The IDEAS clinic included a teen group run by the social worker and a simultaneous parent group run by an endocrinologist. There were six 90-minute sessions with 4–15 families participating in the sessions. There was a short diabetes education portion at the beginning of each session, run by a diabetes educator. The curriculum for the IDEAS clinic was based on cognitive-behavioral strategies. The teen group had a curriculum covering (1) emotional reactions and stages of change; (2) healthy coping; (3) stress management; (4) communication skills; (5) time management; and (6) motivational strategies. The teens also saw the endocrinologist for a brief individual appointment at each session.

IDEAS Clinic

Ashley participated in six sessions over the course of 7 months. She participated in groups that covered communication skills, time management, motivational strategies, and coping skills and in repeat sessions on communication skills and motivational strategies. The family decided to transition to an adult endocrinologist at the end of the IDEAS clinic.

The education and support group allowed Ashley to interact with other teens with DM1, giving her an opportunity for peer social support. Social support interventions that integrate friends into adolescents' diabetes management have been effective in improving psychosocial outcomes (Greco et al., 2001) and glycemic control (Pendley et al., 2002). Although these participants were not Ashley's friends and regular peer group, it may have been beneficial to have some peer support from other teens experiencing the same problems.

The transition to adult care is an important developmental milestone for teens with diabetes but often represents a challenge. During this transition period, there appears to be a subgroup of young adults with DM1, especially females, who are at increased risk for mental health issues, poor glycemic control, and development of complications (Weissberg-Benchell, Wolpert, & Anderson, 2007). Pediatric psychologists can be valuable in preparing families for this transition to adult medical care.

CONCLUSIONS

This case represents a fairly typical course of therapy for a teenager with DM1. Although it would be ideal for families to participate in weekly or biweekly sessions consistently until the treatment goals are met, this is not often reality. Families often are so busy and stressed that they cannot follow through with consistent therapy sessions. It is important to balance comprehensive treatment with reasonable time limits. Perhaps the time-based nature of the IDEAS group (just six sessions) made it easier for this family to follow through with than were individual therapy sessions. Short-term problem-focused therapy is likely the most useful approach with this population. Families can return at different points in their child's development to address new issues that arise with adjusting to diabetes.

In many clinics, doctoral-level pediatric psychologists are not available; it is more likely that master's-level therapists (social workers, mental health counselors) would be on staff. It is advantageous for a mental health provider to be in the endocrinology clinic and see families in conjunction with their scheduled medical appointments. This reduces the need for additional appointments and makes a multidisciplinary approach to care more feasible. In this case, Ashley and her mother did not think that they had time to follow up again with the psychologist (who had an office in a different part of the building), but they were willing to see the social worker and to be involved in the IDEAS group. The increased contact with her endocrinologist (monthly instead of quarterly) may also have helped the family to stay on track. Parents were able to problem-solve issues with the endocrinologist running the parent portion of the group.

Often a pediatric psychologist will be part of the multidisciplinary team (see Conroy & Logan, Chapter 7, this volume) and will provide service in a number of ways at various points in the care of a youth's diabetes. In addition to providing direct psychological intervention and support, a pediatric psychologist may serve in a consultative role, educating other health professionals who may act in supportive psychological roles for youth with diabetes. They also may be instrumental in advocating for the needs of children with chronic illness in school settings, involving extended family members and peers, or assisting in the transition to adult medical care.

ACKNOWLEDGMENTS

I would like to thank Kathleen Kerins, LCSW, for sharing materials and information about the IDEAS clinic and Tim Wysocki, PhD, ABPP, for his assistance with Figure 18.1. The case material presented in this chapter has been disguised.

REFERENCES

American Diabetes Association. (2002). Care of children with diabetes in the school and day care setting. *Diabetes Care, 26*, S131–S135.

Bobrow, E. S., AvRuskin, T. W., & Siller, I. (1985). Mother-daughter interactions and adherence to diabetes regimens. *Diabetes Care, 8*, 146–151.

Carney, R. M., Schechter, K., & Davis, T. (1983). Improving adherence to blood glucose monitoring in insulin-dependent diabetic children. *Behavior Therapy, 14*, 247–254.

Channon, S. J., Huws-Thomas, M. V., Rollnick, S., Hood, K., Cannings-John, R. L., Rogers, C., et al. (2007). A multicenter randomized controlled trial of motivational interviewing in teenagers with diabetes. *Diabetes Care, 30*, 1390–1395.

Chase, H. P. (2006). *Understanding diabetes* (11th ed.). Denver, CO: Children's Diabetes Foundation.

Dantzer, C., Swendsen, J., Maurice-Tison, S., & Salamon, R. (2003). Anxiety and depression in juvenile diabetes: A critical review. *Clinical Psychology Review, 23*, 787–800.

Delamater, A. M., Davis, S., Bubb, J., Smith, J., White, N. H., & Santiago, J. V. (1988). Self-monitoring of blood glucose by adolescents with diabetes: Technical skills and utilization of date. *Diabetes Educator, 15*, 56–61.

Diabetes Control and Complications Trial Research Group. (1994). Effect of intensive treatment on the development and progression of long-term complications in adolescents with insulin-dependent diabetes mellitus. *Journal of Pediatrics,* *125,* 177–188.

Ellis, D. A., Frey, M., Naar-King, S., Templin, T., Cunningham, P., & Cakan, N. (2005). Use of multisystemic therapy to improve regimen adherence among adolescents with Type 1 diabetes in chronic poor metabolic control: A randomized controlled trial. *Diabetes Care, 28,* 1604–1610.

Ellis, D. A., Podolski, C., Frey, M., Naar-King, S., Wang, B., & Moltz, K. (2007). The role of parental monitoring in adolescent health outcomes: Impact of regimen adherence in youth with type 1 diabetes. *Journal of Pediatric Psychology, 32,* 907–917.

Ellis, D. A., Templin, T., Naar-King, S., Frey, M. A., Cunningham, P. B., Podolski, C. L., et al. (2007). Multisystemic therapy for adolescents with poorly controlled Type 1 diabetes: Stability of treatment effects in a randomized controlled trial. *Journal of Consulting and Clinical Psychology, 75,* 168–174.

Epstein, L. H., Beck, S., Figueroa, J., Farkas, G., Kazdin, A. E., Daneman, D., et al. (1981). The effects of targeting improvement in urine glucose on metabolic control in children with insulin-dependent diabetes mellitus. *Journal of Applied Behavior Analysis, 14,* 365–375.

Gage, H., Hampson, S., Skinner, T. C., Hart, J., Storey, L., Foxcroft, D., et al. (2004). Educational and psychosocial programmes for adolescents with diabetes: Approaches, outcomes, and cost-effectiveness. *Patient Education and Counseling, 53,* 333–346.

Greco, P., Pendley, J. S., McDonell, K., & Reeves, G. (2001). A peer group intervention for adolescents with Type 1 diabetes and their best friends. *Journal of Pediatric Psychology, 26,* 485–490.

Grey, M., Boland, E. A., Davidson, M., Li, J., & Tamborlane, W. V. (2000). Coping skills training for youth with diabetes mellitus has long-lasting effects on metabolic control and quality of life. *Journal of Pediatrics, 137,* 107–114.

Grey, M., Lipman, T., Cameron, M. E., & Thurber, F. W. (1997). Coping behaviors at diagnosis and in adjustment one year later in children with diabetes. *Nursing Research, 46,* 312–317.

Heidgerken, A. D., Merlo, L., Williams, L. B., Lewin, A. B., Gelfand, K., Malasanos, T., et al. (2007). Diabetes Awareness and Reasoning Test: A preliminary analysis of development and psychometrics. *Children's Health Care, 36,* 117–136.

Mendez, F. J., & Belendez, M. (1997). Effects of a behavioral intervention on treatment adherence and stress management in adolescents with IDDM. *Diabetes, Care, 24,* 1286–1292.

Pendley, J. S., Kasmen, L. J., Miller, D. L., Donze, J., Swenson, C., & Reeves, G. (2002). Peer and family support in children and adolescents with Type 1 diabetes. *Journal of Pediatric Psychology, 27,* 429–438.

Reynolds, C. R., & Kamphaus, R. W. (2004). *Behavior Assessment System for Children—2nd edition manual.* Bloomington, MN: Pearson Assessments.

Thomas, A. M., Peterson, L., & Goldstein, D. (1997). Problem solving and diabetes regimen adherence by children and adolescents with IDDM in social pressure situations: A reflection of normal development. *Journal of Pediatric Psychology, 22,* 541–561.

U.K. Prospective Diabetes Study Group. (1998). Intensive blood glucose control with sulphonylureas or insulin compared with conventional treatment and risk of complications in patients with type 2 diabetes (UKPDS 33). *Lancet, 352*, 837–853.

Weissberg-Benchell, J., Wolpert, H., & Anderson, B. (2007). Transitioning from pediatric to adult care: A new approach to the post-adolescent young person with type 1 diabetes. *Diabetes Care, 30*(10), 2441–2446.

Wiebe, D. J., Berg, C. A., Korbel, C., Palmer, D. L., Beveridge, R. M., Upchurch, R., et al. (2005). Children's appraisals of maternal involvement in coping with diabetes: Enhancing our understanding of adherence, metabolic control, and quality of life across adolescence. *Journal of Pediatric Psychology, 30*(2), 167–178.

Winkley, K., Landau, S., Eisler, I., & Ismail, K. (2006). Psychological interventions to improve glycaemic control in patients with Type 1 diabetes: Systematic review and meta-analysis of randomized controlled trials. *British Medical Journal, 333*, 65–69.

Wysocki, T. (2006). Behavioral assessment and intervention in pediatric diabetes. *Behavior Modification, 30*, 1–21.

Wysocki, T., Buckloh, L. M., & Greco, P. (2009). The psychological context of diabetes mellitus in youth. In M. C. Roberts & R. G. Steele (Eds.), *Handbook of pediatric psychology* (4th ed.; pp. 287–302). New York: Guilford Press.

Wysocki, T., Harris, M. A., Buckloh, L. M., Mertlich, D., Lochrie, A. S., Mauras, N., et al. (2007). Randomized controlled trial of behavioral family systems therapy for diabetes: Maintenance of effect on diabetes outcomes in adolescents. *Diabetes Care, 30*, 555–560.

Wysocki, T., Harris, M. A., Buckloh, L. M, Mertlich, D., Lochrie, A. S., Taylor, A., et al. (2008). Randomized controlled trial of behavioral family systems therapy for diabetes: Maintenance and generalization of effects on parent-adolescent communication. *Behavior Therapy, 39*, 33–46.

Wysocki, T., Harris, M. A., Greco, P., Mertlich, D., & Buckloh, L. M. (2001). *Behavioral family systems therapy (BFST) for adolescents with chronic illness: Treatment and implementation manual.* Unpublished manual.

Wysocki, T., Iannotti, R., Weissberg-Benchell, J., Hood, K., Laffel, L., Anderson, B. J., et al. (2008). Diabetes problem solving by youths with Type 1 diabetes and their caregivers: Measurement, validation, and longitudinal associations with glycemic control. *Journal of Pediatric Psychology, 33*(8), 875–884.

CHAPTER 19

Pediatric Obesity

CHRISTOPHER C. CUSHING
KELSEY BORNER
RIC G. STEELE

Childhood overweight and obesity affect approximately one-third of children and adolescents in the United States (Ogden, Carroll, Curtin, Lamb, & Flegal, 2010). It is well established that children with overweight and obesity are at increased risk for physical illness, as well as psychosocial problems, such as internalizing symptoms, health-related quality of life impairments, and increased risk for teasing and victimization by peers (see Jelalian & Hart, 2009; Zeller & Modi, 2008, for reviews). As outlined in greater detail in this chapter, expert recommendations for outpatient treatment of pediatric obesity/overweight include lifestyle interventions that incorporate behavioral techniques such as self-monitoring, rewards, and goal setting to increase physical activity and decrease caloric intake. The following case provides one example of how a multicomponent lifestyle intervention might be conducted.

CASE EXAMPLE: NORA

Nora was an 11-year, 9-month-old girl in the sixth grade who resided with her parents and her younger sister, Kaitlyn. Nora was referred to the clinic by her school nurse following a routine health and wellness assessment. At the time of the referral, Nora weighed 147.6 pounds (> 97th percentile for age and sex) and was 64.75 inches tall (> 97th percentile for age and sex), placing her body mass index (BMI) at the 94th percentile for age and sex, or in the "overweight" category, as outlined by the Centers for Disease Control and Prevention (CDC; Ogden et al., 2010). Both of Nora's parents reported their own long-standing weight problems. At 5 feet 4 inches and 156 pounds, Nora's mother also fell into the CDC's overweight category (BMI = 26.2). Nora's father reportedly struggled with weight issues for most of his adult life. Nora's mother reported a family income of approximately $72,000 per year.

Nora reported some physical activity during structured physical education at school but very limited physical activity during unstructured "free" time (e.g., during recess, after school, in the evenings). Nora reported no instances of moderate or vigorous physical activity (MVPA) during the most recent consecutive 5 school days, and neither Nora nor her mother reported significant MVPA as a family (e.g., going on walks). Regarding diet, Nora reported that she was unsure of her ability to use food labels to determine which foods were "good for her" but more confident of her ability to "eat a balanced diet." Margine, Nora's mother, was confident of her ability to identify and choose healthy foods for herself and for her daughter and in her ability to help Nora eat a balanced diet. Margine reported at intake that she felt obligated to control or manage Nora's choices of foods and beverages.

Complicating Nora's referral and treatment were a number of specific psychosocial considerations, including specific internalizing symptoms (e.g., depressive symptoms, sense of inadequacy, social stress), as well as significant school problems. Nora also reported problematic relationships with her parents. Consistent with Nora's self-report of depressive symptoms, Margine reported that Nora evidenced elevated symptoms of social withdrawal, as well as significant symptoms of conduct problems (e.g., disobedience, deceitfulness, "sneaking").

Both Nora and Margine's reports indicated that Nora experienced significantly impaired health-related quality of life (HRQOL). At intake Nora's total score of 36 on the PedsQL (Varni, Seid, & Kurtin, 2001) indicated HRQOL well below the measure's recommended clinical cutoff of 76 (Huang et al., 2009). In terms of her self-reported physical health, Nora indicated body aches, low energy, and difficulty engaging in sports or exercise. Nora's self-reported social HRQOL was significant for poor peer interactions, teasing, and inability to "keep up" with her peers. Margine's report of Nora's HRQOL was also significant for problems with physical activity (e.g., trouble doing chores around the house), emotional symptoms (e.g., anger), social functioning (e.g., getting along with others), and school functioning.

CONSIDERATION OF POSSIBLE
TREATMENT APPROACHES

A number of recent meta-analyses and reviews have established family-based lifestyle interventions as effective treatments for pediatric overweight and obesity (Wilfley et al., 2007; Kitzmann et al., 2010). In line with these research findings, Barlow (2007) and the Expert Committee for the Assessment, Prevention, and Treatment of Pediatric Obesity established specific treatment guidelines, recommending that lifestyle interventions be considered the first line of treatment for pediatric overweight and obesity.

Lifestyle interventions are generally characterized by a holistic approach to weight change, targeting multiple factors to reduce dietary intake and increase energy expenditure. These interventions are founded on behavioral strategies to change the whole family's approach to eating and physical activity, including educational components and behavior modification techniques such as stimulus control, self-monitoring, and reinforcement (Dalton & Kitzmann, 2012). In the context of energy expenditure, stimulus control involves helping families identify and remove unhealthy foods entirely from their home environment and develop family-specific systems of healthy snack reminders, such as a fruit and vegetable list posted on the refrigerator. Many programs also include brief parent training skills to help establish external reinforcement for healthy behavior, such as positive attending. Generally speaking, interventions that use a larger number of behavioral techniques, such as self-monitoring, rewards, stimulus control, and goal setting, can be thought of as having greater impact.

The importance of the role of parents in treatment cannot be overstated (Kitzmann et al., 2010), with some evidence indicating that it may be possible to confer a significant treatment effect on children even when the intervention is delivered exclusively to parents (Janicke et al., 2008). In addition, it has been postulated that family contextual factors, such as parenting style, conflict, and stress, may moderate the effect of treatment, issues that are well known to the practicing clinical child and pediatric psychologist (Kitzmann, Dalton, & Buscemi, 2008).

A group-based family lifestyle intervention appeared most appropriate for Nora and her family given Nora's BMI percentile at presentation, her family's apparent willingness to be involved in treatment, the need to address environmental factors (food availability and family activity level), and a constellation of psychosocial concerns and challenges that could be addressed during group sessions. Further, this was Nora's first attempt at losing weight, and there were no reported medical comorbidities.

Although Nora's treatment was delivered in a group format, it is possible to deliver the same type of lifestyle intervention in an individual format.

Our team prefers to do this with both the parent and child in attendance—assuming that the child does not suffer from some significant psychopathology (e.g., depressive or anxious symptoms). When psychopathology is a concern, an individual format with a sequenced treatment approach may prove useful. Such a format would prioritize any acute concerns before initiating the lifestyle intervention. It is our observation that the absence of the group structure can limit family motivation to perform key components of treatment, such as self-monitoring. As such, it is critical that an individualized plan promote at least 75% completion of self-monitoring records (the value supported by the empirical literature as being associated with weight loss) for each target family member.

IMPLEMENTATION

Although Nora was referred by her school nurse, it is important to remember that the empirical literature supports direct discussions with families about their child's weight and that families prefer that clinicians speak plainly and use clinical language, such as *overweight* and *obese,* when discussing weight. A thorough biopsychosocial assessment should also include quality of life as a means of helping the family understand the day-to-day impact of the excess weight on the child.

Upon referral to the clinic, Nora and her mother (the only two of their family who elected to attend sessions) were assigned to a group of five families of children between the ages of 7 and 13. The group was composed of 3 girls (including Nora) and 2 boys. Treatment in the selected program follows a 10-week course in which children and parents each receive 40 minutes of weekly consultation with a master's-level treatment provider who guides behavioral groups in goal setting and review, psychoeducation, administration of homework assignments (self-monitoring), identification of barriers, and problem solving.

Families also received 40 minutes each week of consultation and education from a nutritionist/dietician. Consistent with the general model demonstrated in the literature (e.g., the Stoplight Diet; Epstein, 1998), a primary goal of the nutrition sessions was to help families increase availability and intake of foods that are low in fat and high in nutrient density and decrease availability and intake of foods that are high in fat and sugar and low in nutrient density.

As per the treatment protocol chosen, children and adults attended separate but parallel group sessions to allow the content to be delivered in a developmentally appropriate manner. Although groups are structured around specific topics, the groups allow the flexibility to address specific concerns and issues that are brought up by the youth and their families. Following the parallel behavior and nutrition groups, youth and families meet together with the behavior therapists to discuss goals for the coming week.

ATTENDANCE AND OUTCOMES

Nora and her mother attended 6 of 10 sessions. Missed sessions were due, in part, to conflicts in schedules (e.g., school activities) and to forgetfulness. They completed five of the weekly self-monitoring homework tasks. Content from missed sessions was briefly reviewed either before or after the next session attended. Due to the group nature of the intervention, missed sessions could not be rescheduled.

Nora's treatment response is summarized in Table 19.1. At the 1-year follow-up, Nora's BMI had further decreased to the 92nd percentile. It is important to remember that, at 12 years old, Nora's 1-year follow-up outcomes were measured during her transition to adolescence, a developmental period that can lead to weight gain and reduced levels of physical activity, especially in females.

Consistent with the "whole family" approach outlined previously, Nora's mother, Margine, had also started responding to treatment. Specifically, she lost 4.8 pounds postintervention (156.4 to 151.6), which placed her BMI at 26. Although Margine's BMI fell in the overweight category postintervention, she evidenced a slight reduction from her initial BMI of 26.2. However, at 1-year follow-up, Margine's weight had rebounded to her baseline level (156.6 pounds).

TABLE 19.1. Baseline and Outcome Measures for Nora

	Initial	Posttreatment	12-month follow-up
Weight (pounds)	147.6	145.2	156.0
BMI percentile	94th	93rd	92nd
Health-related quality of life			
Child report	36	47	73
Parent report	63	67	82
Perception of teasing (*child report*)	104	52	70
Depressive symptoms			
Child report	67	55	43
Parent report	59	50	56

Over the course of the intervention, Nora experienced a substantial and clinically significant improvement in HRQOL, as demonstrated in Table 19.1 by the significant increases in her scores. At follow-up, Nora's HRQOL values were no longer impaired, using the values identified by Varni and colleagues (2001). Importantly, this suggests that the program had an immediate impact on HRQOL and may have set Nora on a "trajectory" of improved functioning following treatment. Margine also noted an improvement in Nora's HRQOL at follow-up, but not immediately post-treatment.

Consistent with her HRQOL scores, other indices of Nora's psychosocial functioning demonstrated some improvement. For example, Nora's perception of teasing by her peers and her self-report of depressive symptoms decreased over treatment. It appears that both the frequency of teasing and the degree of upset that such events caused Nora decreased. Improvements in mood have been reported among children who become more physically active (Ahn & Fedewa, 2011), perhaps due to increased opportunities for reinforcement, as well as to enhanced neurological factors (i.e., release of beta-endorphins) and behavioral activation.

Finally, Nora reported changes in physical activity from baseline to postintervention and again at 1-year follow-up. Immediately postintervention, Nora had increased her vigorous physical activity during the weekdays, especially after school and during the evenings. Prior to the intervention, Nora had reported being physically active only on the weekends. Nora's physical activity declined over the year following the intervention. Some improvements may be traced to systemic changes in access to physical activity: At the time that she received treatment, Nora was in sixth grade (elementary school, in her school district) with daily recess and twice-weekly physical education. With the transition to junior high 1 year later, Nora no longer participated in recess and reported less physical education. At the 1-year follow-up, Nora reported being moderately active on most days of the week, engaging in activities such as walking and biking, but she was no longer active on the weekends.

In many ways Nora's pattern of physical activity reflects the struggle against sedentary activity that accompanies aging into later adolescence and adulthood and should serve as a reminder to the clinician of the increasing barriers to physical activity and the expected decrease in physical activity as structured activity declines with age. Although her overall physical activity decreased, it is encouraging that Nora continued to be physically active while at home. This finding may be due to her mother's increase and maintenance of physical activity as a result of the treatment program. Margine increased her physical activity postintervention and maintained that increase at the 1-year follow-up. Margine reported engaging in more physical activities, including aerobics classes, in the afternoons and evenings.

CLINICAL SIGNIFICANCE

The program chosen for Nora conferred a number of salutary benefits on her psychological well-being, while providing modest benefits with regard to weight and BMI. At the age of 18, an average girl of Nora's height should weigh no more than approximately 159 pounds to have a BMI in the "normal" or healthy range. In Nora's case this means that her weight at the follow-up period may not necessarily represent a clinical problem, provided that Nora remains in control of excess weight gain throughout the remainder of adolescence. Exemplifying one of the ways that weight management differs in pediatric relative to adult populations, this case demonstrates that the objective is not necessarily always weight loss but rather arresting out-of-control weight gain and establishing healthful life-long behaviors. Moreover, the pediatric psychologist working in the area of weight management must be prepared for cases such as Nora's in which the initial, posttreatment, and follow-up phases all see the patient in the overweight category. This case underscores the importance of a broad and systemic view of treatment outcome, with a special emphasis on psycho-social variables.

SPECIFIC CHALLENGES
AND HOW THESE WERE ADDRESSED

This case highlights a number of specific challenges to the successful treatment of pediatric obesity. As noted previously, adherence to treatment recommendations was problematic for Nora and her family, and several factors may have affected treatment adherence. First, Nora's internalizing symptoms may have served as a barrier to treatment due to low energy and motivation. Equally important was a low propensity for physical activity at baseline and high levels of weight-related teasing. Some data indicate that girls are particularly susceptible to attenuated physical activity in the presence of weight-related criticism, making it difficult to complete the necessary energy expenditure to change weight-related health outcomes. Further, some studies indicate that symptoms of anxiety and depression, low baseline physical activity, and low socioeconomic status are particular risk factors for poor performance in treatment. Given Nora's presentation of at least two of these risk factors, her outcome of rather modest improvement on BMI percentile is not surprising. We believe it is important for clinicians to carefully screen patients at baseline and consider appropriately sequencing treatment to meet the individual's needs. In Nora's case, the family may have been better served to have been referred for a brief course of behavioral activation and structured physical activity outside of school (e.g., club swimming, volleyball, running club) before initiating the treatment program.

Nora and her family also struggled to turn in self-monitoring homework. Self-monitoring of health behavior is among the most important components of treatment in adults and appears to also play a large role among adolescents. In fact, studies of adolescents reveal a significant correlation between consistently monitoring behavioral outcomes and both initial weight loss (Kirschenbaum, Germann, & Rich, 2005) and post-treatment success (Germann, Kirschenbaum, & Rich, 2007). This fact, combined with our anecdotal observations of Nora's difficulty completing our assigned self-monitoring homework, led our team to explore e-health and m-health solutions for encouraging self-monitoring. For example, the use of personal electronic devices (e.g., iPod, smartphone, tablet) rather than a paper-based logs has been shown to increase self-monitoring in adolescents in treatment for obesity and overweight (e.g., Cushing, Jensen, & Steele, 2010). More broadly, e-health interventions have demonstrated efficacy for modifying a number of child and adolescent health behaviors (Cushing & Steele, 2010). The use of commercially available activity and caloric intake monitoring applications (e.g., MyPlate Calorie Tracker) may be of clinical benefit to many adolescents who struggle with self-monitoring.

SUMMARY AND CONCLUSIONS

Overall, this case represents a typical family presenting to an outpatient pediatric clinic for weight-management treatment and illustrates typical challenges to implementing well-established behavioral treatment components. The use of a group-based therapeutic approach may have supported the patient's improved QOL and decreased depressive symptoms, while the behavioral and educational components likely helped establish healthier behaviors. Although BMI outcomes were modest, the case illustrates the importance of establishing healthier lifestyles for consistent long-term health improvement and the potential for more substantial changes in HRQOL.

REFERENCES

Ahn, S., & Fedewa, A. L. (2011). A meta-analysis of the relationship between children's physical activity and mental health. *Journal of Pediatric Psychology,* *36*(4), 385–397.

Barlow, S. E. (2007). Expert committee recommendations regarding the prevention, assessment, and treatment of child and adolescent overweight and obesity: Summary report. *Pediatrics, 120*(4), 164–192.

Cushing, C. C., Jensen, C. D., & Steele, R. G. (2010). The impact of a personal electronic device on self-monitoring compliance in the context of a weight-management program: A multiple baseline design. *Journal of Pediatric Psychology, 36,* 301–307.

Cushing, C. C., & Steele, R. G. (2010). A meta-analytic review of eHealth interventions for pediatric health promoting and maintaining behaviors. *Journal of Pediatric Psychology, 35,* 937–949.

Dalton, W. T., III, & Kitzmann, K. T. (2012). A preliminary investigation of stimulus control, self-monitoring, and reinforcement in lifestyle interventions for pediatric overweight. *American Journal of Lifestyle Medicine, 6*(1), 75–89.

Epstein, L. H., & Squires, S. (1998). The stoplight diet for children: An eight-week program for parents and children. Boston, MA: Little, Brown.

Germann, J. N., Kirschenbaum, S., & Rich, B. H. (2007). Child and parental self monitoring as determinants of success in the treatment of morbid obesity in low-income minority children. *Journal of Pediatric Psychology, 32,* 111–121.

Huang, I., Thompson, L. A., Chi, Y. Y., Knapp, C. A., Revicki, D. A., Seid, M., et al. (2009). The linkage between pediatric quality of life and health conditions: Establishing clinically meaningful cutoff scores for the PedsQL. *Value in Health, 12*(5), 773–781.

Janicke, D. M., Sallinen, B. J., Perri, M. G., Lutes, L. D., Huerta, M., Silverstein, J. H., et al. (2008). Comparison of parent-only vs. family-based interventions for overweight children in underserved rural settings: Outcomes from project STORY. *Archives of Pediatrics and Adolescent Medicine, 162*(12), 1119–1125.

Jelalian, E., & Hart, C. N. (2009). Pediatric obesity. In M. C. Roberts & R. G. Steele (Eds.), *Handbook of pediatric psychology* (4th ed., pp. 446–463). New York: Guilford Press.

Kirschenbaum, D. S., Germann, J. N., & Rich, B. C. (2005). Treatment of morbid obesity in low-income adolescents: Effects of parental self-monitoring. *Obesity Research, 13,* 1527–1529.

Kitzmann, K. M., Dalton, W. T., III, & Buscemi, J. (2008). Beyond parenting practices: Family context and the treatment of pediatric obesity. *Family Relations, 57*(1), 13–23.

Kitzmann, K. M., Dalton, W. T., III, Stanley, C. M., Beech, B. M., Reeves, T. P., Buscemi, J., et al. (2010). Lifestyle interventions for youth who are overweight: A meta-analytic review. *Health Psychology, 29*(1), 91.

Ogden, C. L., Carroll, M. D., Curtin, L. R., Lamb, M. M., & Flegal, K. M. (2010). Prevalence of high body mass index in U.S. children and adolescents 2007–2008. *Journal of the American Medical Association, 303*(3), 242–249.

Varni, J. W., Seid, M., & Kurtin, P. S. (2001). PedsQL 4.0: Reliability and validity of the Pediatric Quality of Life Inventory Version 4.0 generic core scales in healthy and patient populations. *Medical Care, 39,* 800–812.

Wilfley, D. E., Tibbs, T. L., Van Buren, D., Reach, K. P., Walker, M. S., & Epstein, L. H. (2007). Lifestyle interventions in the treatment of childhood overweight: A meta-analytic review of randomized controlled trials. *Health Psychology*, 26(5), 521–532.

Zeller, M. H., & Modi, A. C. (2008). Psychosocial factors related to obesity in children and adolescents. In E. Jelalian & R. G. Steele (Eds.), *Handbook of childhood and adolescent obesity* (pp. 25–42). New York: Springer.

CHAPTER 20

Pediatric Cancer

LAUREN C. DANIEL
MATTHEW C. HOCKING
LAMIA P. BARAKAT

Children facing cancer and their families experience profound changes to their lives as they confront mortality and disrupted child and family development. Intense and often lengthy multimodal treatments, as well as long-term consequences of cancer and its treatment, all pose unique challenges, acutely affecting parent and child distress, family functioning, parenting stress, and child and parent quality of life (see Vannatta, Salley, & Gerhardt, 2009, for a summary). Although distress at diagnosis is normative and generally attenuates over time for most families, it may persist through treatment into survivorship and manifest as posttraumatic stress symptoms (PTSS; Sawyer, Antoniou, Toogood, Rice, & Baghurst, 2000). Additionally, cancer and treatment late effects may continue to strain families after treatment ends (Friedman & Meadows, 2002). However, most children and families adapt well (Kazak et al., 2007) and even exhibit positive outcomes (Zebrack et al., 2011), including posttraumatic growth (Barakat, Alderfer, & Kazak, 2006).

Typical roles for pediatric psychologists in oncology include consulting to the health care team or being part of a multidisciplinary team assessing psychological and neuropsychological functioning; conducting individual, family, and/or group psychological intervention; and collaborating to support families and teams in communication and decision making. A survey of Children's Oncology Group (COG) institutions revealed that in 62% of

257

hospitals, more than half of families are offered psychosocial services in the first 30 days after diagnosis (Selove, Kroll, Coppes, & Cheng, 2012). Consistent with other centers (Clerici et al., 2008), the most common reason for referral in our cancer center is adaptation to diagnosis and treatment (25%), followed by symptoms of depression (22%), neuropsychological/psychoeducational assessment (21%), anxiety (18%), and family issues (15%). Unfortunately, psychosocial service provision is not always matched to child and family need or consistent across cancer centers (Selove et al., 2012).

Understanding specific risks and resiliencies guides the provision of psychosocial services to match child and family needs. Because childhood cancer is addressed in the context of the family, health care, and school systems, family psychosocial risks and resources may be identified at each level of the child's social ecology (Kazak et al., 2007). Specific risk factors include lower socioeconomic status, maladaptive parental coping (Kupst et al., 1995), and treatment-related factors. Protective factors related to better outcomes include child self-esteem (Anholt, Fritz, & Keener, 1993), perceived social support, and family cohesion (Varni, Katz, Colegrove, & Dolgin, 1994). The pediatric psychosocial preventative health model (PPPHM; Kazak et al., 2007) is a three-tiered model of risk used at our cancer center to direct psychosocial care to families. The *universal* level encompasses most families; at this level families are appropriately distressed but have resources and exhibit an ability to adapt. Examples of universal interventions given to all families include social workers and child life specialists who provide psychoeducation and connect families with educational, financial, and social support resources. The *targeted* level includes families at risk for poor adaptation largely due to preexisting risk factors or potential treatment late effects. Assessment and intervention approaches for families at this level target their specific risks and include such things as coping strategies to manage procedural distress or neuropsychological evaluations subsequent to cranial radiation therapy. The *clinical* level comprises families at the highest level of risk (e.g., preexisting psychiatric disorders, substance use, physical or sexual abuse) and few skills and resources for managing distress. Services for families at the clinical level typically include psychological consultation and intervention with referral to psychiatry or community mental health providers when appropriate. Psychology interventions are intended to be brief and strength focused. Care coordination among the various teams also is central to intervention.

ASSESSMENT

Assessment in childhood cancer consists of either a psychological evaluation of the child and family as part of a consultation or a neuropsychological evaluation. In addition to the standard tools available to assess child psychological adjustment and adaptive functioning (e.g., self-reports, parent rating scales, interviews), such as the Children's Depression Inventory (CDI; Kovacs, 1992) and the Behavior Assessment System for Children—Second Edition (BASC-2; Reynolds & Kamphaus, 2004), there are oncology-specific measures available. For example, the Psychosocial Assessment Tool 2.0 (PAT2.0; Pai et al., 2008) is a screener of family psychosocial risks that has been validated at diagnosis in pediatric cancer and offers information related to family risks, child and sibling behavioral adjustment, caregiver distress, and available social supports. Scores from the PAT2.0 map directly onto the levels of PPPHM and offer guidance on the appropriate level of intervention for families. Additional relevant domains to assess include child health-related quality of life and PTSS. The Pediatric Quality of Life Inventory (PedsQL) measurement model (Varni, Burwinkle, Katz, Meeske, & Dickinson, 2002) offers general and cancer-specific modules to assess domains relevant to this population (e.g., fatigue). PTSS is another important domain given its potential impact on school and community reintegration, caregiving, and engagement in health care. Available assessment tools include clinical interviews, such as the Impact of Traumatic Stressors Interview Schedule (Kazak et al., 2001), or self-report scales, such as the Impact of Event Scale—Revised (Weiss & Marmar, 1997).

COG (2007) recommends continued medical care for surveillance and management of long-term adverse health outcomes, or late effects, for childhood cancer survivors, including neurocognitive changes, psychosocial adjustment, organ dysfunction, and secondary cancers (Friedman & Meadows, 2002). Neuropsychological evaluations are indicated for certain groups at risk for neurodevelopmental late effects (Nathan et al., 2007). For example, children with central nervous system disease or treatments are at risk for difficulties with attention, processing speed, executive function, and memory (Hocking & Alderfer, 2012) and should undergo assessment at the end of medical treatment, with reevaluations occurring as clinically indicated to facilitate appropriate educational plans and accommodations (Nathan et al., 2007). Assessment of ongoing or emerging psychosocial late effects, self-management and health education needs, and educational or financial challenges are also important (Friedman, Fryer, & Levitt, 2006).

INTERVENTION

Clinical practice in pediatric oncology draws on clinical child and adolescent psychology, together with family systems approaches (Kazak, Simms, & Rourke, 2002). Given the impact of childhood cancer on the child's family, pediatric psychologists in oncology often work with the entire family or portions of the family system (i.e., siblings or parents only), in addition to or instead of the child with cancer. Psychological interventions successfully evaluated in pediatric cancer target reducing PTSS (Kazak et al., 2004), social skills training for children (e.g., Barakat et al., 2003; Barrera & Schulte, 2009), enhancing maternal problem solving (Sahler et al., 2002), improving child adjustment (e.g., Hinds et al., 2000), and cognitive remediation (e.g., Butler et al., 2008; Hardy, Willard, & Bonner, 2011). Cognitive-behavioral techniques for pain management and procedural distress are well established across pediatric conditions, including several randomized controlled trials in oncology (Uman, Chambers, McGrath, & Kisely, 2006). Recently, the Cellie Coping Kit for school-age children with cancer was found to be relevant and useful to families of school-age children (Marsac et al., 2012). Frequently, evidence-based treatments from clinical child psychology are applied to address common presenting concerns of children with cancer (i.e., symptoms of anxiety or depression associated with treatment, inconsistent parenting). Flexibility in approach is important given the heterogeneity of cancer diagnoses, treatments, and treatment stages (e.g., diagnosis through palliative care or survivorship); the wide range in developmental levels of children; and variable psychosocial needs.

Several models have been applied to clinical care in pediatric oncology. Along with the PPPHM and medical traumatic stress models, family systems theory (Kazak et al., 2002) and biopsychosocial models (Armstrong, 2006) highlight the role of early screening and targeted intervention. A family systems approach emphasizes a strength-based model focused on joining with the family to facilitate collaboration among systems within the child's social ecology to address the presenting problem (Kazak et al., 2002). Biopsychosocial models also are integral to understanding the complex interrelationships between physical functioning, psychological adjustment, and systems responses to cancer (Armstrong, 2006). Continuing to integrate psychosocial services into multidisciplinary teams (Carlson et al., 2008) and offering a tiered approach to intervention (Kazak et al., 2007) can support patients through transition to long-term survival and eventually adult health care. The cases presented demonstrate implementation of evidence-based assessment, consultation, and intervention targeted to common presenting problems in childhood cancer and tailored to disease, developmental, and family factors.

CASE EXAMPLE 1: ABBY

Abby was a 16-year-old Caucasian adolescent diagnosed with high-risk acute myeloid leukemia (AML) resulting in fatigue, diffuse pain, and chemotherapy-related nausea. She lived with her mother, Ms. Jones, and two younger siblings. The family moved to Philadelphia after her parents divorced the prior year. Abby's father lived in Florida and was minimally involved in her care. The medical team (oncologist, social worker) consulted the psychologist shortly after diagnosis due to Abby's increased irritability and withdrawal, sleep disturbances, and depressed mood and to concerns related to her adjustment to the intense and lengthy AML treatment, including hematopoietic stem cell transplantation.

During the psychology consultation, Abby was reserved and deferred to her mother in responding to interview questions. Ms. Jones was tearful as she described Abby's diagnosis, the family's adjustment, and future treatment. She reported that Abby had been lonely and irritable and had had difficulty coping with pain. Ms. Jones also acknowledged significant stress in balancing demands between caring for Abby and her other children and work. Individually, Abby reported difficulties related to isolation, reduced autonomy, sleep, and self-consciousness. She reported watching television until falling asleep late at night, waking several times during the night, and sleeping most of the day. The family denied mental health diagnoses in the immediate family, although Ms. Jones reported "some anxiety" on her side of the family. On the PAT2.0, Ms. Jones's responses indicated many risk factors, including family structure, limited social support, maternal distress, family conflict, and a history of child emotional distress, suggesting a need for clinical-level intervention. On the BASC-2 and CDI, Abby self-reported elevated internalizing symptoms, specifically anxiety and depression. Other psychosocial team members reported difficulty engaging the family in activities and minimal involvement from Abby in treatment discussions and revealed that Ms. Jones often made excuses to allow Abby to miss school at the hospital.

Abby's presenting problems were conceptualized as difficulty adjusting to her diagnosis, with mixed features of anxiety and depression due to reduced social support, prediagnosis emotional difficulties, high parental distress, and health-related hindrance affecting her academic and social goal pursuit (Schwartz & Drotar, 2009). Twice-weekly individual and family psychology intervention was recommended to achieve the following aims.

1. Reduce Abby's distress over pain and procedures through behavioral stress management techniques (i.e., guided imagery, deep breathing, distraction; Uman et al., 2006).
2. Reduce Ms. Jones's distress, increase her adaptive coping skills, and challenge her distorted thoughts about Abby's prognosis using a problem-solving framework (Sahler et al., 2002).
3. Help Abby identify meaningful goals for treatment, school, future plans, and social relationships (Weersing & Brent, 2003). Cognitive

restructuring techniques, together with behavioral activation, helped Abby start leaving her room when medical status allowed, visit with friends in person and through electronic means, and challenge her negative thoughts.

4. Reduce family conflict through family therapy with Abby and Ms. Jones focused on identifying and achieving common goals (i.e., Abby's completing tenth grade), as well as ways that Ms. Jones can support Abby while allowing Abby to retain some independence.

5. Address Abby's insomnia with cognitive-behavioral strategies (Mindell & Owens, 2009).

Abby, in collaboration with her child life specialist, was supported in maintaining a daily schedule, reducing her daytime sleep, creating a relaxing bedtime routine, and learning strategies to challenge distorted cognitions about sleep. With Abby's medical team we discussed strategies to support Abby's autonomy during treatment planning, specifically by including Abby in all treatment decisions and providing information about procedures, medications, and treatments to both Abby and her mother. As Abby transitioned into transplant, treatment focused on expectations for transplant, changes in her mood and physical status, and coping strategies for the prolonged hospitalization and isolation. Despite new physical symptoms in transplant, Abby continued to utilize coping strategies, improving her sense of control and autonomy. Abby and her mother reported fewer internalizing symptoms, reduced conflict, and more interest in social activities and schoolwork. Sleep disturbances persisted as Abby's transplant treatment included steroids; however, continuing to apply cognitive-behavioral insomnia strategies helped Abby return to regular sleep habits after completing steroids.

CASE EXAMPLE 2: SAM

Sam was a 5-year-old African American male diagnosed with a fibrillary astrocytoma of the posterior fossa at 18 months of age. He had a partial resection and a ventriculoperitoneal shunt placed due to hydrocephalus at presentation. This was followed by 13 months of chemotherapy for continued tumor growth. Recurrence was noted shortly after his third birthday, and Sam underwent a second surgical resection and began another chemotherapy regimen that lasted approximately 2 years. At the time of the psychology referral, Sam was approximately 3 months past completion of chemotherapy. Sam had speech dysarthria, ataxia, and mild right hemiparesis. Sam lived with his biological parents, Mr. and Mrs. Smith, and his 7-year-old brother, James. He currently attended half-day kindergarten through cyberschool as well as a half-day program at the preschool where his mother works. Sam transitioned to these placements due to parental perceptions that the public school did not adequately address his needs.

The family had been referred for a psychological consultation by Sam's neuro-oncologist on multiple occasions over the previous 2 years but did not engage in treatment consistently. Current referral concerns included emotional and behavioral outbursts, aggressive and oppositional behaviors, anxiety, and social difficulties. Sam presented with flat affect, and he was shy and difficult to engage. During the initial session, he frequently interrupted his parents and became upset and noncompliant at the end of the session when his mother asked him to clean up the room. On the BASC-2, parents reported elevated levels of aggression, conduct problems, anxiety, and withdrawal, as well as low levels of adaptive behaviors. Mr. and Mrs. Smith also described increased negative attention-seeking behaviors in their other son, James, including temper tantrums. They acknowledged moderate levels of marital conflict between them due to the difficulties related to parenting their children and consistently implementing consequences. Mrs. Smith described herself as feeling "robotic" due to the demands of managing Sam's medical, educational, and behavioral needs and angry when presented with reminders of Sam's brain tumor. Additionally, Mr. Smith indicated that his father had died from a brain tumor and described intense fear related to his son's medical status and avoidance of Sam's medical appointments.

Sam's behavioral and emotional disturbances were conceptualized as the result of an interaction between his neurodevelopmental sequelae secondary to treatment-related central nervous system insult and his parents' difficulties managing his behavior and coping with his uncertain medical status. In particular, parental PTSS, including intrusive thoughts about Sam's cancer history, hypervigilance about Sam's health, and avoiding reminders of Sam's cancer, was viewed as a significant factor impeding their ability to consistently balance the demands of parenting a child with serious medical and behavioral issues with the different needs of a healthy child. The family was presented with the recommendations of (1) regular family therapy to address parents' behavioral management skills and their coping with traumatic stressors and (2) neuropsychological evaluation to facilitate the development of an appropriate educational plan and to inform psychological intervention. Sessions occurred sporadically during the initial phase of therapy and the endorsement and encouragement of the medical team were critical to family engagement. Family therapy integrated typical components associated with evidence-based behavior management interventions (e.g., positive reinforcement, ignoring) with elements of the Surviving Cancer Competently Intervention Program (SCCIP; Kazak et al., 2004) in order to address the parents' PTSS. Sessions focused on increasing parents' awareness of their PTSS and its effect on parenting, on enhancing their communication related to their stressors and parenting strategies, on reducing the impact of PTSS by implementing cognitive-behavioral strategies (e.g., problem solving, relaxation, reframing), and on putting their medical stressors "in their place." Parents' perceptions of Sam's behaviors and functioning were also targeted so that they could adjust their expectations of him and reduce the potential for continued frustration. Recommendations from the neuropsychological report were integrated into treatment by collaborating with school personnel to develop an individualized education plan that included behavioral strategies as Sam transitioned back to public school. Parental reports of externalizing symptoms declined over treatment. Both parents improved their ability to recognize and restructure automatic responses to traumatic stressors and child behaviors, helping them to be more present to manage their sons' challenging behaviors and set reasonable expectations for each child based on his unique needs.

SUMMARY AND CONCLUSIONS

There is a well-defined and growing literature on medical and psychosocial late effects of childhood cancer and treatment (Friedman & Meadows, 2002), as well as an established literature outlining responses to diagnosis, child coping and adaptation, and family functioning during treatment (Vannatta et al., 2009). Yet gaps in our understanding of the pediatric cancer experience for children, their parents, and their siblings remain, evidence-based assessment and intervention specific to pediatric oncology is limited, and assessment and intervention are inconsistently applied across children's cancer centers (Selove et al., 2012). Importantly, attention is turning to defining the period as children move off treatment in terms of increased anxiety among parents, heightened school reintegration challenges, and educational needs in terms of medical late effects and the need for follow-up care (Vannatta et al., 2009). Interventions to prevent negative consequences of cancer, including distress (Stuber, Schneider, Kassam-Adams, Kazak, & Saxe, 2006) and neurocognitive late effects (Hardy et al., 2011), are emerging. Initial steps in linking psychosocial screening to evidence-based intervention to develop guidelines for intervention have been taken (Kazak et al., 2011). In addition, there are important efforts to structure communication and psychosocial interventions at diagnosis (Yap et al., 2009) and in palliative and end-of-life care (Kang et al., 2005). These advances will allow the development of assessment approaches to identify at-risk children and families, the application of treatments targeted to families at critical junctures in the treatment continuum, and the implementation of preventive strategies to reduce distress and mitigate late effects.

REFERENCES

Anholt, U. V., Fritz, G.K., & Keener, M. (1993). Self-concept in survivors of childhood and adolescent cancer. *Journal of Psychosocial Oncology, 11,* 1–16.

Armstrong, F. D. (2006). Cancer and blood disorders in childhood: Biopsychosocial-developmental issues in assessment and treatment. In R.T. Brown (Ed.), *Comprehensive handbook of childhood cancer and sickle cell disease: A biopsychosocial approach* (pp. 17–34). New York: Oxford University Press.

Barakat, L. P., Alderfer, M. A., & Kazak, A. E. (2006). Posttraumatic growth in adolescent survivors of cancer and their families. *Journal of Pediatric Psychology, 31,* 413–419.

Barakat, L. P., Hetzke, J. D., Foley, B., Carey, M. E., Gyato, K., & Phillips, P. C. (2003). Evaluation of a social skills training group intervention with children treated for brain tumors. *Journal of Pediatric Psychology, 28,* 299–307.

Barrera, M., & Schulte, F. (2009). A group social skills intervention program for survivors of childhood brain tumors. *Journal of Pediatric Psychology, 35,* 1108–1118.

Butler, R. W., Copeland, D. R., Fairclough, D. L., Mulhern, R. K., Katz, E. R., Kazak, A. E., et al. (2008). A multicenter, randomized clinical trial of a cognitive remediation program for childhood survivors of a pediatric malignancy. *Journal of Consulting and Clinical Psychology, 76,* 367–378.

Carlson, C. A., Hobbie, W. L., Brogna, M., & Ginsberg, J. P. (2008). A multidisciplinary model of care for childhood cancer survivors. *Journal of Pediatric Oncology Nursing, 25,* 7–13.

Children's Oncology Group. (2007). *Long-term follow-up guidelines for survivors of childhood, adolescent and young adult cancers.* Retrieved from *www.survivorshipguidelines.org*

Clerici, C. A., Massimino, M., Casanova, M., Cefalo, G., Terenziani, M., Vasquez, R., et al. (2008). Psychological referral and consultation for adolescents and young adults with cancer treated at pediatric oncology unit. *Pediatric Blood and Cancer, 51,* 105–109.

Friedman, D. L., Freyer, D. R., & Levitt, G. A. (2006). Models of care for survivors of childhood cancer. *Pediatric Blood and Cancer, 46,* 159–168.

Friedman, D. L., & Meadows, A. T. (2002). Late effects of childhood cancer therapy. *Pediatric Clinics of North America, 49,* 1083–1106.

Hardy, K. K., Willard, V. W., & Bonner, M. J. (2011). Computerized cognitive training in survivors of childhood cancer: A pilot study. *Journal of Pediatric Oncology Nursing, 28,* 27–33.

Hinds, P. S., Quargnenti, A., Bush, A., Pratt, C., Fairclough, D., Rissmiller, G., et al. (2000). An evaluation of the impact of a self-care coping intervention on psychological and clinical outcomes in adolescents with newly diagnosed cancer. *European Journal of Oncology Nursing, 4,* 6–17.

Hocking, M. C., & Alderfer, M.. (2012). Neuropsychological sequelae of childhood cancer. In S. Kreitler, M. W. Ben Arush, & A. Martin (Eds.), *Pediatric psycho-oncology: Psychosocial aspects and clinical interventions* (2nd ed., pp. 177–186). Chichester, UK: Wiley.

Kang, T., Hoehn, K. S., Licht, D. J., Mayer, O. H., Santucci, G., Carroll, J. M., et al. (2005). Pediatric palliative, end-of-life, and bereavement care. *Pediatric Clinics of North America, 52*, 1029–1046.

Kazak, A. E., Alderfer, M., Streisand, R., Simms, S., Rourke, M., Barakat, L.P., et al. (2004). Treatment of posttraumatic stress symptoms in adolescent survivors of childhood cancer and their families. *Journal of Family Psychology, 18*, 493–504.

Kazak, A. E., Barakat, L. P., Alderfer, M. A., Rourke, M. T., Meeske, K., Gallagher, P. R., et al. (2001). Posttraumatic stress in survivors of childhood cancer and mothers: Development and validation of the Impact of Traumatic Stressors Interview Schedule (ITSIS). *Journal of Clinical Psychology in Medical Settings, 8*, 307–323.

Kazak, A. E., Barakat, L. P., Hwang, W. T., Ditaranto, S., Biros, D., Beele, D., et al. (2011). Association of psychosocial risk screening in pediatric cancer with psychosocial services provided. *Psycho-Oncology, 20*, 715–723.

Kazak, A. E., Rourke, M. T., Alderfer, M. A., Pai, A., Reilly, A. F., & Meadows, A. T. (2007). Evidence-based assessment, intervention and psychosocial care in pediatric oncology: A blueprint for comprehensive services across treatment. *Journal of Pediatric Psychology, 32*, 1099–1110.

Kazak, A. E., Simms, S., & Rourke, M. (2002). Family systems practice in pediatric psychology. *Journal of Pediatric Psychology, 27*, 133–143.

Kovacs, M. (1992). *Manual for the Children's Depression Inventory.* North Tonawanda, NJ: Multi-Health Systems.

Kupst, M. J., Natta, M. B., Richardson, C.C. Schulman, J. L., Labigne, J. V., & Das, L. (1995). Family coping with pediatric leukemia: Ten years after treatment. *Journal of Pediatric Psychology, 20*, 601–617.

Marsac, M. L., Hildenbrand, A. K., Clawson, K., Jackson, L., Kohser, K., Barakat, L. P., et al. (2012). Acceptability and feasibility of family use of the Cellie Cancer Coping Kit. *Supportive Care in Cancer, 20*, 3315–3324.

Mindell, J. A., & Owens, J. A. (2009). *A clinical guide to pediatric sleep: Diagnosis and management of sleep problems.* Philadelphia: Lippincott Williams & Wilkins.

Nathan, P. C., Patel, S. K., Dilley, K., Goldsby, R., Harvey, J., Jacobson, C., et al. (2007). Guidelines for identification of, advocacy for, and intervention in neurocognitive problems in survivors of childhood cancer: A report from the Children's Oncology Group. *Archives of Pediatrics and Adolescent Medicine, 161*, 798–806.

Pai, A. L. H., Patino-Fernandez, A. M., McSherry, M., Beele, D., Alderfer, M. A., Reilly, A. T., et al. (2008). The Psychosocial Assessment Tool (PAT2.0): Psychometric properties of a screener for psychosocial distress in families of children newly diagnosed with cancer. *Journal of Pediatric Psychology, 33*, 50–62.

Reynolds, C. R., & Kamphaus, R. W. (2004). *Manual for the Behavior Assessment System for Children* (2nd ed.). Circle Pines, MN: AGS.

Sahler, O. J. Z., Varni, J. W., Fairclough, D. L., Butler, R. W., Noll, R. B., Dolgin, M. J., et al. (2002). Problem-solving skills training for mothers of children with newly diagnosed cancer: A randomized trial. *Journal of Developmental and Behavioral Pediatrics, 23*, 77–86.

Sawyer, M., Antoniou, G., Toogood, I., Rice, M., & Baghurst, P. (2000). Childhood cancer: A 4-year prospective study of the psychological adjustment of children and parents. *Journal of Pediatric Hematology/Oncology, 22*, 214–220.

Schwartz, L. A., & Drotar, D. (2009). Health-related hindrance of personal goal pursuit and well-being of young adults with cystic fibrosis, pediatric cancer survivors, and peers without a history of chronic illness. *Journal of Pediatric Psychology, 34*, 954–965.

Selove, R., Kroll, T., Coppes, M., & Cheng, Y. (2012). Psychosocial services in the first 30 days after diagnosis: Results of a web-based survey of Children's Oncology Group (COG) member institutions. *Pediatric Blood and Cancer, 58*, 435–440.

Stuber, M. L., Schneider, S., Kassam-Adams, N., Kazak, A. E., & Saxe, G. (2006). The Medical Traumatic Stress Toolkit, *CNS Spectrums, 11*, 137–142.

Uman, L. S., Chambers, C. T., McGrath, P. J., & Kisely, S. (2006). Psychological interventions for needle-related procedural pain and distress in children and adolescents. *Cochrane Database of Systematic Reviews*, CD005179.

Vannatta, K., Salley, C. G., & Gerhardt, C. A. (2009). Pediatric oncology: Progress and future challenges. In M. C. Roberts & R. G. Steele (Eds.), *Handbook of pediatric psychology* (4th ed., pp. 319–333). New York: Guilford Press.

Varni, J. W., Burwinkle, T. M., Katz, E. R., Meeske, K., & Dickinson, P. (2002). The PedsQL™ in pediatric cancer. *Cancer, 94*, 2090–2106.

Varni, J. W., Katz, E. R., Colegrove, R., & Dolgin, M. (1994). Perceived [0]stress and adjustment of long-term survivors of childhood cancer. *Journal of Psychosocial Oncology, 12*, 1–16.

Weersing, V. R., & Brent, D. A. (2003). Cognitive-behavioral therapy for adolescent depression. In A. E. Kazdin & J. R. Weisz (Eds.), *Evidence-based psychotherapies for children and adolescents* (pp. 135–147). New York: Guilford Press.

Weiss, D., & Marmar, C. (1997). The Impact of Event Scale—Revised. In J. Wilson & T. Keane (Eds.), *Assessing psychological trauma and PTSD* (pp. 399–411). New York: Guilford Press.

Yap, T. Y., Yamokoski, A., Noll, R., Drotar, D., Zyzanski, S., & Kodish, E. (2009). A physician-directed intervention: Teaching and measuring better informed consent. *Academic Medicine, 84*, 1036–1042.

Zebrack, B. J., Stuber, M. L., Meeske, K. A., Phipps, S., Krull, K. R., Liu, Q., et al. (2011). Perceived positive impact of cancer among long-term survivors of childhood cancer: A report from the childhood cancer survivor study. *Psycho-Oncology, 21*, 630–639.

CHAPTER 21

Pediatric Seizure Disorders

AVANI C. MODI
SHANNA M. GUILFOYLE

Epilepsy, one of the most common neurological disorders of childhood, is characterized by two or more unprovoked seizures. Approximately 1% of children under the age of 20 are diagnosed with epilepsy.
Self-management is a critical component of any chronic medical condition, including epilepsy. Children and their families are required to make
clinic appointments, adhere to prescribed treatments, obtain prescrip-
tions and refills, and manage symptoms (Modi et al., 2012). Antiepileptic drugs (AEDs) are the primary treatment for epilepsy, as well as good
sleep hygiene, stress management, and avoidance of known seizure triggers. Unfortunately, adherence to AEDs in children is quite poor, with 58%
of young children with epilepsy exhibiting nonadherence (Modi, Rausch,
& Glauser, 2011). Nonadherence can lead to significant negative consequences, including continued seizures (Simard-Tremblay & Shevell, 2009),
mortality (Faught, Weiner, Guerin, Cunnington, & Duh, 2009), and higher
health care costs (Faught et al., 2009). Several factors have been shown to
contribute to nonadherence in children with epilepsy (Modi & Guilfoyle,
2011), including psychological comorbidities.

Children with epilepsy are at high risk for psychological comorbidities, which can be attributed to multiple factors, including underlying brain
pathology, seizures, AED side effects, or a combination of these (Jensen,

268

2011). These comorbidities significantly compromise health-related quality of life (Baca, Vickrey, Caplan, Vassar, & Berg, 2011). Disruptive behavioral disorders (e.g., behavioral and attentional problems) are the most prevalent comorbidity in children with epilepsy, ranging from 23 to 34% (Austin et al., 2011). Prevalence of depressive and anxiety symptoms in pediatric epilepsy is also high, 23 and 36%, respectively (Jones et al., 2007). This is of particular concern because a recent study has established a relationship between internalizing symptoms and suicidal ideation (27% of youth endorsed suicidal ideation; Wagner, Ferguson, & Smith, 2012). Notably, children with epilepsy often experience subclinical symptoms (Dunn, Austin, & Perkins, 2009) and may benefit from proactive assessment and intervention prior to symptom deterioration and functional impairment.

EVIDENCE-BASED ASSESSMENT AND TREATMENT

Assessment

Despite the increased risk for psychological comorbidities and a common desire by families for integrated medical and psychosocial health care (Shore, Buelow, Austin, & Johnson, 2009), a gap exists between epilepsy expert recommendations (Barry et al., 2008; Kerr et al., 2011) and clinical practice. This is likely due to lack of resources (e.g., psychologists, social workers) to conduct routine psychological screenings (Gilliam, 2002; Shore et al., 2009). Efforts to integrate psychological services (i.e., routine screening) into clinic visits have increased (Wagner, Modi, & Smith, 2011), with a focus on using reliable and valid assessment measures, such as the Pediatric Quality of Life Inventory (PedsQL; Varni, Burwinkle, Seid, & Skarr, 2003) and the Pediatric Epilepsy Side Effects Questionnaire (Morita, Glauser, & Modi, 2012).

Given elevated learning and academic issues in pediatric epilepsy, neuropsychological testing can also lead to better understanding of the impact of seizures and AED treatment on higher cortical functions (Jones-Gotman et al., 2010), along with providing recommendations for academic planning and accommodations (e.g., individualized education and 504 plans).

Intervention

Few pediatric epilepsy interventions have been developed or tested to address psychological comorbidities or self-management. Two recent Cochrane reviews suggest a need for better self-management interventions in pediatric epilepsy (Al-aqeel & Al-sabhan, 2011) that can be implemented in standard clinical practice (Lindsay & Bradley, 2010). Similarly, a review of psychosocial interventions in pediatric epilepsy indicated mixed results, as these trials were fraught with significant limitations (Wagner & Smith, 2006). However, several interventions have recently been developed that show significant promise; for example, Coping Openly and Personally with Epilepsy (COPE; Wagner, Smith, Ferguson, Van Bakergem, & Hrisko, 2010) and a cognitive-behavioral prevention program for adolescents with epilepsy at risk for depression (Martinovic, Simonovic, & Djokic, 2006). Standard behavioral, cognitive-behavioral, and family-based interventions are often used in pediatric epilepsy but have yet to be tested in a rigorous manner.

CASE EXAMPLES

The following are two case examples of patients diagnosed with epilepsy at various stages of epilepsy management. The first example is of a young girl newly diagnosed with epilepsy seen in a seizure clinic for three clinic-based consultations. The second example is of an adolescent male who managed epilepsy for a number of years and recently had an unsuccessful wean from his AED. He participated in four behavioral appointments with a psychologist outside of the clinic (see Table 21.1 for an overview).

Case Example 1: Jasmine

Jasmine was a 3-year-old African American female newly diagnosed with idiopathic localization-related epilepsy and prescribed carbamazepine. During Jasmine's diagnostic epilepsy visit with the epileptologist, her parent completed a Behavioral Assessment System for Children–Second Edition (BASC-2; Reynolds & Kamphaus, 2004), a "well-established" (Holmbeck et al., 2008) broadband measure of psychological functioning, to assess baseline behavioral functioning prior to AED initiation. The BASC-2 generates individual psychological subscales, along with composite subscales that offer summary scores. Scores fall within three potential categories: within normative limits, at risk, and clinically elevated. These data are used as a diagnostic tool to help determine potential behavioral side effects to AEDs. For example, if aggression was noted on the BASC-2 prior to AED initiation but a parent returns to clinic and states that aggression is secondary to recent AED initiation, this information is used by the medical team to determine whether an AED should be continued.

Consultation 1

During the 1-month follow-up clinic visit, the pediatric psychologist shared the BASC-2 data with Jasmine's family, which indicated that composite

TABLE 21.1. Case Examples: Intervention Overview

Session (location)	Content
Jasmine	
Consultation 1 (seizure clinic)	• Review BASC-2 data • Behavioral principles and contingency management for medication side effects and cosleeping with parents • Cognitive modification for anxiety
Consultation 2 (seizure clinic)	• Cognitive and behavioral modification to address anxiety
Consultation 3 (seizure clinic)	• Behavioral modification to address cosleeping: Positive reinforcement
Michael	
Interview (behavioral medicine)	• CDI-2 administration and clinical interview
Session 1 (behavioral medicine)	• Clinical interview and CDI-2 administration • Cognitive-behavioral treatment: Cognitive triad and behavioral activation
Session 2 (behavioral medicine)	• CDI-2 administration • Cognitive-behavioral treatment: Cognitive modification
Session 3 (behavioral medicine)	• CDI-2 administration • Cognitive-behavioral treatment: Behavioral activation and cognitive modification
Session 4 (behavioral medicine)	• CDI-2 administration • Relapse prevention: Behavioral activation, cognitive modification, and adherence promotion

scores were within normative limits (see Figure 21.1). However, she exhibited at-risk anxiety symptoms, which suggested closer monitoring. Clinical interview data from Jasmine's mother indicated that Jasmine had experienced significant behavioral changes following AED initiation, including increased fatigue, noncompliance, hyperactivity, aggression, and irritability. Her mother corroborated BASC-2 anxiety findings, but she minimized functional impairment. When anxious, Jasmine was reported to engage in excessive reassurance seeking and clinginess to her parents. Transitions between activities, frequent nighttime awakenings, and attempts to sleep with her parents were identified as minor concerns. However, externalizing behaviors were of primary concern during this visit.

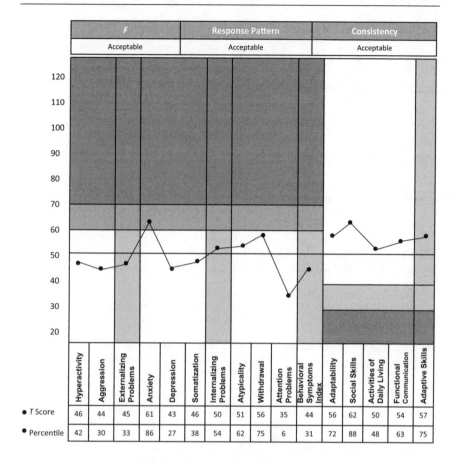

FIGURE 21.1. Jasmine's BASC-2 Parent Rating Scale scores: *T score profile.*

Consultation 2

Jasmine and her mother had three additional consultations with the psychologist at routine clinic visits. In response to the increased externalizing symptoms described by Jasmine's mother and significant changes from the BASC-2 data, an extended release formulation of carbamazepine was recommended by the medical team to minimize dose and behavioral side effects. This AED change was likely to help Jasmine in the next few weeks, but it was also felt that Jasmine's mother might benefit from receiving evidence-based behavioral recommendations to manage acute noncompliance, aggression, hyperactivity, fatigue, and irritability. Broadly, psychoeducation on behavioral principles and contingency management, along with identification of emotional triggers (e.g., behavioral compliance when fatigued), was provided. Although these symptoms appeared to be related to AED side effects, the family was advised to manage the behaviors so that maladaptive behaviors did not persist. Specific strategies reviewed included clear behavioral expectations, consistency, proactive planning around emotional triggers (e.g., ensuring consistent sleep so that the child would be more compliant with behavioral commands, such as accepting the word "no"), positive attending, planned ignoring, and time-out for aggressive behaviors. Some broader cognitive modification strategies were outlined to target anxiety symptoms, such as proactive review of scheduled activities, sleep hygiene (e.g., a consistent return to her own bed to avoid co-sleeping), and positive reinforcement of adaptive coping methods. The medical team recommended a 3-month follow-up appointment in clinic. Jasmine was evaluated twice over the next 7 months as part of routine clinical care.

Consultation 3

Jasmine's mother reported a positive benefit from extended release carbamazepine. Concerns of noncompliance, hyperactivity, aggression, fatigue, and irritability had decreased and had minimal impact on daily functioning. Although her mother identified medication adjustment as particularly beneficial, she also noted that she had made efforts to attend to positive behaviors and to consistently use time-out for aggression. However, anxiety (e.g., poor transitioning, extreme preferences related to clothing) and co-sleeping were of increasing concern. Her mother reported that Jasmine's frequent rumination about transitions (e.g., doctor's visits, blood draws) and limited clothing preferences (e.g., refusing to wear anything other than one of three short-sleeved shirts in the winter) had been challenging and caused functional impairment. In turn, psychoeducation on evidence-based anxiety treatment (e.g., modification of cognitions and behaviors, parental management) was provided. Specific strategies reviewed included systematic exposure and positive reinforcement for engaging in new behaviors (e.g., providing immediate rewards for wearing long-sleeved clothes). A behavioral chart to promote compliance with more varied clothing options was provided. Due to limited clinic time, the issue of co-sleeping with parents was deferred.

Consultation 4

At the last consultation, Jasmine's mother reported implementing behavioral strategies and described improvement with transitions and clothing preferences. Co-sleeping persisted, however, which led to a review and generalization of behavioral principles and strategies discussed during the initial consultation. Specifically discussed was the importance of consistency and how positive reinforcement (i.e., rewards) can be used to progressively increase independent sleep.

Case Example 2: Michael

Michael was a 17-year-old Caucasian male referred for outpatient assessment and treatment to the psychology division for depressive symptoms and passive suicidal ideation identified by his medical provider at a follow-up seizure clinic visit. The initial diagnostic interview was attended by Michael and his stepmother. Michael stated that he was graduating from high school soon and was registered to attend an out-of-state college in the fall. Michael reported that he had been diagnosed with epilepsy at 13 years of age and treated for idiopathic generalized epilepsy for 3.5 years but was weaned off of his AED medication after being seizure free for 2 years. Seven months following his AED discontinuation, Michael experienced a seizure, and an AED was reinitiated. Michael described the onset of depressive symptoms, including increased appetite, lethargy, hopelessness, frequent tearfulness, and passive suicidal ideation experienced over the past several months since his epilepsy relapse. He noted that he had not wanted to spend time with friends, who had also commented on his changed personality. His stepmother confirmed these behavioral changes and noted that Michael had stopped running cross-country after having his last seizure. A Children's Depression Inventory—Second Edition (CDI-2; Kovacs, 2003) was administered. The CDI-2 has subscales that reflect feelings of ineffectiveness, disruptions to sleep/appetite, negative mood and self-esteem, and interpersonal difficulties. Scores fall within four categories: average, high average, elevated, and very elevated. Results reflected clinically elevated depressive symptoms (T score ≥ 65; see Figure 21.2) across all subscales. Michael attributed the onset of his depressive symptoms to the unsuccessful AED weaning and not to reinitiation of the AED. He described having the belief that he had outgrown epilepsy and that it was in his past. His seizure recurrence was disappointing to him, and he felt it would have a negative impact on his college life. During the risk assessment for suicidal ideation, he denied active suicidal ideation or intent to harm himself or others, but he did describe having thoughts that things would be easier if he were not living. When discussing epilepsy self-management, Michael reported that he relied on his parents to provide reminders, which he appreciated given frequent forgetfulness when he took his AED independently. Collectively, data obtained from the clinical interview and CDI-2 suggested a diagnosis of adjustment disorder with depressed mood given that Michael's depressed mood was directly linked to his recent unsuccessful AED weaning.

Michael participated in four sessions of evidence-based cognitive-behavioral treatment (see Table 21.1) over a 10-week period to address his adjustment difficulties and depressed mood. The CDI-2 was completed at the beginning of each session (see Figure 21.2).

Session 1

This appointment occurred 2 weeks following the diagnostic interview in which Michael's CDI-2 scores remained clinically elevated (see Figure 21.2). Treatment content consisted primarily of behavioral activation and cognitive modification, including identification of thought distortions, thought stopping, and cognitive reframing. This session was dedicated to education on the cognitive triad and how behavioral activation can aid in increasing positive thoughts and emotions. Homework from this session included engaging in positive activities to improve his mood daily and monitoring his mood before, during, and after activities using a scale of 1 (low mood) to 10 (high mood).

Sessions 2 and 3

Homework was reviewed, and Michael acknowledged that when he forced himself to hang out with friends, he often felt better than when he was staying at home and sleeping. These appointments introduced cognitive modification strategies and a discussion of how Michael's experiences were influenced by his thoughts and how he responded to his thoughts. Michael described that he engaged in catastrophic thinking and that he ultimately felt that his college experience would be ruined if he had to manage epilepsy during college. Cognitive reframing exercises to identify his thoughts about college and epilepsy were reviewed and assigned as homework. Michael specifically worried that others, such as dormitory roommates, would judge him for having epilepsy and that his social activities would be compromised. When these maladaptive thoughts were challenged, he recognized that his current friends were aware of his epilepsy and did not judge him. He also became cognizant that his social activities were not limited in high school when his seizures were well controlled and thus would not be limited in college.

Session 4

Behavioral activation and cognitive modification strategies that were particularly effective for Michael were reviewed. Based on CDI-2 data, Michael was told that his depressive symptoms were now in the average range. He said that he believed that epilepsy would likely have a minimal impact on

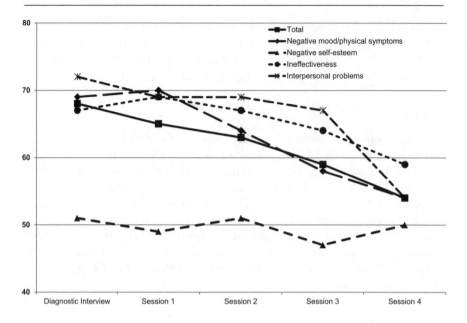

FIGURE 21.2. Michael's CDI-2 scores over time.

college, but he inquired about the interaction between his AED and alcohol use. Alcohol abstinence was recommended. Relapse prevention and strategies to optimize medication adherence independently to maximize seizure control were reviewed (e.g., a consistent dosing routine, medication was easily accessible even if he was away from his dorm, use of a cell phone alarm). Michael was also encouraged to work with his parents to progressively begin "practicing" increased responsibility for his medication taking for the 2 months before college so that he could develop a consistent routine and strategies that helped with dosing (e.g., pairing dosing with meals or brushing teeth). This "trial" period would allow Michael to also identify personal barriers that could be problem-solved before he was independent at college.

CONCLUSIONS AND FUTURE DIRECTIONS

These two cases illustrate the psychological comorbidities often associated with epilepsy and its treatment in youth with epilepsy. Although there is a paucity of literature about evidence-based assessment and treatment approaches specific to children with epilepsy, standard approaches used in pediatric psychology appeared to work well in both cases presented. The psychologist's knowledge of epilepsy and the ability to provide standard psychological assessment and treatment for Jasmine within the clinic setting were critical to Jasmine's positive outcome. Similarly, although the psychologist used broad cognitive-behavioral treatment approaches, she was able to recognize the epilepsy-specific aspects of Michael's depressive symptoms that needed to be discussed during therapy (e.g., relapse after weaning). In general, our experience suggest that pediatric psychology trainees would benefit from training in pediatric epilepsy, an area that has been relatively neglected (Wagner et al., 2011). Such training would highlight the biopsychosocial framework and the value of clinic-based care, which is the foundation of pediatric psychology. Overall, the future of best-practice epilepsy care requires (1) testing of existing evidence-based assessment and interventions, (2) the development of new epilepsy-specific assessment and treatment approaches that can be provided during routine clinical care, and (3) providing epilepsy training opportunities for the next generation of pediatric psychologists.

REFERENCES

Al-aqeel, S., & Al-sabhan, J. (2011). Strategies for improving adherence to antiepileptic drug treatment in patients with epilepsy. *Cochrane Database of Systematic Reviews,* Issue 1, Art. No. CD008312.

Austin, J. K., Perkins, S. M., Johnson, C. S., Fastenau, P. S., Byars, A. W., deGrauw, T. J., et al. (2011). Behavior problems in children at time of first recognized seizure and changes over the following 3 years. *Epilepsy and Behavior, 21,* 373–381.

Baca, C. B., Vickrey, B. G., Caplan, R., Vassar, S. D., & Berg, A. T. (2011). Psychiatric and medical comorbidity and quality of life outcomes in childhood-onset epilepsy. *Pediatrics, 128,* e1532–e1543.

Barry, J. J., Ettinger, A. B., Friel, P., Gilliam, F. G., Harden, C. L., Hermann, B., et al. (2008). Consensus statement: The evaluation and treatment of people with epilepsy and affective disorders. *Epilepsy and Behavior, 13,* S1–S29.

Dunn, D. W., Austin, J. K., & Perkins, S. M. (2009). Prevalence of psychopathology in childhood epilepsy: Categorical and dimensional measures. *Developmental Medicine and Child Neurology, 51,* 364–372.

Faught, R. E., Weiner, J. R., Guerin, A., Cunnington, M. C., & Duh, M. S. (2009). Impact of nonadherence to antiepileptic drugs on health care utilization and costs: Findings from the RANSOM study. *Epilepsia, 50,* 501–509.

Gilliam, F. (2002). Optimizing health outcomes in active epilepsy. *Neurology, 58,* S9–S20.

Holmbeck, G. N., Thill, A. W., Bachanas, P., Garber, J., Miller, K. B., Abad, M., et al. (2008). Evidence-based assessment in pediatric psychology: Measures of psychosocial adjustment and psychopathology. *Journal of Pediatric Psychology, 33,* 958–980.

Jensen, F. E. (2011). Epilepsy as a spectrum disorder: Implications from novel clinical and basic neuroscience. *Epilepsia, 52*, 1–6.

Jones, J. E., Watson, R., Sheth, R., Caplan, R., Koehn, M., Seidenberg, M., et al. (2007). Psychiatric comorbidity in children with new onset epilepsy. *Developmental Medicine and Child Neurology, 49*, 493–497.

Jones-Gotman, M., Smith, M. L., Risse, G. L., Westerveld, M., Swanson, S. J., Giovagnoli, A. R., et al. (2010). The contribution of neuropsychology to diagnostic assessment in epilepsy. *Epilepsy and Behavior, 18*, 3–12.

Kerr, M. P., Mensah, S., Besag, F., de Toffol, B., Ettinger, A., Kanemoto, K., et al. (2011). International consensus clinical practice statements for the treatment of neuropsychiatric conditions associated with epilepsy. *Epilepsia, 52*, 2133–2138.

Kovacs, M. (2003). *The Children's Depression Inventory (CDI): Technical Manual.* North Tonawanda, NY: Multi-Health Systems.

Lindsay, B., & Bradley, P. M. (2010). Care delivery and self-management strategies for children with epilepsy. *Cochrane Database of Systematic Reviews*, Issue 12. Art. No. CD006245.

Martinovic, Z., Simonovic, P., & Djokic, R. (2006). Preventing depression in adolescents with epilepsy. *Epilepsy and Behavior, 9*, 619–624.

Modi, A. C., & Guilfoyle, S. M. (2011). Adherence to antiepileptic drug therapy across the developmental life-span. In J. Pinikahana & C. Walker (Eds.), *Society, Behaviour and Epilepsy* (pp. 175–205) New York: Nova Science.

Modi, A. C., Pai, A. L., Hommel, K. A., Hood, K. K., Cortina, S., Hilliard, M. E., et al. (2012). Pediatric self-management: A framework for research, practice, and policy. *Pediatrics, 129*, e473–e485.

Modi, A. C., Rausch, J. R., & Glauser, T. A. (2011). Patterns of non-adherence to antiepileptic drug therapy in children with newly diagnosed epilepsy. *Journal of the American Medical Assocation, 305*, 1669–1676.

Morita, D. A., Glauser, T. A., & Modi, A. C. (2012). Development and validation of the Pediatric Epilepsy Side Effects Questionnaire. *Neurology, 79*(12), 1252–1258.

Reynolds, C. R., & Kamphaus, R. W. (2004). *Behavior Assessment System for Children—Second Edition.* Circle Pines, MN: American Guidance Service.

Shore, C. P., Buelow, J. M., Austin, J. K., & Johnson, C. S. (2009). Continuing psychosocial care needs in children with new-onset epilepsy and their parents. *Journal of Neuroscience Nursing, 41*, 244–250.

Simard-Tremblay, E., & Shevell, M. (2009). A profile of adolescent-onset epilepsy. *Journal of Child Neurology, 24*, 1243–1249.

Varni, J. W., Burwinkle, T. M., Seid, M., & Skarr, D. (2003). The PedsQL 4.0 as a pediatric population health measure: Feasibility, reliability, and validity. *Ambulatory Pediatrics, 3*, 329–341.

Wagner, J. L., Ferguson, P. L., & Smith, G. (2012). The relationship of coping behaviors to depressive symptoms in youth with epilepsy: An examination of caregiver and youth proxy report. *Epilepsy and Behavior, 24*, 86–92.

Wagner, J., Modi, A. C., & Smith, G. (2011). Commentary: Pediatric epilepsy: A good fit for pediatric psychologists. *Journal of Pediatric Psychology, 36*(4), 461–465.

Wagner, J. L., & Smith, G. (2006). Psychosocial intervention in pediatric epilepsy: A critique of the literature. *Epilepsy and Behavior, 8,* 39–49.

Wagner, J. L., Smith, G., Ferguson, P., Van Bakergem, K., & Hrisko, S. (2010). Pilot study of an integrated cognitive-behavioral and self-management intervention for youth with epilepsy and caregivers: Coping openly and personally with epilepsy (COPE). *Epilepsy and Behavior, 18,* 280–285.

CHAPTER 22

Pediatric Organ Transplantation

REBECCA J. JOHNSON

$\mathbf{A}$s pediatric organ transplant has become more prevalent and long-term survival has improved, the presence of a psychologist on the transplant team has become routine. Solid organ transplant encompasses heart, liver, kidney, lung, and small intestine transplant and in some instances involves multiple organs. Multidisciplinary transplant teams consist of physicians, nurses, social workers, transplant coordinators, dieticians, child life specialists, and others, in addition to psychologists. The psychologist's role on the transplant team is diverse and encompasses a variety of services, including pretransplant psychological evaluation, posttransplant support and monitoring, inpatient consultation–liaison during the hospitalizations, brief consultation in medical clinics, and outpatient assessment and psychotherapy, both pre- and posttransplant. Psychologists provide services to patients, families, and other caregivers and also provide education and consultation to medical teams with regard to adherence and patient and family adjustment, coping, and quality of life. Psychologists on transplant teams are often asked to provide information regarding psychological, developmental, behavioral, and familial strengths and weaknesses that may affect recipient selection and future health outcomes. This information is obtained during the pretransplant psychological evaluation (Fung & Shaw, 2008; Pai, Tackett, Ittenbach, & Goebel, 2011; Rodrigue, Gonzalez-Peralta, & Langham, 2004; Streisand & Tercyak, 2001). The *Handbook of Pediatric Psychology* provides an excellent overview of the literature pertaining to clinical issues that are commonly addressed by pediatric psychologists working within the field of organ transplantation (Rodrigue & Zelikovsky, 2009).

Many presenting concerns are addressed using evidence-based treatments common to clinical child psychology, often adapted to address health-related stressors and issues. Some presenting concerns are more specific to pediatric psychology and transplant. Three of these—needle-related pain and distress, pill-swallowing difficulty, and nonadherence—are illustrated in the following case examples.

CASE EXAMPLE 1: NEEDLE-RELATED PROCEDURAL PAIN AND DISTRESS

Background

Children with chronic health conditions are often exposed to frequent, aversive, and sometimes painful medical experiences and procedures, many involving needles. Needle-related procedures elicit significant fear and distress for many children (Humphrey, Boon, van Linden van den Heuvell, & van de Wiel, 1992), but too often evidence-based strategies to prevent or manage pain and distress are not applied to these so-called "minor" procedures, despite the fact that the effects of poorly managed pain and distress can be negative and long-lasting (Taddio et al., 2009; Walco, 2008). If pain and distress are well managed early and consistently, significant anxiety and pain can be reduced and related complications (e.g., refusal) avoided. Following organ transplant, the ability to tolerate needle-related procedures is very important, not only to promote the patient's health but also to reduce or avoid patient, caregiver, and staff distress, as routine venipuncture and other procedures will be necessary indefinitely.

Many empirically supported strategies are available to address procedural pain and anxiety, including topical anesthetics, sucrose, and breastfeeding (Shah, Taddio, & Rieder, 2009) and distraction, hypnosis, information/preparation, and combined cognitive-behavioral interventions (Cohen, 2008; Uman, Chambers, McGrath, & Kisely, 2008). As demonstrated in the following case, these strategies can be applied to or adapted for medical procedures experienced by transplant patients and their families.

Case

A 10-year-old male with cystic fibrosis (CF) who had recently completed evaluation for a lung transplant was referred to psychology for treatment of needle-related distress. The lung transplant team was concerned about posttransplant care that would involve not only blood draws but also routine injections. In addition, the patient needed several immunizations prior to being eligible for transplant. This patient lived with his parents and two younger siblings. The patient and his parents explained that he had always been somewhat anxious about procedures involving needles and that his anxiety had progressively worsened over time, particularly for immunizations and blood draws. During the patient's most recent immunization, parents initially bargained and pleaded with him to cooperate, then became tearful and upset when he did not. The patient had eventually required restraint by multiple adults while he screamed and was combative. This experience had raised concern regarding the patient's ability to tolerate pre- and posttransplant medical care.

The treatment plan for this patient incorporated several evidence-based strategies, including psychoeducation, teaching active coping skills (including relaxation training and positive self-talk), distraction, positive reinforcement of desired behaviors, and parent training. The first session focused on building rapport with the patient, gathering information from his parents, and providing parents with psychoeducation regarding needle-related pain and distress, including what parent behaviors (e.g., staying calm and matter-of-fact) would promote the child's coping. The patient reported that he did not feel anxious talking or thinking about needles, experienced mild distress waiting for the immunization, and then experienced high distress when approached with the needle. He reported fear of pain as his only fear and appeared to understand that his fear was excessive but felt helpless to modulate his response. I introduced diaphragmatic breathing, and we generated and rehearsed coping self-statements (e.g., "I can do this," "I will be calm"). The patient and parent agreed to practice breathing and the coping statements two times per day for the next week. The patient used a child-friendly tracking application on his mobile electronic device to track the frequency of his practice. At our next session, he proudly showed me the results, which indicated that he had practiced the interventions daily.

We then developed, based on his interests, a superhero-themed coping plan that included application of topical 4% lidocaine cream, relaxation (diaphragmatic breathing), coping self-statements, behavioral distraction (board games), comfort positioning (Kurfis Stephens, Barkey, & Hall, 1999), and positive reinforcement of desired behaviors. Our child life staff provided a variety of small, tangible rewards, and the patient and his parents also generated a list of available activity and tangible rewards. The patient was instructed that he must follow the steps of his coping plan and maintain a "calm body" during the immunization, which was defined as "no hitting, kicking, biting, or pinching" the parent holding him, in order to access his rewards.

The patient's CF nurse was consulted and was willing to administer the topical anesthetic and support the coping plan. At the patient's next CF clinic visit, we rehearsed all of the steps of the coping plan, with a "pretend" immunization at the end and a small reward following the patient's cooperation. The next week, the patient and his parent successfully completed all steps of the coping plan, the patient remained calm during the immunization, and he earned his reward. Over the next 3 weeks, he received three more immunizations, remaining calm throughout and continuing to earn rewards. Later, we were able to adapt the patient's coping plan to include venipuncture, and his successful coping behaviors generalized across multiple procedures.

Discussion

This patient experienced significant needle-related procedural pain and distress that had not been adequately addressed. His symptoms presented a potential barrier to lung transplant and were distressing not only for him but also for his parents and staff. There are a number of cognitive-behavioral and pharmacological strategies available to manage needle-related pain, anxiety, and distress, including many for immunizations (Schechter et al., 2007; Shah, Taddio, & Rieder, 2009). The current intervention targeted multiple pathways relevant to the presenting concern, including nociceptive pain (4% lidocaine cream), emotional distress (comfort positioning, diaphragmatic breathing, and coping self-statements), and behavioral expression of pain and distress (increasing positive reinforcement of desired behaviors). Parents were trained to remain calm and matter-of-fact during the procedure, and positive expectations that the patient could be successful with this task were communicated to the patient and family. An important element of the patient's success was the multidisciplinary relationship that existed between the psychologist, the medical providers, and the nursing staff. The CF team initially recognized that the patient could benefit from psychology services and placed the referral, and the patient's CF nurse was flexible with her time and the immunization process.

CASE EXAMPLE 2: PILL SWALLOWING

Background

Arguably the most important aspect of the posttransplant treatment regimen is getting immunosuppressive medications into the patient (whether orally in pill or liquid form, or via a gastrostomy or nasogastrostomy tube) consistently and on time. This involves the patient's having access to medications, remembering to take medications, and (most often) swallowing medications. A common presenting concern that can arise either before or after transplant is pill-swallowing difficulty. Ideally, pill-swallowing difficulties are absent or completely resolved prior to transplant. However, this is not always the case, and new difficulties can emerge when new medications are introduced or the number of pills that must be swallowed increases. During the pretransplant evaluation process, pill swallowing must be carefully assessed. Simply asking whether or not the patient can swallow pills is insufficient. Rather, the interview should include the following questions:

1. What number of pills is the patient currently swallowing, and when?
2. Does anyone directly observe the patient swallowing pills?
3. How many pills can the patient swallow at one time?
4. How long does it take the patient to swallow the prescribed pills? Must he/she pause between pills, and for how long?
5. Does the patient have any aversions to or difficulties with size, taste, shape, or texture of pills?
6. Does the patient need specific circumstances, people, or beverages to swallow pills successfully?
7. Does the patient ever gag or vomit when taking pills, and if so, how often?
8. What are the patient's feelings with regard to taking medication (e.g., does the patient ever state "I hate taking medicine" or "I am sick of taking medicine")?
9. Has the caregiver ever observed or discovered that the patient has hidden or disposed of pills?

Any answers to these questions that raise concern should prompt further assessment and discussion. Given the number of medications that must be swallowed posttransplant and the fact that the patient will likely need to take these medications for the rest of his or her life, it is imperative that the patient can swallow medications quickly and fluently. Pill swallowing can be effectively taught or improved through the use of behavioral strategies and operant conditioning, including modeling pill swallowing, shaping, positive reinforcement, and parent training (Anderson, Ruggiero, & Adams, 2000; Blount, Dahlquist, Baer, & Wuori, 1984; Walco, 1986). Varying sizes of candy or placebo pills can be used to approximate the posttransplant medication regimen and assess the patient's ability to successfully take his or her medications.

Case

A 15-year-old female with end-stage renal disease and other comorbid chronic health conditions was admitted to the inpatient nephrology service and referred to psychology for nonadherence to oral medications. She lived at home with her mother, who worked full time; her parents were divorced, and the patient had little contact with her father. The patient was on home peritoneal dialysis. The family lived a considerable distance from the hospital. The patient was first seen by a psychologist at age 11 for pill-swallowing difficulties and negative parent–child interactions over medication administration. At that time, the patient's pill swallowing rapidly improved following a straightforward behavioral approach (see Blount et al., 1984), and parent–child interactions improved following brief behavioral parent training that focused on positive reinforcement of desired behaviors, ignoring undesired behaviors, and maintaining a calm, matter-of-fact approach to the child's pill swallowing.

When the family followed up 4 years later, the situation had markedly deteriorated. Although the medical team had recommended psychology follow-up during the interim, the family had struggled to attend follow-up. As the patient's nonadherence had increased, so had the number and dosages of the medications prescribed. At the initial meeting with the psychologist, it was determined that the patient was prescribed more than 40 pills per day and was taking none of them consistently. When the patient attempted to swallow pills, she often gagged and vomited. Parent–child interactions were frequently negative, as the patient's mother was both worried and angry that the patient "refused" to take care of herself. In addition, the patient's nonadherence had resulted in increased health care costs for the family. The patient was distressed for a number of reasons, including the fact that her nonadherence was a barrier to kidney transplant.

Detailed assessment followed, including asking the medical team to identify "priority" medications; the current medication administration routine at home; and information from child life and nursing staff, who had both been working with the patient. The patient reported significant anxiety that taking, or attempting to take, her medications would cause nausea and vomiting. Psychology staff observed the patient attempt to take medication in various ways: in pill form, as liquid, crushed and placed in food, or sprinkled on food. The patient's behavior (vomiting) did not change as a function of medication form or amount, and she expressed anxiety that she would feel nausea and/or vomit regardless of how the medication was presented. She did not vomit following eating food or drinking beverages. A consistent consequence following gagging and vomiting was escape from medication administration. Thus the intervention was conceptualized in terms of negative reinforcement; in other words, vomiting was being reinforced via escape from medication administration. Following discussion, the patient agreed to an intervention that included eliminating the escape contingency following vomiting (i.e., escape extinction) and positive reinforcement contingent upon on the patient continuing with the intervention, even if she vomited. Given that the patient had the same response regardless of the form of medication (e.g., liquid or pills), it was agreed that she would take all medication in pill form, as this would be the most convenient method of medication administration in the long term. Positive reinforcement was contingent on the patient swallowing a progressively greater number of pills over several sessions. Child life staff provided a variety of attractive items from which the patient could choose when she met criteria for a reward. The medical team approved the intervention and provided guidance regarding when it was safe to readminister medications if she vomited (e.g., if she vomited within 15 minutes of swallowing the pill, it could be administered again). Relaxation training and positive self-talk to address her anxiety regarding vomiting were also included as part of the intervention.

During the first session incorporating escape extinction, she vomited twice but persisted until she had swallowed one pill successfully. During the second session, she initially vomited once, but then swallowed two pills successfully. During subsequent sessions she did not gag or vomit and swallowed an increasing number of pills during each session, earning rewards for meeting her goals. Because negative parent–child interactions surrounding medication administration had been identified as contributing to the patient's anxiety, several sessions of behavioral parent training were completed prior to discharge. They included providing psychoeducation, modeling the procedure and coaching the mother to stay calm and matter-of-fact during medication administration, and identifying a clear plan for ongoing positive reinforcement of desired behaviors at home.

At the time of discharge, the patient was swallowing all of the medications prioritized by the medical team. Over the next few weeks, many of her medication dosages were reduced and some medications eliminated, as her improved adherence allowed the medical team to make more informed decisions regarding her care.

Discussion

This case illustrates the importance of having a solid understanding of applied behavior analysis and the application of behavioral strategies. This knowledge informs assessment, case conceptualization, and selection of interventions. In this case, a clear understanding of the consequences of the identified behavior (vomiting) led to the selection of an effective intervention. The literature on feeding disorders (see Volkert & Piazza, 2012) was useful in terms of guiding intervention.

In this case, the intervention took place within an inpatient setting. The benefits of this setting included readily available medical and pharmacological consultation, frequent opportunities for patient and parent training and intervention, and close monitoring by nursing staff. Some of the challenges of the inpatient setting can include effective communication among all members of the treatment team, ensuring that all staff follow the treatment plan, and generalizing treatment gains to the home setting. A typical approach to addressing the third concern, in addition to outpatient follow-up, is to have the patient and/or parent complete all health care tasks on their own during the last day or two of admission, while consultation and support are still available.

This patient's most recent difficulties could have been prevented with periodic follow-up or booster sessions, but the family faced challenges with regard to follow-up, primarily due to distance and transportation. The increasing availability of telemedicine and e-health applications has the potential to improve access to behavioral health care for many patients, including those who would benefit from the services of a pediatric psychologist.

CASE EXAMPLE 3: NONADHERENCE

Background

As anyone who has experience working with children who have chronic health conditions knows very well, nonadherence is a common concern, affecting 50–75% of children and adolescents with chronic health conditions (Rapoff, 2011). Children who are candidates for organ transplant typically have time-consuming and demanding treatment regimens, including clinic appointments, oral medications, dietary restrictions or supplements, and tasks specific to their health condition, such as airway clearance and nebulized medications for CF or dialysis for kidney failure. A "simple" list of prescribed treatments does not take into account cleaning equipment, scheduling appointments, filling pillboxes, going to the pharmacy, or the myriad other tasks involved in managing a chronic health condition. Post-transplant, the patient and his or her caregivers can expect, at minimum, to continue multiple oral medications, appointments, and frequent blood draws, as well as other care specific to the patient's condition. As is often emphasized to patients and their families, organ transplant is a treatment, not a cure. Evidence-based treatment of nonadherence may include education, organizational strategies, self-management strategies, and behavioral parent training (Rapoff, 2011).

Case

A 16-year-old male with CF and CF-related liver disease was referred to psychology for a liver pretransplant psychological evaluation. He lived with his mother, a single parent, and two younger siblings, one of whom also had CF. His mother worked two jobs, and the family had limited resources. The patient was largely responsible for his own care, as his mother was often working, had two younger children to care for, and expressed the belief that, at 16, he should be independent regarding his care. The patient was hospitalized frequently and often for extended periods of time, with his mother on site infrequently. The medical team had expressed concern that the patient was not adherent to all aspects of his treatment regimen, frequently refused medical care or procedures, and was argumentative with staff. All felt these issues needed to be resolved before moving forward with a liver transplant.

The first step was to ascertain the patient's current adherence. Information was gathered from pharmacy refill records, lab results, and matter-of-fact, detailed interviews with the patient and parent separately. The information gathered suggested that the patient was generally adherent to oral medications and nutrition recommendations but struggled with nebulized medications and airway clearance treatments. The patient often completed one of two prescribed treatments early in the day, but by evening he felt fatigued and unmotivated, and his nonadherence typically was not noticed (or not addressed) by his mother.

The importance of parental monitoring was discussed with the patient and his mother, and the patient's mother was encouraged to base decisions about monitoring on the patient's current performance rather than on his chronological age. For example, he was adherent to his oral medications with almost no parental oversight, so only periodic monitoring was necessary. With regard to CF treatments, however, more monitoring was needed. The patient's mother agreed to "check in" with the patient each evening and assist him with initiating his CF treatment. She also agreed to exempt him from an assigned household chore that he found aversive if he had completed the previous night's treatment. A written agreement of what the parental reminder, assistance, and monitoring would "look like" and the criteria for earning his reward was created. During follow-up 1 week later, both parent and patient reported that he had been adherent to his CF treatment every night except one.

In addition to adherence at home, another priority of treatment was decreasing the patient's treatment refusals and argumentative behavior while he was admitted to the hospital. In general, the patient was adherent to his typical treatment regimen, but he would refuse "new" treatments or procedures (e.g., an unfamiliar procedure or new medication). The psychologist validated his frustration regarding the sheer amount of treatment he was being asked to do and his desire to exert some control over his own care. He agreed to the following "rule" that would balance his desire for more control with the medical team's desire for more positive interactions: When presented with a new treatment or procedure, he did not have to agree immediately, but his first response could not contain the word "no." Rather, he would ask a question instead (e.g., "Can you tell me more about why you want me to do that?" or "Why is that necessary?"). A succinct, written version of this language was taped to his bedside table, and the patient and psychologist rehearsed a variety of scenarios and requests. Our intervention was described to all members of the medical team during multidisciplinary team meetings, and staff members were asked to respond as positively as possible to the patient's efforts. Although it was not possible to obtain objective information with regard to the patient's interactions with staff, physician and nursing feedback was elicited during a weekly team meeting both prior to and following the intervention, and it indicated that the number of patient refusals had improved from several per week to zero for several weeks in a row. It appeared that eliminating the charged word "no" from the patient's initial response decreased staff defensiveness, improved interactions between the patient and staff, and resulted in improved adherence for the patient.

Discussion

Unfortunately, decisions to decrease parental monitoring of adherence are often related to chronological age (regardless of the adolescent's current adherence) rather than actual performance, or they occur subsequent to repeated, frustrating interactions between caregivers and adolescents, with caregivers ultimately "giving up." However, appropriate and disease-specific parental monitoring is related to adherence (Ellis et al., 2007; Ellis, Templin, Naar-King, & Frey, 2008), and, rather than being withdrawn abruptly, it should evolve over the course of the child's development and be faded gradually.

When assessing adherence, the psychologist will obtain information from a variety of sources, including pharmacy refill records, lab results, staff reports, and, rarely, electronic monitoring. The bulk of adherence information is often obtained during patient and parent interviews. Although research shows that patients often overestimate adherence (see Rapoff, 2011, for a review), an interview that is matter-of-fact, free of reprimands and judgment, and includes carefully worded questions (e.g., avoiding "Did you take your medications?" in favor of "Thinking about the last week, how often did you forget to take a dose of your medication?") can promote the acquisition of more accurate information. In addition, questionnaires and structured interviews exist that can assist with assessment of adherence and barriers to adherence (Modi & Quittner,

2006; Simons & Blount, 2007; Zelikovsky, Schast, Palmer, & Meyers, 2008).

With regard to the patient's adherence while admitted to the hospital, in the preceding case a number of factors had contributed to the development of treatment refusal and negative patient–staff interactions, including a system in which—too often—compliance had been demanded, rather than adherence elicited through discussion and collaboration. It is understandable that the medical team was reluctant to allow the allocation of a scarce resource (an organ) to a patient who, at times, refused treatment. By asking both sides to alter their communication styles, the psychologist was able to promote more positive communication and interactions between the patient and the staff and facilitate an interaction style that continued posttransplant.

CONCLUSION

As the preceding case examples illustrate, the role of a psychologist on a multidisciplinary transplant team involves collaboration with many other disciplines to improve patient care and health outcomes. Perhaps most important, the transplant setting presents many opportunities to apply evidence-based psychological interventions across a variety of concerns and contexts, with the goals of reducing distress and improving quality of life for children with organ failure and their families.

REFERENCES

Anderson, C. M., Ruggiero, K. J., & Adams, C. D. (2000). The use of functional assessment to facilitate treatment adherence: A case of a child with HIV and pill refusal. *Cognitive and Behavioral Practice, 7,* 282–287.

Blount, R. L., Dahlquist, L. M., Baer, R. A., & Wuori, D. (1984). A brief, effective method for teaching children to swallow pills. *Behavior Therapy, 15,* 381–387.

Cohen, L. L. (2008). Behavioral approaches to anxiety and pain management for pediatric venous access. *Pediatrics, 122*(Suppl. 3), S134–S139.

Ellis, D. A., Podolski, C., Frey, M., Naar-King, S., Wang, B., & Moltz, K. (2007). The role of parental monitoring in adolescent health outcomes: Impact on regimen adherence in youth with type 1 diabetes. *Journal of Pediatric Psychology, 32,* 907–917.

Ellis, D. A., Templin, T. N., Naar-King, S., & Frey, M. A. (2008). Toward conceptual clarity in a critical parenting construct: Parental monitoring in youth with chronic illness. *Journal of Pediatric Psychology, 33,* 799–808.

Fung, E., & Shaw, R. J. (2008). Pediatric Transplant Rating Instrument: A scale for the pretransplant psychiatric evaluation of pediatric organ transplant recipients. *Pediatric Transplantation, 12,* 57–66.

Humphrey, G. B., Boon, C. M., van Linden van den Heuvell, G. F., & van de Wiel, H. B. (1992). The occurrence of high levels of acute behavioral distress in children and adolescents undergoing routine venipunctures. *Pediatrics, 90,* 87–91.

Kurfis Stephens, B., Barkey, M. E., & Hall, H. R. (1999). Techniques to comfort children during stressful procedures. *Accident and Emergency Nursing, 7,* 226–236.

Modi, A. C., & Quittner, A. L. (2006). Barriers to treatment adherence for children with cystic fibrosis and asthma: What gets in the way? *Journal of Pediatric Psychology, 31,* 846–858.

Pai, A. L. H., Tackett, A., Ittenbach, R. F., & Goebel, J. (2011). Psychosocial Assessment Tool 2.0_General: Validity of a psychosocial risk screener in a pediatric kidney transplant sample. *Pediatric Transplantation, 16,* 92–98.

Rapoff, M. A. (2011). *Adherence to pediatric medical regimens* (2nd ed.). New York: Springer.

Rodrigue, J. R., Gonzalez-Peralta, R., & Langham, M. (2004). Solid organ transplantation. In R. T. Brown (Ed.), *Handbook of pediatric psychology in school settings* (pp. 679–699). Mahwah, NJ: Erlbaum.

Rodrigue, J. R., & Zelikovsky, N. (2009). Pediatric organ transplantation. In M. C. Roberts & R. G. Steele (Eds.), *Handbook of pediatric psychology* (2nd ed., pp. 392–402). New York: Guilford Press.

Schechter, N. L., Zempsky, W. T., Cohen, L. L., McGrath, P. J., McMurtry, C. M., & Bright, N. S. (2007). Pain reduction during pediatric immunizations: Evidence-based review and recommendations. *Pediatrics, 119,* 1184–1198.

Shah, V., Taddio, A., & Rieder, M. J. (2009). Effectiveness and tolerability of pharmacologic and combined interventions for reducing injection pain during routine childhood immunizations: Systematic review and meta-analyses. *Clinical Therapeutics, 31*(Suppl. B), S104–S151.

Simons, R. E., & Blount, R. L. (2007). Identifying barriers to medication adherence in adolescent transplant recipients. *Journal of Pediatric Psychology, 32,* 831–844.

Streisand, R. M., & Tercyak, K. P. (2001). Evaluating the pediatric transplant patient: General considerations. In J. R. Rodrigue (Ed.), *Biopsychosocial perspectives on transplantation* (pp. 71–92). New York: Kluwer Academic/Plenum Press.

Taddio, A., Chambers, C. T., Halperin, S. A., Ipp, M., Lockett, D., Rieder, M. J., et al. (2009). Inadequate pain management during routine childhood immunizations: The nerve of it. *Clinical Therapeutics, 31*(Suppl. 2), S152–S167.

Uman, L. S., Chambers, C. T., McGrath, P. J., & Kisely, S. (2008). A systematic review of randomized controlled trials examining psychological interventions for needle-related procedural pain and distress in children and adolescents: An abbreviated Cochrane review. *Journal of Pediatric Psychology, 33,* 842–854.

Volkert, V. M., & Piazza, C. C. (2012). Pediatric feeding disorders. In P. Sturmey & M. Hersen (Eds.), *Handbook of evidence-based practice in clinical psychology: Vol. 1. Child and adolescent disorders.* Hoboken, NJ: Wiley.

Walco, G. A. (1986). A behavioral treatment for difficulty in swallowing pills. *Journal of Behavior Therapy and Experimental Psychiatry, 17,* 127–128.

Walco, G. A. (2008). Needle pain in children: Contextual factors. *Pediatrics, 122*(Suppl. 3), S125–S129.

Zelikovsky, N., Schast, A. P., Palmer, J. A., & Meyers, K. A. C. (2008). Perceived barriers to adherence among adolescent renal transplant candidates. *Pediatric Transplantation, 12,* 300–308.

CHAPTER 23

Pediatric Feeding Disorders

LORETTA A. MARTIN-HALPINE

Pediatric feeding disorders occur in children in a variety of populations, ranging from typically developing children with concerns such as gastroesophageal reflux to children with mild developmental delays and those with complex medical and developmental histories (Linscheid, Budd, & Rasnake, 2003). Commonly identified feeding concerns include not consuming enough calories for growth and development; feeding selectivity (e.g., eating a limited variety, particular preferences about brand or appearance of foods); difficulty transitioning to foods of higher texture; and lack of progression in skills relating to feeding, such as self-feeding, cup drinking, or chewing.

One commonality across populations with feeding disorders involves negative learning associated with feeding (Babbitt, et al, 1994). In addition to examples of more direct learning, such as physical discomfort that occurs during feeding, patterns of inadvertent reinforcement of behaviors also develop. These patterns may begin in an attempt to find effective strategies to feed a child who is otherwise not thriving or not demonstrating typical feeding development. Although these strategies may be somewhat effective in the short term, they often interfere with positive, developmentally appropriate feeding in the long term. These patterns of behaviors often persist even when the source of discomfort is managed.

As feeding is a complex, developmental skill rather than a natural intuitive process, a multidisciplinary approach to assessment and treatment is important (Eicher, 1998; Kedesky & Budd, 1998; Miller, Burlow, Santoro, Mason, & Rudolph, 2001). Multiple factors need to be working together well for a child to develop effective feeding (Linscheid et al., 2003), and it is important to assess these factors within the global development of the specific child and typical feeding development (Schroeder & Gordon, 2002). A multidisciplinary approach addresses feeding within a biopsychosocial model including organic, mechanical, and psychosocial factors (Burlow, Phelps, Schultz, McConnell, & Rudolph, 1998).

Within a multidisciplinary setting, intensive behavioral models of treatment in day hospital or inpatient settings have been shown to be effective for treatment of feeding disorders (Kedesky & Budd, 1998; Kerwin, 1999; Linscheid, 2006; Sharp, Jaquess, Morton, & Herzinger, 2010).

CASE EXAMPLE OF FEEDING REFUSAL: JOE

Joe was a 25-month-old, full-term boy evaluated for concerns relating to limited intake of volume and variety and slow weight gain. Joe had a history of back-arching, projectile emesis, and multiple formula changes starting around age 3 months. Symptoms of discomfort and disruptive behaviors during feeding decreased with gastroesophageal reflux medications. Weight gain slowed after discontinuation of these. Around age 15 months, medication was restarted, and supplementation with a calorically dense beverage led to improvement in reflux symptoms, increased willingness to eat one food only, and weight gain.

At the time of the evaluation, Joe's weight was within the normal range. However, his oral intake was meeting only 82% of his estimated caloric needs, with a calorically dense supplemental beverage providing the majority of calories.

Feeding Joe was reported to be stressful and very effortful. Joe was fed every 2–3 hours while being held in a caretaker's arms and being distracted within a specific location outside the family home. Meals lasted longer than 30 minutes for smaller-than-age-typical portions. Joe drank 3–4 ounces of a nutritious beverage in 10–15 minutes between meals. Drinking larger amounts or drinking more quickly consistently led to symptoms of discomfort. Every few weeks, an exacerbation of reflux symptoms occurred without any change in feeding practices. Appetite and interest in feeding was limited even for highly preferred foods and with longer periods between meals. Joe's parents also reported concerns related to refusal to drink from a cup, limited interest in self-feeding, and the impact of feeding on participation in activities such as preschool. Parents had no developmental or behavioral concerns outside of feeding, and Joe received no developmental therapies.

Joe's caregivers had tried a wide variety of strategies with limited success. Offering smaller, more frequent meals, increasing liquids, giving preferred foods, and using distractions while feeding were identified as strategies that maximized intake. However, there were very few effective distractions. Accordingly, the family's ability to be away from the home was very limited, and caregivers spent most of the day focused on feeding. Mealtime behaviors included Joe's refusing to eat, blocking his mouth, turning away, spitting out food, whining, gagging, coughing, vomiting, holding food on his tongue and in his cheeks, swatting at the feeder, pushing away the spoon, and closing his mouth. These behaviors occurred throughout meals when no distraction was used and at the start and end of all meals even with distraction.

During the meal observation, Joe played with preferred foods, self-fed small amounts at a slow pace, and accepted a limited number of bites of a highly preferred food fed by his mother. Parents reported that the meal observation was typical of home meals.

MULTIDISCIPLINARY ASSESSMENT OF FEEDING DISORDERS

The most comprehensive multidisciplinary teams often include the following disciplines: medical practitioners, nutritionists, speech pathologists, occupational therapists, and psychologists. Assessment involves a range of factors that affect feeding and frequently involves direct observation of feeding.

The psychologist on these teams may assess a wide range of factors, including a comprehensive behavioral history of feeding (e.g., history, structure, and scheduling of mealtimes, parent and child behaviors and interaction, previous strategies and outcomes). Additional areas of assessment might include psychosocial factors (e.g., stressors related to feeding practices), child temperament, and match between a child's general development and current feeding. In addition to determining whether the child is medically and nutritionally stable, it is important to identify potential limiting factors and to establish appropriate treatment goals for each child.

Impressions and Recommendations

Joe's refusal of feeding and the resulting growth concerns appeared to be negatively affected by ongoing gastrointestinal discomfort. Based on his long history of early satiety and small amounts consumed, there was a concern about gastroparesis (a disorder of motility of the gastrointestinal system), which was confirmed by further testing. Joe had learned that feeding led to discomfort and attempted to refuse feeding accordingly. Joe's parents did whatever they needed to do maintain his growth. Over time, patterns of disruptive behaviors had developed around feeding, due to negative associations between feeding and discomfort and inadvertent reinforcement of these behaviors.

Although self-feeding was limited and the parents indicated that Joe preferred softer foods, these concerns appeared related to limited motivation for and comfort in swallowing rather than fine motor or oral motor skill deficits. Neither the speech pathologist nor the occupational therapist identified any additional significant concerns related to Joe's feeding. Due to concern that Joe was not meeting his caloric needs, the nutritionist recommended that his parents prioritize intake of the supplemental beverage over solids until time of admission to an intensive feeding program.

INTERVENTION

Intensive feeding programs generally occur in inpatient or day hospital settings. Length of such programs typically ranges from 4 to 8 weeks. Intervention generally continues to occur within multidisciplinary teams, although the unifying treatment in most programs is behaviorally based. Behavioral strategies used often include contingency management, differential social attention, positive and negative consequences, and stimulus control. An excellent discussion of these factors can be found in Linscheid et al. (2003). Qualitative and quantitative information guide treatment decisions over time. Treatment components generally include direct intervention with the child and parent training. Follow-up postdischarge varies by program. Typical goals for follow-up include maintaining behavioral changes in the home setting, expanding on changes established during the treatment program, and making changes in the behavioral feeding plan over time.

Joe in a Day Hospital Feeding Program

Direct Intervention with the Child

Joe was admitted to a day hospital program, where he received three to four daily meal sessions 5 days weekly for 4 weeks. Over the course of the admission, a set of behavioral strategies was created to target goals of increased oral acceptance of volume and variety during meals. After discussion with Joe's parents, feeding goals were prioritized in the following order: (1) increasing volume of intake to promote weight gain, (2) decreasing reliance on a supplemental beverage and testing the impact of increased intake of solids on symptoms related to gastroparesis, (3) cup drinking of a nutritious beverage rather than using an infant bottle, and (4) increasing dietary variety. Caregiver training (i.e., proficiency in use of the behavioral strategies) was also a primary goal.

During meal sessions, a differential reinforcement protocol was used to increase behaviors that supported feeding. Social attention and toy play were used to reward acceptance. Positive and negative reinforcement and shaping were the behavioral strategies most frequently used during Joe's admission.

Although self-feeding was not a primary goal of the admission, the opportunity to self-feed was provided as part of the mealtime strategies, using a three-step presentation for each bite presented. First, Joe was given the opportunity to self-feed the bite for 5 seconds. Second, hand-over-hand assistance with the utensil was provided if the utensil was not picked up in 5 seconds. Third, the feeder presented the bite if hand-over-hand assistance was resisted for 5 seconds.

Treatment began with offering what Joe was most consistently accepting so that he received the reinforcement, learned the expectations of the sessions, and began to establish momentum in the behaviors of picking up the utensil and putting it in his mouth consistently. As Joe was not taking any food consistently and was refusing all spoon feeding, five presentations of a spoon with nothing on it were offered. Demand gradually increased over time, so that Joe was next introduced to the familiar supplemental beverage by spoon. Purees were introduced on the spoon quickly, as the percentage of bites consumed was high and the number of disruptive behaviors remained low. Dry spoons and spoons of supplemental beverage were faded from the meals as purees were introduced.

Introduction of soft, chewable foods was well accepted but was associated with decreased mouth clearance (i.e., swallowing in the interval before the next bite is offered). As bite sizes of chewable foods remained small to promote clearance and facilitate practice, a limited number of chewable foods were introduced to maximize total volume in each meal. To facilitate cessation of the use of the infant bottle, cup drinking of the supplemental beverage was introduced in both the meal sessions and in separate, additional cup drinking sessions, using the same behavioral strategies.

Multidisciplinary Coordination of Care

Intervention during a multidisciplinary program involves coordination among multiple areas, including behavioral and nutritional changes and gastrointestinal symptoms. The starting behavioral plan for any child is affected by his or her medical and nutritional status. As changes are made over time, patterns may be identified that inform ongoing medical and nutritional care as well. Components of behavioral programs, such as systematic changes, review of data collected, and control of the behavioral contingencies often provide information that might be difficult to gather otherwise on an outpatient basis. For Joe, mealtime schedule, volume and content of meals, and medication use were three examples of multidisciplinary coordination.

At time of admission, Joe was prescribed three medications for his gastrointestinal difficulties (an appetite stimulant, a reflux medication, and a medication to facilitate motility). Because the appetite stimulant effect can wear off with continued use, this medication is often cycled to be taken on and off over a several-week period. At the start of the admission, the timing of the dosage plan was altered so that the medication would have maximum effect at the point in the admission when parent training was occurring.

Initially, the use of the prokinetic agent resulted in decreased vomiting with increased volumes in meals. However, vomiting increased when it was given at full doses. Changes in dosages and resulting changes in vomiting were recorded as part of the data regularly collected. Working together with the team and the family, a schedule of titration of the dosage was designed that preserved the beneficial effect without increased vomiting. Over time, the effectiveness of the medication was demonstrated to decrease, and it was discontinued shortly before discharge.

A schedule for drinking between meal therapy sessions was designed at admission in coordination with the nutritionist to maintain hydration and maximize motivation from hunger during the program. For Joe, very small changes in volume consumed at or between meals significantly affected symptoms such as vomiting and, accordingly, his meal plan. Working with the nutritionist, several alterations to the schedule of liquids and solids were tried systematically over the course of the admission to promote weight gain, despite frequent vomiting. Although calorie boosting, most often with fats, is frequently recommended for children with slow weight gain, these strategies were specifically avoided in Joe's diet because increased fat tends to slow gastrointestinal motility.

Although not relevant for Joe, if disruptive behaviors had limited the ability of the speech pathologist to assess oral motor skill, further evaluation could have occurred after oral acceptance had been established using the behavioral strategies. If there were concerns during the meal sessions about oral motor skill level limiting intake or ability to progress, the speech pathologist would have been consulted at that point in the admission.

If sensory processing had been identified as a concern, coordination between the psychologist and the occupational therapist would have occurred for introduction of new foods. The psychologist might identify several new foods that would be introduced in meals in the near future, and the occupational therapist would use those in food play and simple food preparation activities to provide exposure to those foods without the demand to eat them. After exposure, these would be introduced into the structured meal sessions for consumption. Alternatively, if the occupational therapist in her treatment sessions had identified foods that Joe interacted with more easily, those might have been introduced next.

The removal of parents from the feeding setting at the start of the program, the intensity of intervention and repeated trials, and the changing of behavioral contingencies promoted development of new patterns of behavior prior to reintroducing the parents into the meal.

Parent Education and Support

Education for parents and other caregivers is a crucial factor in changing the patterns of interaction during feeding. In addition to education regarding rationale for use of the behavioral strategies, any potential limiting factors specifically affecting a particular child, family, or medical condition are important to discuss.

The parent training component might include observation of meal sessions via a two-way mirror, education and support from the psychologist, and in vivo training. This training process is a gradual transition from clinical staff to parent as feeder. Independent practice in both clinic and home settings is ideal prior to discharge. Some programs also offer family support groups and provide an opportunity for parents to meet other families whose children have feeding challenges.

Joe's parents demonstrated a good understanding of the need for behavioral intervention and a strong commitment to participate in treatment. In Joe's case, there were several challenges specific to gastroparesis that were discussed prior to and throughout the admission. As refusal of feeding decreases and intake increases, symptoms such as vomiting and signs of discomfort may increase rather than decrease. The amount that Joe would be able to consume at one time was likely to continue to be smaller than age-typical and might require more frequent meals. There was also the possibility that Joe might not be able to consume all the calories needed for growth in his waking hours and could require overnight supplemental tube feeding.

During week 3 of treatment, once high, consistent levels of oral acceptance were established (i.e., > 80%), Joe's mother and father were trained to maintain this acceptance and to manage disruptive behaviors during structured meals. Acceptance remained high throughout parent training with the predicted increase in disruptive behaviors, which again decreased over time. An increase in the behaviors previously displayed with parents is expected as parents act as cues to the previous set of behaviors. Effective management of these behaviors teaches the child that the contingencies have changed. Additional training was also provided in meal composition and making a pureed diet. After being fully trained, both parents completed practice meals in the home using various foods and training to make a pureed diet environment to assist with transition home. Joe's parents reported that intake remained high and disruptive behaviors remained low and manageable.

Therapy Outcomes

Joe exceeded his admission goals and was consuming sufficient calories to maintain age-typical growth. Over the course of the admission, a meal schedule of food and calorically dense nutritious beverages was designed that maximized intake and minimized vomiting. This included four smaller, more frequent meals and two "snacks" of a drink. Joe's mother and father were proficient in use of established mealtime protocol. Joe gained 1.64 pounds, compared with an age-typical rate of gain of 1/4 to 5/8 pounds for this period. Percentage of total calories from a supplemental beverage decreased from 96% to 54%. Use of the bottle was discontinued, as all fluid was now consumed via cup. Joe's variety increased by nine foods. At discharge, Joe's parents reported significant decrease in distress related to feeding.

Follow-up Care

Intervention with Joe's family continued in multidisciplinary, follow-up appointments. Follow-up was designed to build on the behavioral platform established within the day hospital. Short-term goals included successful maintenance of treatment gains in the transition to the home environment and continued progress toward increased variety as volume goals had been reached. Longer term goals can include progress toward other feeding-related goals that may not have been prioritized in the day hospital (e.g., transition to foods of higher texture, increased self-feeding). Additionally, for many children, the ultimate goals are to facilitate developmentally appropriate mealtimes for each child and to maximize positive associations with feeding for the child and family. For some children, long-term use of some version of a behavioral program is necessary at mealtimes.

Consistent with his history, periods of ongoing vomiting continued after discharge even without changes to intake or scheduling. Joe's parents did a commendable job using the behavioral strategies to maintain his oral acceptance and growth throughout these periods. Ongoing discomfort and limited appetite were barriers to the development of more positive associations with feeding. This affected Joe's progress toward goals such as increased independence at mealtimes and willingness to self-feed.

Joe's parents understood that there was no certainty that his gastrointestinal challenges and the resulting limited internal motivation to eat would change. Accordingly, the typical plan to fade use of the external reinforcement over time was not recommended. Changes were made to the feeding plan over time to maximize ease of implementation within family mealtimes.

After several months of close follow-up with the team, a plan for the long term was developed with Joe's family to continue to shape progress toward his feeding goals. The family was educated regarding ways to systematically make and assess effectiveness of any changes and how to integrate effective changes into a comprehensive feeding plan.

At the time of most recent follow-up, Joe continued to grow in weight and height. Meals were more positive, less effortful, and less stressful. Although Joe's motility had improved, both gastroparesis and gastroesophageal reflux continued to have a significant impact on his feeding. Due to his ongoing discomfort and limited inherent enjoyment of eating, his parents continued to utilize the behavioral strategies to provide external motivation for continued successful feeding.

SUMMARY

Joe is one excellent example of the transaction among various factors affecting the development and maintenance of feeding disorders and the effectiveness of multidisciplinary assessment and treatment. Determining an optimal meal schedule for Joe, changing his behavior, maximizing his nutrition, managing his gastrointestinal symptoms, and providing his parents with a way of feeding him that decreased the stress and set the stage for more typical feeding could not have been accomplished without multidisciplinary collaboration. The set of strategies designed during the day hospital admission enabled Joe's parents to maintain intake and growth despite ongoing gastrointestinal obstacles, and Joe continues to show successful feeding and growth over time.

REFERENCES

Babbitt, R. L., Hoch, T. A., Coe, D. A., Cataldo, M. F., Kelly, K. J., Stackhouse, C., et al. (1994). Behavioral assessment and treatment of pediatric feeding disorders. *Developmental and Behavioral Pediatrics, 15*(4), 278–291.

Burlow, K. A., Phelps, A., Schultz, J. R., McConnell, K., & Rudolph, C. (1998). Classifying complex pediatric feeding disorders. *Journal of Pediatric Gastroenterology and Nutrition, 27*, 143–147.

Eicher, P. S. (1998). Nutrition and feeding. In J. P. Dormas & L. Pelligrino (Eds.), *Caring for children with cerebral palsy: A team approach* (pp. 243–279). Baltimore: Brookes.

Kedesky, J. H., & Budd, K. S. (1998). *Childhood feeding disorders: Biobehavioral assessment and intervention*. Baltimore: Brookes.

Kerwin, M. E. (1999). Empirically supported treatments in pediatric psychology: Severe feeding problems. *Journal of Pediatric Psychology, 24*(3), 193–214.

Linscheid, T. R. (2006). Behavioral treatments for pediatric feeding disorders. *Behavior Modification, 30*(1), 6–23.

Linscheid, T. R., Budd, K. S., & Rasnake, L. K. (2003). Pediatric feeding problems. In M. C. Roberts (Ed.), *Handbook of pediatric psychology* (3rd ed., pp. 481–498). New York: Guilford Press.

Miller, C. K., Burlow, K. A., Santoro, K., Mason, D., & Rudolph, C. (2001). An interdisciplinary team approach to management of pediatric feeding and swallowing disorders. *Children's Health Care, 30,* 201–218.

Schroeder, C. S., & Gordon, B. N. (2002). *Assessment and treatment of childhood problems*. New York: Guilford Press.

Sharp, W. G., Jaquess, D. L., Morton, J. F., & Herzinger, C. V. (2010). Pediatric feeding disorders: A quantitative synthesis of treatment outcomes. *Clinical Child and Family Psychology Review, 13*(4), 348–365.

CHAPTER 24

Pediatric Elimination Disorders

SUSANA R. PATTON
MARTHA U. BARNARD

Elimination disorders include disorders of repeated voiding of urine (enuresis) or stool (encopresis) outside of the toilet beyond the age when continence is expected (e.g., 5 years for enuresis and 4 years for encopresis; American Psychiatric Association, 2013). In both disorders, the voiding can be intentional or involuntary and needs to have occurred for at least 3 months. Most children with these disorders may have a medical or physiological reason for the disorder (American Psychiatric Association, 2013; Felt, Brown, Harrison, Kochhar, & Patton, 2008), which needs to be addressed in the context of behavioral treatments. Additionally, these disorders are often associated with family stress, embarrassment, and conflict, which will require treatment. In this chapter, we present case studies followed by a review of the evidence-based treatments for each disorder.

CASE EXAMPLE OF ENURESIS: JON

Presentation

Jon, a 6-year-old boy, was referred by his pediatrician for behavioral treatment. Jon achieved daytime control of urine and stool when he was 3 years old. However, he continues to have wetting accidents at least 5 nights per week. Nighttime wetting accidents are described as "complete and drenching." Jon will sometimes awaken on his own following an accident, but more often the accidents are discovered when his mother awakens him at midnight. In an attempt to stop the accidents, Jon's family had tried planned sitting on the toilet at nighttime (sits), limiting fluid intake after dinner, having him empty his bladder several times between dinner and bedtime, and restricting his diet (e.g., eliminating caffeine and dairy). None of these strategies had resulted in change. More frustrating, Jon's mother reported that he had begun to have daytime wetting accidents during the past 4 months. They happened at school, on the way home from school, and on the weekends, especially if Jon was busy playing outside or on the computer. He averaged three small to complete accidents per week. A recent trip to the pediatrician ruled out the presence of a urinary tract infection, diabetes, or constipation. There was no concern for sexual abuse. Jon had a history of attention problems, but his attention problems were well controlled with stimulant medication.

Evidence-Based Treatment

Jon met criteria for both nocturnal and diurnal enuresis. Prevalence rates suggest that between between 5 to 10% of 5-year-olds and 3 to 5% of 10-year-olds, more boys than girls, struggle with enuresis (American Psychiatric Association, 2013; Graham & Levy, 2009). Children with nocturnal enuresis tend to have an impaired ability to wake up when their bladders are full. Additionally, there may be a discrepancy between urine production and bladder capacity (Sureshkumar, Jones, Caldwell, & Craig, 2009). There is emerging evidence suggesting that nocturnal enuresis can also be a symptom of obstructive sleep apnea (Bascom et al., 2011; Kovacevic et al., 2012). Thus sleep apnea should be ruled out at diagnosis.

Medication and behavioral treatments are available for nocturnal enuresis. Medications treat the symptoms by controlling the production or retention of urine overnight, but they do not achieve a cure. The first line of medication is desmopressin acetate (DDAVP), an antidiuretic hormone that increases reabsorption of urine in collecting ducts of the kidney, thus reducing urine output at night (Neveus, 2011a, 2011b). DDAVP is effective within 1 hour and completely cleared from the system within 9 hours of administration, limiting its effect only to the night of administration. Imipramine, a tricyclic antidepressant, is another medication that may be prescribed for nocturnal enuresis once cardiac risks have been ruled out (Graham & Levy, 2009; Reiner, 2008). Imipramine is thought to work by promoting urine retention, decreasing bladder contractions, and by increasing arousal. Similar to DDAVP, imipramine can have a high relapse rate once it is stopped. In addition, imipramine can cause uncomfortable side effects and is considered highly toxic if ever taken as an overdose, thus making it a second line intervention (Graham & Levy, 2009; Reiner, 2008).

If a parent is seeking to cure nighttime enuresis, the evidence clearly supports the use of the bed-wetting alarm, which has a 78% cure rate (Mellon & McGrath, 2000). This therapy draws from classical conditioning theory. The child wears a device to bed that has an alarm that is triggered by moisture. If the child has a urine accident, the alarm will sound and alert the child (and/or parent) of the accident so the child can go to the bathroom. It is hypothesized that the child becomes conditioned to the sensation of having a full bladder and thus learns to wake up on his or her own to use the toilet. This treatment may take up to 4 months for a child to achieve complete dry nights and can be stressful and tiring for families (Graham & Levy, 2009). Several studies have incorporated basic urine alarm treatment within a multicomponent program. One example, dry-bed training, combines the urine alarm with a behavioral plan consisting of overnight toilet sits, positive practice, and punishment for accidents (e.g., child assisting with cleanup; Azrin, Sneed, & Foxx, 1974). This 4-week multicomponent treatment program has an average success rate of 75% (Azrin et al., 1974; Mellon & McGrath, 2000). Follow-up studies suggest that without the bed-wetting alarm, success rates are lower (Mellon & McGrath, 2000).

With respect to diurnal enuresis, behavior therapy (monitoring, scheduled toilet sit times, double voiding, and reinforcement) is the first line of treatment. Daytime enuresis can occur if children ignore or become desensitized to the sensation of having a full bladder, leading to problems with urgency and leaking. Children diagnosed with attention-deficit/hyperactivity disorder (ADHD) can be vulnerable to daytime wetting related to their attention problems (Baeyens et al., 2004; Graham & Levy, 2009; Joinson et al., 2008). Also, daytime wetting can be a symptom of constipation, which should be ruled out (Felt et al., 2008; Graham & Levy, 2009). Monitoring and scheduled toilet sit times can help to ensure that the child takes time to empty his or her bladder throughout the day and before activities when the child may be most at risk for an accident (Graham & Levy, 2009). Scheduled toilet sits should last about 5 minutes, but the exact duration can be adjusted either up or down depending on the child's success in passing urine. Children should not bring a toy, book, or game with them into the bathroom during a scheduled toilet sit, as these may prove too distracting. However, to help with children's cooperation and motivation, a structured incentive program for completed sit times may be effective. Double voiding is simply asking the child to void, wait a short time (e.g., count of 20), and then void a second time (Graham & Levy, 2009). This procedure can be helpful if it is suspected that the child is not completely emptying during scheduled toilet sits. Other recommendations include dietary restriction and limiting the intake of known bladder irritants such as caffeine, carbonated beverages, beverages with a high citrus content, and foods with artificial red dyes (Graham & Levy, 2009).

Analysis

Jon's treatment initially focused on his daytime enuresis, as the family considered it most stressful. The family was trained to complete a daily log to monitor the frequency and timing of accidents throughout treatment. Jon and his mother agreed to a behavioral toileting plan wherein he would void in the toilet every 2 hours. Because accidents were happening at school, appropriate measures were taken so that the psychologist could contact the teacher to seek her support with the behavioral plan. At a follow-up appointment, Jon's accident log revealed that he was most at risk for an accident in the early afternoon. The psychologist learned that Jon had a scheduled toilet sit between lunch and recess and that he was rushing through this sit so that he could go outside with his friends. The school agreed to move the toilet sit so that Jon would not miss recess. With the addition of monitoring and the behavioral plan, Jon decreased his wetting accidents to less than one time per week within 6 weeks of treatment initiation. In a follow-up appointment, the toileting plan was modified to reduce the number of prompted toilet sits and to reinforce Jon for using the toilet independently. Because of Jon's comorbid attention problems, the psychologist recommended that the school day include at least two prompted toilet sits for a consistent voiding.

To address Jon's nocturnal enuresis, the family purchased a bed-wetting alarm, and the psychologist trained them to use the alarm, along with a scheduled overnight sit plan. Again, the family completed a monitoring log recording the frequency and timing of nighttime accidents. Jon's family was advised that treatment would take several weeks of consistent alarm use and not to become discouraged if the nighttime accidents persisted. Two weeks into using the bed-wetting alarm, Jon's monitoring log revealed no change in his accident frequency. The family said that Jon was able to sleep through the alarm and that he was difficult to awaken. The psychologist normalized these concerns and encouraged the family to stick to the program. In addition, Jon's mother agreed to an incentive plan wherein Jon earned a token each night for cooperating with his scheduled sits. He could save these tokens to trade in for a larger prize each weekend (e.g., a video game rental). Three weeks later, Jon's monitoring log revealed a modest decrease in the frequency of accidents and new success in passing urine in the toilet following an alarm, suggesting that Jon was becoming more alert to the alarm and able to stop the urine flow. Jon attained consistently dry nights after using the bed-wetting alarm for 10 weeks.

A challenge to the treatment was Jon's predisposition to heavy sleeping. Also, Jon's parents were divorced, and he spent every other weekend with his father. At first, Jon did not take the alarm with him to his dad's home. However, in a phone call to Jon's dad, the psychologist discussed the treatment approach and the necessity for consistent alarm use, and Jon's father agreed to participate. There was a discussion of using DDAVP. However, the family opted not to use DDAVP because Jon was already on stimulant medication. Using DDAVP might have helped to relieve some of the stress related to the alarm treatment. However, from a classical conditioning perspective, the DDAVP would also have limited Jon's experience with accidents, which are important to forming the conditioned response. Jon was successful in treatment because he was motivated to reduce his daytime and nighttime wetting accidents. Yet the addition of a formal incentive plan for his positive toileting behaviors appeared to be beneficial. In designing these incentive plans, it is important to keep the goals realistic and to encourage families to incentivize behavior (e.g., cooperating with toilet sits) and not outcomes (e.g., dry days or nights), which may be less under the child's immediate control.

CASE EXAMPLE OF ENCOPRESIS: WILL

Presentation

Will, a 4-year, 6-month-old boy, was referred for behavioral treatment by his pediatrician. Will was first noted to have constipation when he transitioned to solid food at 10 months of age and started to pass small, pebble-like stools in his diaper. However, because he passed a stool at least once every other day, his parents did not seek treatment for his constipation. When he was 3 years old, Will started toilet training. By report, Will attained daytime urine control within about 4 weeks but resisted using the toilet for stools. Moreover, he started to have loose stool accidents in his underwear multiple times during the day. An appointment with his pediatrician revealed a stool impaction. The pediatrician recommended a clean-out regimen using polyethylene glycol (PEG 3350) and, following the clean-out, a daily dose of 1 capful of PEG 3350 mixed in 8 ounces of water. The clean-out regimen led to a large amount of stool excretion. However, the parents noted that within 10 days of the clean-out, the accidents resumed. Will's parents continued to give him the PEG 3350 for another month and then discontinued it because he continued to have accidents. At the first appointment, Will was passing a stool in a pull-up 3–4 times per day. Typical stools were described as very soft or liquidy. However, every 2 weeks, Will passed a very large, hard, and painful stool. The parents openly shared their frustration. Because of the soiling and the necessity of putting Will back in pull-ups, he was not allowed to attend their local prekindergarten program. They also had to withdraw him from swim lessons.

Evidence–Based Treatment

Will met criteria for encopresis (American Psychiatric Association, 2013). He also met criteria for functional constipation based on the Rome III guidelines, the gold-standard diagnostic tool for physicians (Felt et al., 2008; Rasquin et al., 2006). In many cases, children who present with encopresis will also have a history of constipation, and it is important to determine whether the constipation has resolved (Felt et al., 2008; Rasquin et al., 2006). Another medical condition to rule out at diagnosis is Hirschsprung's disease, which is a congenital disorder of the colon that can lead to chronic constipation (Felt et al., 2008).

Medication plus behavioral treatment is the standard of care for encopresis (Felt et al., 2008). Table 24.1 provides a summary of common medications available for children. Although all of these medications are available over the counter, a psychologist may wish to work with a physician to ensure that children are taking the correct medication and dose. All of these medications have general dosing guidelines. However, small variations (e.g., 20%) on these guidelines should be considered to ensure that the medication response is optimal (Felt et al., 2008).

Behavioral intervention includes monitoring of accidents (Felt et al., 2008). In particular, it is helpful for parents to record the frequency, time, size, and consistency of stool accidents, as well as any excreted stools in the toilet. Frequency and timing of accidents is important for determining a toilet sit schedule, optimizing the medication dose, and identifying stool withholding. Consistency and size of the stool and current stool pattern will help to inform whether the medication dose is optimal. For example, a record showing multiple small outputs and only intermittent large outputs can suggest the child is withholding stool. Parents and children should monitor stool output daily until the problem is completely resolved. Training should focus on increasing children's appropriate toileting behavior. As part of the training, a toilet sit schedule should be developed. It is optimal to target prompted sit times at about the times when children may be most at risk for an accident (Felt et al., 2008). In the absence of a specific pattern of soiling, it is helpful to target sit times first thing in the morning (e.g., orthocolic reflex), 30 minutes after meals (e.g., gastrocolic reflex), and/or during natural transition times. If children are afraid to sit on the toilet, a shaping program may be needed. Parents should expect children to sit on the toilet for at least 5 minutes at each sit; however, this time can be adjusted up or down based on the child's resistance or stool production

TABLE 24.1. Common Medications for Constipation

Medication	Comments/side effects
Osmotics (retains water in the stools)	
Polyethylene glycol (also known as PEG 3350, Glycolax, Miralax)	Tasteless; adherence typically very good; side effects: diarrhea, bloating
Magnesium hydroxide (also known as Milk of Magnesia)	Multiple flavors; adherence varies; side effects: hypermagnesemia
Lactulose	Typically reserved for infants and toddlers; side effects: abdominal cramping, gas
Sorbitol	May be less expensive than lactulose; side effects: abdominal cramping, gas
Lubricants (lubricate hard stools)	
Mineral oil	Chill or give with juice; adherence can be problematic; side effects: leakage if dose is too high or impaction is present
Kondrumel (plain emulsion)	Sweet taste; adherence may be improved over straight mineral oil; side effect: leakage if dose is too high or impaction is present

(Felt et al., 2008). Children should not be allowed to bring toys, books, or other distractions with them for these toilet sits. About 50% of children with constipation and encopresis can also have paradoxical sphincter control, meaning that they have the tendency to constrict versus relax their sphincters during defecation (van der Plas et al., 1996). For these children, behavioral treatment needs to include teaching relaxation in an attempt to reverse this learned response (van der Plas et al., 1996). Likewise, many children with encopresis may have become accustomed to passing stool in a nonsitting position (e.g., squatting) and will need to learn how to sit on the toilet correctly (viz., foot support, hands on their knees, slightly leaning forward, and bending at the waist; Felt et al., 2008). A structured incentive program can help with children's cooperation and motivation. Finally, there is some support for making dietary changes, including increasing children's daily intake of fiber and clear fluids (Felt et al., 2008; Loening-Baucke, Miele, & Staiano, 2004). The standard fiber guideline for children with encopresis is 5 grams + child age in years. For children who also have constipation, the guideline is 10 grams + child age in years (Felt et al., 2008). It is recommended that children's daily clear fluid intake double in fluid ounces their fiber intake. Clear fluids include water and other nondairy, noncaffeinated beverages (Felt et al., 2008). On average, treatment can take up to 6 months and during this time children are at risk for relapse. If the child is taking medication for constipation, parents should be advised not to wean the medication too quickly, as this can increase the risk of relapse. For children with underlying constipation, recovery is achieved when children have achieved a pattern of at least three stools per week with no soiling (Felt et al., 2008).

Different service delivery formats exist for behavior therapy for encopresis. Stark and colleagues have had success treating encopresis in a group format (Stark et al., 1997). The specific content of the treatment is very similar to standard behavioral care. Parents and children participate in their own simultaneous groups to review the curriculum. Research has shown this program is successful, with an average decrease in soiling of 84%. Moreover, several advantages exist because of the group format. Parents and children have the chance for peer support, which may help to reduce feelings of isolation. Children can benefit from the added incentive of earning a weekly prize in front of their "poop group" friends. Finally, this format can be very efficient in treating a larger number of families simultaneously (Stark et al., 1997). Recently, Ritterband and colleagues (2008) have instituted a trial of an Internet-based program. In this trial, 95% of youth experienced at least a 50% improvement in soiling. An advantage of using the Internet for treatment delivery is that it extends behavioral therapy beyond a medical center and to families who might otherwise be unable to access care.

Analysis

Will's stool frequency suggested that he was constipated. Therefore, the psychologist referred the family back to the pediatrician to restart the PEG 3350, but at a slightly higher dose (2 T), to ensure that the stools were soft and easy to pass and to make it harder for Will to withhold. The psychologist also normalized the parents' feelings of frustration and explained why rectal distention and accommodation may account for Will's unawareness of accidents. Will's parents were taught to monitor his stool frequency. The psychologist also developed an incentive program wherein Will earned stickers for reporting a soiling accident. These stickers could be turned in for a larger prize each week. Will's parents reported that he had been very resistant to past attempts to sit on the toilet. Thus, as a next step, a shaping program was used, gradually reinforcing Will for behavioral approximations until he was able to sit on the toilet, pants down, for a minimum of 5 minutes. Once Will had achieved this goal and was passing soft stools daily, the psychologist implemented toileting practice. Will was instructed to sit on the toilet for a minimum of 5 minutes at least four times daily (30 minutes after each meal and before bedtime). An incentive program was established wherein Will could earn a sticker for passing stool in the toilet during these prompted toilet sits. The first week of this plan, Will complied with the toilet sits but did not pass any stool in the toilet. At the next appointment, the psychologist reviewed the steps for a toilet sit (see previous discussion) and consulted with Will's pediatrician to ensure that medication was optimal. Will had a success the following week, passing one small stool in the toilet but still soiling. Will's parents were instructed to praise him for his success and to allow Will to trade in his sticker chart for a larger prize. This initial success led to more outputs in the toilet, and finally, by the 9th week of treatment (fifth session), Will was in a pattern of passing all stools in the toilet during a prompted sit time. Concomitant to working on the behavioral toileting plan, the psychologist taught Will and his parents how to recognize foods containing fiber and recommended that Will consume at least 14 grams of fiber and 28 ounces of water daily. At the last appointment, Will was in a pattern of daily stool excreted in the toilet, some even during self-initiated toilet sits. Will was consuming an average of 10 grams of fiber and 20 ounces of water daily. Will's parents were advised to continue with the PEG 3350 and were referred back to their pediatrician for medication management. Finally, they were taught how to recognize early symptoms of a relapse.

The most significant challenge to Will's recovery was his past history with constipation, which had reinforced a perception that stools were hard and uncomfortable to pass. This, in turn, reinforced Will's withholding behaviors and his resistance to sitting on the toilet. Will had developed a pattern of passing stools while standing on his tiptoes, often hiding behind a piece of furniture. Thus he needed specific instruction on how to sit on the toilet and how to relax the anal sphincter to allow stools to pass. Will was compliant with his medication, and he was a good eater, which made it easier when it came time to modify his diet and increase his fiber intake. However, for picky eaters, it is possible to use fiber supplements in order to reach the daily fiber goal. Also, within the past 5 years, greater variety of fiber-rich foods have become available in grocery stores, which may help if children are not fond of fruits or vegetables. PEG 3350 is a well-tolerated medication that is tasteless when mixed in most beverages. Older osmotics are still available should children object to PEG 3350 and want to try another form of medication (see Table 24.1). Will lived in an intact family that received support from extended family. Likewise, Will's day care program was willing to participate in the program. Treatment for encopresis can be more challenging if there is no consistency in the behavioral schedule across multiple settings. Thus it is beneficial, when treating children for encopresis, to seek permission from parents to involve other caregivers, teachers, and school nurses in the behavioral program.

CONCLUSION

Elimination disorders are common in childhood and can be developmentally, behaviorally, and emotionally disruptive for families. In some cases, these problems have an underlying medical concern that needs to be addressed or ruled out within the scope of treatment. The good news for families and children struggling with these disorders is that for both enuresis and encopresis, evidence-based behavioral treatments exist with very high rates of success, suggesting that children do not need to suffer needlessly from the stress or embarrassment related to having urine or stool accidents.

REFERENCES

American Psychiatric Association. (2013). *Diagnostic and statistical manual of mental disorders* (5th ed.).Arlington, VA: Author.

Azrin, N. H., Sneed, T. J., & Foxx, R. M. (1974). Dry-bed training: Rapid elimination of childhood enuresis. *Behavior Research Therapy, 12,* 147–156.

Baeyens, D., Roeyers, H., Hoebeke, P., Verte, S., Van Hoecke, E., & Walle, J. V. (2004). Attention-deficit/hyperactivity disorder in children with nocturnal enuresis. *Journal of Urology, 171,* 2576–2579.

Bascom, A., Penney, T., Metcalfe, M., Knox, A., Witmans, M., Uweira, T., et al. (2011). High risk of sleep disordered breathing in the enuresis population. *Journal of Urology, 186,* 1710–1713.

Felt, B. T., Brown, P. I., Harrison, R. V., Kochhar, P. K., & Patton, S. R. (2008). Functional constipation and soiling in children. *Guidelines for Clinical Care.* Retrieved June 7, 2012, from *www.med.umich.edu/1info/fhp/practiceguides/newconstipation.html*

Graham, K. M., & Levy, J. B. (2009). Enuresis. *Pediatric Review, 30,* 165–172.

Joinson, C., Heron, J., von Gontard, A., Butler, U., Golding, J., & Emond, A. (2008). Early childhood risk factors associated with daytime wetting and soiling in school-age children. *Journal of Pediatric Psychology, 33,* 739–750.

Kovacevic, L., Jurewicz, M., Dabaja, A., Thomas, R., Diaz, M., Madgy, D. N., et al. (2012). Enuretic children with obstructive sleep apnea syndrome: Should they see otolaryngology first? *Journal of Pediatric Urology, 9*(2), 145–150.

Loening-Baucke, V., Miele, E., & Staiano, A. (2004). Fiber (glucomannan) is beneficial in the treatment of childhood constipation. *Pediatrics, 113,* e259–e264.

Mellon, M. W., & McGrath, M. L. (2000). Empirically supported treatments in pediatric psychology: Nocturnal enuresis. *Journal of Pediatric Psychology, 25,* 193–214.

Neveus, T. (2011a). Nocturnal enuresis: Theoretic background and practical guidelines. *Pediatric Nephrology, 26,* 1207–1214.

Neveus, T. (2011b). Sleep enuresis. *Handbook of Clinical Neurology, 98,* 363–369.

Rasquin, A., DiLorenzo, C., Forbes, D, Guiraldes, E., Hyams, J. S., Staiano, A., et al. (2006). Childhood functional gastrointestinal disorders: Child/adolescent. *Gastroenterology, 130,* 1527–1537.

Reiner, W. G. (2008). Pharmacotherapy in the management of voiding and storage disorders, including enuresis and encopresis. *Journal of the American Academy of Child and Adolescent Psychiatry, 47,* 491–498.

Ritterband, L. M., Ardalan, K., Thorndike, F. P., Magee, J. C., Saylor, D. K., Cox, D. J., et al. (2008). Real world use of an Internet intervention for pediatric encopresis. *Journal of Medical Internet Research, 10,* e16.

Stark, L. J., Opipari, L. C., Donaldson, D. L., Danovsky, M. B., Rasile, D. A., & DelSanto, A. F. (1997). Evaluation of a standard protocol for retentive encopresis: A replication. *Journal of Pediatric Psychology, 22,* 619–633.

Sureshkumar, P., Jones, M., Caldwell, P. H., & Craig, J. C. (2009). Risk factors for nocturnal enuresis in school-age children. *Journal of Urology, 182,* 2893–2899.

van der Plas, R. N., Benninga, M. A., Buller, H. A., Bossuyt, P. M., Akkermans, L. M., Redekop, W. K., et al. (1996). Biofeedback training in treatment of childhood constipation: A randomised controlled study. *Lancet, 348,* 776–780.

CHAPTER 25

Pediatric Traumatic Brain Injury

SHARI L. WADE

CLINICAL PRESENTATION
AND COMMON FEATURES
OF PEDIATRIC TRAUMATIC BRAIN INJURY

Traumatic brain injury (TBI) in children can result in significant cognitive, behavioral, and social impairment. Common cognitive consequences include impaired attention, slowed processing speed, perseveration, and deficits in inhibition, planning, and problem solving. Emerging behavior problems occur in up to three-quarters of children who have sustained a severe TBI (Schwartz et al., 2003). Although there is a high incidence of secondary attention-deficit/hyperactivity disorder (SADHD), problems with emotional lability, aggression, and anxiety and/or obsessive–compulsive symptoms are also possible. These cognitive and behavioral changes are often accompanied by impairments in social interactions due to difficulties reading social cues, maintaining the thread of a conversation, inhibiting inappropriate responses, and planning or implementing an appropriate response. Children with TBI are also at high risk for legal difficulties because of their slowed processing and impaired judgment; they are drawn into schemes by peers and then get caught because they are unable to respond as quickly or as easily as others (Williams, Cordan, Mewse, Tonks, & Burgess, 2010).

Although behavioral and social consequences are often the most troubling problems for families, children with TBI often struggle academically as well (Ewing-Cobbs et al., 2004). Academic difficulties can be puzzling for parents and teachers because IQ and achievement test scores often fall within the normal range while the child is failing in the classroom. This discrepancy between ability and performance may be attributable to difficulties processing and integrating information amid typical classroom distractions. Difficulties with shifting attention, slowed processing speed, impaired working memory, and poor problem solving may all adversely affect classroom performance. Given that the effects of such executive function deficits may be less apparent in the context of an office-based assessment, it is critical to couple traditional neuropsychological assessments with classroom observations.

PREDICTORS OF RECOVERY

There is wide variability in outcomes even among children with similar injury severity. Premorbid functioning, earlier age at injury, and family dysfunction and disadvantage all are associated with poorer behavioral outcomes (Gerring & Wade, 2012); however, their relationship to postinjury cognitive deficits is less clear-cut. Assessing these factors can aid in treatment planning and can suggest avenues for interventions. The psychologist can also play an important role in family adjustment by sharing with the family, early in recovery, the facts that child and family outcomes vary greatly and are difficult to predict.

THE ROLE
OF NEUROPSYCHOLOGICAL ASSESSMENT

Comprehensive neuropsychological assessment can be very helpful in evaluating the effects of the injury on cognitive and academic abilities and in developing treatment recommendations tailored to the child's unique strengths and needs. Any assessment should include measures of attention and executive function skills, because they are frequently affected by TBI and play a role in academic and social functioning. Evaluations of speech and language abilities (including pragmatic language and discourse) to identify communication deficits can also be helpful, whether conducted by a neuropsychologist or speech language pathologist. It is critical to evaluate how the child's performance is affected in everyday settings, such as the classroom or the community. Given the impact of behavioral factors on cognitive performance, it is also critical to assess the child's emotional and behavioral functioning to identify factors that promote optimal functioning. Given the close association between parent/family functioning and the child's recovery post-TBI, the evaluating psychologist should also assess parental distress and coping, as well as family strengths and dysfunction.

EVIDENCE-BASED APPROACHES TO TREATMENT

Emerging evidence supports the potential utility of several different approaches to address the cognitive, behavioral, and family consequences of TBI, depending on the child's age and injury severity. Single-case studies and uncontrolled trials provide tentative evidence that behavioral approaches, particularly those that focus on the antecedents of problem behaviors and on structuring the environment to support optimal functioning, can be effective in reducing disruptive behaviors (Feeney & Ylvisaker, 1995). Three recent studies also support the utility of parent skills training to reduce behavior problems, particularly in younger children (Wade, Oberjohn, Burkhardt & Greenberg, 2009; Wade, Oberjohn, Conaway, Osinska, & Bangert, 2011; Woods, Catroppa, Giallo, Matthews, & Anderson, 2012).

Several randomized trials provide support for the utility of family problem-solving therapy in reducing child behavior problems (Wade, Carey & Wolfe, 2006a, 2006b; Wade, Walz, Carey, et al.; 2010; Wade, Walz, et al., 2011) and parental distress (Wade et al., 2006b). Findings suggest that older children and adolescents and those from economically disadvantaged families may be particularly likely to benefit from these approaches. Problem-solving training may also serve as a metacognitive heuristic for adolescents with TBI, contributing to improvements in executive dysfunction and behavior, particularly when combined with self-regulation training and metacognitive strategies (Catroppa, Anderson, & Muscara, 2009; Wade, Walz, Carey, et al., 2010; Wade, Walz, et al., 2011).

Thus standard behavioral and cognitive-behavioral approaches are likely to be helpful if applied in the context of knowledge of the child's pattern of strengths and deficits and the family's functioning. Given that pediatric TBI is a relatively common condition and that knowledgeable therapists are lacking, a pediatric or child clinical psychologist is likely to be called upon to treat a child with consequences of TBI at some point in his or her career.

CASE EXAMPLE: CARTER

As the following case illustrates, TBI can profoundly alter the course of a child's development at a variety of levels while also affecting family, parent/

caregiver, and sibling functioning. Thus the roles for a pediatric psychologist are varied (assessment, discharge planning, academic planning and consulting with the schools, individual and family therapy) and continue over the course of the child's development to adulthood. Developmental transitions often spark a need for additional evaluation and treatment, particularly as opportunities for greater autonomy (e.g., driving) arise. Although initial assessment and treatment planning are highly interdisciplinary, involving input from various medical specialists (neurosurgeons, physiatrists, neurologists, pediatric neuropsychologists, speech pathologists, physical therapists, occupational therapists, and other allied professionals), most children with TBI (from mild to severe) receive few services of any type beyond the initial year postinjury, despite persistent, and at times intensifying, difficulties.

Carter was 13 years old when he sustained a severe TBI after being struck by a motor vehicle. He spent 2 weeks in the intensive care unit, in critical condition and on a respirator. His injury resulted in substantial white matter shearing, causing disruptions in neural connectivity. Brain stem swelling and focal injuries produced motor weakness and right-sided hemiplegia. As he regained consciousness, the extent of his deficits became apparent. During his subsequent 2-month hospitalization on an inpatient rehabilitation unit, Carter received intensive physical, speech, and occupational therapy to help him learn to walk and talk again. His family worked with a psychologist to assist them in understanding and coping with the cognitive and behavioral effects of Carter's injury.

Carter was the older of two children from a close-knit, financially secure family. Prior to his injury, he was an A student in the seventh grade and involved in numerous extracurricular activities, including scouting and hockey. He was gregarious and well liked by peers and teachers. Thus he benefited from social resources and supports, as well as a high level of premorbid functioning factors that promoted his recovery.

Neuropsychological assessment at the time of hospital discharge revealed deficits in a number of areas, including processing speed, attention, inhibition, and planning. Although his verbal IQ was still solidly in the average range, it was likely lower than before. His performance IQ was adversely affected by physical weakness that affected his right side, as well as by problems inhibiting impulsive responding. He displayed significant language difficulties, including problems with word-finding, rambling, tangential speech, perseveration on certain ideas or thoughts, and difficulties maintaining reciprocity in conversation. Difficulties with inhibition caused him to blurt out rude and inappropriate remarks, a source of embarrassment for his sibling.

Carter's family experienced numerous stresses as a result of his injury. During the lengthy hospitalization, Carter's mother spent most of her time in the hospital, while his father continued to work full time. As a consequence, his 8-year-old sister received limited attention. She was unsure of what was going on at the hospital and whether her brother would survive his injuries. Although she continued to do well in school, she developed anxiety symptoms and began sleeping in her parents' bed.

Carter's mother was a vigorous advocate for Carter's recovery and care during the course of his hospitalization, but she was exhausted and clinically depressed by the time he returned home from the hospital. The marital relationship had also become strained due to limited time together and different styles of coping (Wade, Walz, Cassedy, et al., 2010). As a consequence, the parents weren't able to effectively provide support to one another during this time.

Carter's family would have benefited from both individual and family-centered treatment at this time to address the multiple individual and family level concerns; Carter may have benefited from treatment with stimulant medication for his SADHD symptoms, which included poor concentration, distractibility, excessive talking, and difficulty remaining seated. However, Carter's family did not pursue referrals for psychological services at this time. This is a common response following severe TBI for several reasons. Family resources are directed toward physical recovery while the child typically receives multiple therapies (physical, speech, occupational) each week. Given the focus on medical issues, relatively less attention is given to cognitive and behavioral concerns. Additionally, families are reluctant to acknowledge the possibility of persistent cognitive and/or behavioral deficits. Parents downplay their distress and marital tensions, attributing them to situational stresses. Although parental depression often resolves without treatment, child cognitive–behavioral difficulties and marital tensions may intensify.

Carter returned to school after missing nearly half a year. The pediatric neuropsychologist and school reentry coordinator from the inpatient rehabilitation unit worked together with the school to craft accommodations, such as reduced hours and additional time for tests and assignments. An individualized education plan (IEP) identified specific academic and behavioral goals and plans for achieving them. Because behavioral consequences (such as rewards and punishments) are often not effective in controlling problem behaviors following TBI, the pediatric neuropsychologist worked with the school psychologist and Carter's teachers to adapt the school environment with particular emphasis on structuring the classroom to facilitate successful performance. For example, they moved his seat to the front of the classroom, where distractions were less likely, and planned for breaks during the class period. The teachers were encouraged to ignore disinhibited behavior (such as getting out of his seat) or off-target comments rather than punishing Carter for them.

Carter was fortunate because his school was eager to work with hospital personnel to help him get back to grade-level expectations. Children with less severe injuries or more complicated psychosocial histories may not be identified as eligible for necessary school services, yet they may require even more extensive involvement from a psychologist to recommend accommodations and to advocate for their implementation (Glang et al., 2008). For children with premorbid behavioral issues or ADHD, it may be particularly hard to distinguish the effects of the TBI, although their symptoms are likely to be more intense and less responsive to traditional behavior management strategies.

Carter's social life changed dramatically as a result of his TBI. Before the injury, Carter had been popular with peers. Although many children continued to identify him as a friend after the injury, no one considered him to be a best friend or chose to spend much time with him. As a once avid hockey player, many of his closest friends had been his teammates. Although his neurologist reluctantly allowed him to participate in pre-season camps with the rest of the team, she advised him to never again play contact sports due to the potentially fatal consequences of reinjury. Changes in Carter's personality, coupled with lack of contact with his teammates, caused his friendships with other boys on the team to fall away. Carter's parents responded to these changes by spending more time with him and identifying new activities for him, shifting attention away from their daughter.

Carter's social difficulties were less apparent than they are for many children with TBI because he maintained superficial contacts with previous friends. Often, disinhibition and dysregulation following TBI are manifested in explosive outbursts and physical aggression, particularly in boys. Deficits in self-awareness and difficulties in reading social cues may compound difficulties with peers and authority figures. Peers, parents, and teachers often fail to link the aggressive behavior to the TBI, leading to peer avoidance, rejection, academic suspensions, and expulsions for aggressive behavior.

Eighteen months following Carter's injury, he and his family were enrolled in a family problem-solving therapy program to address some of the unresolved concerns surrounding his injury. This was the first psychological treatment that the family had received since discharge from inpatient rehabilitation. This structured program of 11 sessions delivered by a psychologist over a 6-month period involved the entire family and provided training in problem solving and communication skills, as well as education regarding the common consequences of TBI and behavioral strategies for addressing them (see Wade, Michaud, & Brown, 2006, for a complete description).

Interview and questionnaire data regarding Carter's behavior and functioning at intake revealed continuing difficulties with attention and executive functioning skills. Although he was receiving A's and B's in ninth grade, maintaining these grades required long hours of homework and considerable parental support. His sister continued to report feelings of anxiety, as well as irritation with Carter, over what she perceived as provocative behavior. Carter's mother's depression had not fully resolved. Carter's father reported minimal psychological distress, engaging in active coping strategies and increased involvement in his job. The couple reported a strong marriage although there were conflicts over Carter, with the father perceiving the mother as overly protective. This is a common dynamic following TBI and often results in communication difficulties due to differing perspectives on the injured child's abilities and vulnerabilities.

The initiation of treatment represented the first time that the family had discussed Carter's injury and how it affected them. Although Carter clearly had challenges and limitations that were not present before the injury, the family was reluctant to acknowledge losses, instead focusing on their gratitude for Carter's remarkable recovery. For children with TBI and their families, there is an ongoing tension between realistic hope for further recovery and denial of the extent of disability; this tension was apparent in Carter's family and in how they described his current functioning. For the psychologist working with a child and his or her family following TBI, it is critical to respect their perceptions of recovery while gently pointing out areas for potential growth or accommodation. Otherwise, families are likely to drop out.

The program teaches strategies for cognitive monitoring (e.g., being mindful of self-statements and their effect on one's well-being), reframing (e.g., changing negative or critical beliefs to positive adaptive ones), and relaxation (e.g., deep breathing, positive imagery, and self-care). During the session on cognitive reframing and staying positive, Carter's mother recognized that her self-perception and mood were affected by negative cognitions she had about Carter, herself, her family, and the future. The therapist worked with her to use strategies for cognitive monitoring, reframing, and relaxation to address these negative thoughts. As a result she experienced a significant reduction in depressive symptoms during the initial several weeks of treatment.

As treatment shifted from cognitive reframing to problem solving, each family member identified a range of goals to address using problem-solving strategies. These included reducing conflict between Carter and his sister, helping the sister feel less anxious about being alone, and identifying opportunities for Carter to engage with peers now that he was no longer involved in contact sports. The entire family participated in refining these goals, brainstorming about options, examining the pros and cons of various solutions, and crafting a detailed plan for implementing their agreed-upon solution.

Part of the treatment involved helping both Carter and his family understand that his disinhibited behavior (blurting out offensive comments, dropping his pants in class) represented the effects of TBI and not a need for attention. Linking behavioral changes to the brain insult is critically important following TBI because parents and teachers are likely to misattribute such behaviors to other factors (e.g., being spoiled while in the hospital, laziness), resulting in unhelpful behavior management strategies. Behavioral analysis can be useful in identifying environmental antecedents or triggers of problem behaviors and developing a plan for environmental modifications and supports (Feeney & Ylvisaker, 1995).

In Carter's case, the family brainstormed about how to respond to these inappropriate behaviors and agreed on a hand signal that would remind Carter that his behavior was "out of bounds" and that he should "chill out." The psychologist also worked directly with Carter to help him to stop and think before acting and to watch the reactions of others for feedback about his behavior's effect on them. Together these strategies minimized the inappropriate comments and actions, although it did not eliminate them entirely. The treating psychologist worked with the school psychologist to adapt these behavioral plans for the classroom setting and to incorporate them into Carter's IEP. Ongoing communication between providers and school throughout the course of recovery is critical for ensuring the successful implementation of treatment recommendations as they evolve.

Given Carter's SADHD symptom severity, the psychologist referred him to a psychiatrist for medication evaluation. The use of methylphenidate for treatment of attention problems after pediatric TBI is common in clinical practice; however, evidence regarding its efficacy is limited and contradictory (Pangilinan, Giacoletti-Argento, Shellhaas, Hurvitz, & Hornyak, 2010). For this reason, it is particularly important to closely monitor behavioral response and side effects as the dosage level is titrated. Carter reported an improvement in his ability to focus, and his teachers noted a reduction in off-task and out-of-seat behaviors when he was taking the medication, providing evidence that it was a useful addition to behavioral strategies in his case.

Carter's sister's anxiety continued to be an issue and thus became a focus of treatment. She was able to express her fears about Carter nearly dying as a result of his injury, as well as her own feelings of vulnerability. Together, she and her parents developed a successful behavioral plan to help her feel comfortable being alone, including sleeping in her own bed.

The limited research on the effects of TBI on siblings suggests that siblings may experience disruptions in emotional well-being and self-esteem (Sambuco, Brookes, Catroppa, & Lah, 2012). Changes in family dynamics, such as reductions in parental attention, shifting roles, and increased responsibilities for household chores, may contribute to sibling distress. Siblings who witnessed the injury may also experience symptoms of post-traumatic stress disorder, which may go unrecognized because of the focus on the injured child. Additionally, siblings may become socially isolated because of embarrassment over the injured child's behavior in public. Thus, treating psychologists should always be sensitive to how siblings are coping.

As the time-limited treatment program neared completion, focus turned toward planning for the future and anticipating the difficulties that may accompany developmental transitions, including moving from middle school to high school and beginning to drive, date, and work independently. Carter and his family were encouraged to anticipate potential problems (e.g., starting high school), to use the problem-solving process to identify potential solution(s) that were acceptable to all, and to develop concrete plans for implementation (e.g., meeting with teachers and guidance counselors over the summer to discuss academic needs and potential behavioral concerns). Because issues associated with TBI, such as disinhibited behavior and executive dysfunction, can be lifelong, it is important to consider how these issues may manifest themselves in the future and how to translate current lessons, including the problem-solving process, to future challenges. As Carter's family completed treatment, each family member endorsed an increased understanding of how Carter was affected by his injury and strategies for responding to the ongoing behavioral changes and family stresses. Subsequent treatment will likely be needed in the future to address development transitions and emerging problems.

CONCLUSION

TBI can result in a complex constellation of cognitive, behavioral, and social consequences, as well as persistent medical problems (e.g., seizures) in some cases. The roles for pediatric psychologists are diverse and cycle over the course of recovery, from assessment, treatment planning, and community reintegration to behavior management and family treatment to long-term follow-up. Mounting evidence suggests that individuals who experience TBI may also be at increased risk for later difficulties, including traumatic chronic encephalopathy and dementia (DeKosky, Ikonomovic, & Gandy, 2010). Thus it is important to provide opportunities for follow-up, including updated assessment, proactive problem solving, and treatment throughout the lifespan. The need for ongoing monitoring and follow-up is particularly important following a TBI in early childhood that may be forgotten or minimized as the child reaches adolescence or adulthood.

REFERENCES

Catroppa, C., Anderson, V. A., & Muscara, F. (2009). Rehabilitation of executive skills post-childhood traumatic brain injury (TBI): A pilot intervention study. *Developmental NeuroRehabilitation, 12*, 361–369.

DeKosky, S. T., Ikonomovic, M. D., & Gandy, S. (2010). Traumatic brain injury: Football, warfare, and long-term effects. *New England Journal of Medicine, 363*, 1293–1296.

Ewing-Cobbs, L., Barnes, M., Fletcher, J. M., Levin, H. S., Swank, P. R., & Song, J. (2004). Modeling of longitudinal academic achievement scores after pediatric traumatic brain injury. *Developmental Neuropsychology, 25*, 107–133.

Feeney, T. J., & Ylvisaker, M. (1995). Choice and routine: Antecedent behavioral interventions for adolescents with severe traumatic brain injury. *Journal of Head Trauma Rehabilitation, 10*, 67–86.

Gerring, J., & Wade, S. L. (2012). The essential role of psychosocial risk and protective factors in pediatric TBI research. *Journal of Neurotrauma, 29*, 621–628.

Glang, A., Todis, B., Thomas, C., Hood, D., Bedell, G., & Cockrell, J. (2008). Return to school following childhood TBI: Who gets services? *NeuroRehabilitation, 23*, 477–486.

Pangilinan, P. H., Giacoletti-Argento, A., Shellhaas, R., Hurvitz, E. A., & Hornyak. J. E. (2010). Neuropharmacology in pediatric brain injury: A review. *Physical Medicine and Rehabilitation, 2*, 1127–1140.

Sambuco, M., Brookes, N., Catroppa, C., & Lah, S. (2012). Predictors of long-term sibling behavioral outcome and self-esteem following pediatric traumatic brain injury. *Journal of Head Trauma Rehabilitation, 27*(6), 413–423.

Schwartz, L., Taylor, H. G., Drotar, D., Yeates, K. O., Wade, S. L., & Stancin, T. (2003). Long-term behavior problems following pediatric traumatic brain injury: Prevalence, predictors, and correlates. *Journal of Pediatric Psychology, 28*, 251–263.

Wade, S. L., Carey, J., & Wolfe, C. R. (2006a). The efficacy of an online cognitive-behavioral family intervention in improving child behavior and social competence following pediatric brain injury. *Rehabilitation Psychology, 51*, 179–189.

Wade, S. L., Carey, J., & Wolfe, C. R. (2006b). An online family intervention to reduce parental distress following pediatric brain injury. *Journal of Consulting and Clinical Psychology, 74*, 445–454.

Wade, S. L., Michaud, L., & Brown, T. M. (2006). Putting the pieces together: Preliminary efficacy of a family problem-solving intervention for children with traumatic brain injury. *Journal of Head Trauma Rehabilitation, 21*, 57–67.

Wade, S. L., Oberjohn, K., Burkhardt, A., & Greenberg, I. (2009). Feasibility and preliminary efficacy of a web-based parenting skills program for young children with traumatic brain injury. *Journal of Head Trauma Rehabilitation, 24*, 239–247.

Wade, S. L., Oberjohn, K., Conaway, K., Osinska, P., & Bangert, L. (2011). Live coaching of parenting skills using the Internet: Implications for clinical practice. *Professional Psychology: Research and Practice, 42*, 487–493.

Wade, S. L., Walz, N. C., Carey, J., McMullen, K. M., Cass, J., Mark, E., et al. (2011). Effect on behavior problems of teen online problem-solving for adolescent traumatic brain injury. *Pediatrics, 128,* e947–e953.

Wade, S. L., Walz, N. C., Carey, J., Williams, K. M., Cass, J., Herren, L., et al. (2010). A randomized trial of teen online problem solving for improving executive function deficits following pediatric traumatic brain injury. *Journal of Head Trauma Rehabilitation, 25,* 409–415.

Wade, S. L., Walz, N. C., Cassedy, A., Taylor, H. G., Stancin, T., & Yeates, K. O. (2010). Caregiver functioning following early childhood TBI: Do moms and dads respond differently? *NeuroRehabilitation, 27,* 63–72.

Williams, H. W., Cordan, G., Mewse, A. J., Tonks, J., & Burgess, C. N. W. (2010). Self-reported traumatic brain injury in male young offenders: A risk factor for re-offending, poor mental health and violence? *Neuropsychological Rehabilitation, 20,* 801–812.

Woods, D. T., Catroppa, C., Giallo, R., Matthews, J., & Anderson, V. A. (2012). Feasibility and consumer satisfaction ratings following an intervention for families who have a child with acquired brain injury. *NeuroRehabilitation, 30,* 189–198.

CHAPTER 26

End of Life
in the Pediatric Population

VICTORIA W. WILLARD
VALERIE McLAUGHLIN CRABTREE
SEAN PHIPPS

Approximately 50,000 infants, children, and adolescents die each year in the United States, according to the most recent report from the Health Resources and Services Administration (U.S. Department of Health and Human Services [DHHS], 2011). More than half of these deaths occur during infancy, with congenital malformations and extreme prematurity/low birth weight as the leading causes. Among children and adolescents ages 1–19 years, unintentional injuries are the leading cause of death, followed by congenital anomalies and cancer in children ages 1–14 and by homicide and suicide in adolescents ages 15–19. In adolescents, cancer and heart disease comprise the fourth and fifth leading causes of death, respectively (DHHS, 2011). Recent advances in technology and medical care have resulted in children and adolescents living longer with life-limiting illnesses, creating an increased need for pediatric palliative care services (Friebert, 2009; Himelstein, Hilden, Boldt, & Weissman, 2004). For those pediatric patients who die following a life-threatening or life-limiting illness, high-quality care, both physical and psychological, during their illness and at the end of life is essential.

High-quality palliative care for children is universally described as an integrated team approach to alleviating suffering in children and their families. Within this integrated team approach, the psychological needs of the child and family must be attended to, in addition to physical, spiritual, psychosocial, and practical needs (Committee on Bioethics and Committee on Hospital Care, 2000; European Association for Palliative Care Taskforce for Palliative Care in Children, 2009; Himelstein et al., 2004). According to the American Academy of Pediatrics, "The goal [of palliative care] is to add life to the child's years, not simply years to the child's life" (Committee on Bioethics and Committee on Hospital Care, 2000, p. 353). Quality palliative care must support the family as a whole, involve the child and family in decision making and care planning, relieve pain and other symptoms, ensure continuity of care, provide in-depth psychological support for parents and siblings, and provide grief and bereavement support for the family (Dokken et al., 2001; Friebert, 2009). To provide appropriate guidance in decision making, providers caring for children at the end of life and their families must have an understanding of child development and must be able to communicate sensitive information at developmentally appropriate levels to children (Himelstein et al., 2004).

Quality pediatric palliative care includes the need for interdisciplinary teams to meet psychological needs, to understand child development while including the child and family in decision making, to alleviate symptoms at the end of life, and to provide bereavement care for parents and siblings. This interdisciplinary team approach clearly supports the need for psychologists to integrate into palliative care teams, and psychologists are uniquely qualified to provide this aspect of family-centered care.

PSYCHOLOGICAL CARE
OF CHILDREN AT THE END OF LIFE

The research on pediatric end-of-life care in the past two decades has focused largely on symptoms, symptom management, and medical decision making (Drake, Frost & Collins, 2003; Maurer et al., 2010; Wolfe et al., 2000). Much of this research has focused on reports of parents rather than patients and has utilized retrospective designs that are limited by potential biases in recall (Phipps & Noll, 2010). Nevertheless, these studies suggest that the symptom burden near the end of life is high, that pain and symptom management is not always optimal, and that suboptimal symptom management at the time of death is a risk factor for problematic grief reactions in parents (Kreicbergs et al., 2005).

There are several potential roles for the pediatric psychologist in the end-of-life setting, either as a consultant or as part of a palliative care team.

Although there are no empirically based interventions specifically developed for end of life, there are numerous well-validated approaches, both to intervention and assessment, to which psychologists can provide unique expertise. Certainly, provision of accurate assessment of patient symptoms using empirically supported measures of pain, fatigue, mood disturbance, and other aspects of psychological functioning, are crucial to medical management. Participation in pain management, including direct provision of nonpharmacological pain interventions, as well as education of patients and families regarding appropriate expectations for palliation, are additional areas for psychologists' involvement (see McLaughlin & Gillespie, Chapter 12, and Lynch-Jordan, Chapter 13, in this volume for more information on pain management).

COMMUNICATION AND DECISION MAKING

Parents and families must communicate with the medical team throughout their child's illness. From diagnosis through treatment and perhaps up to and including end of life, conversations between parents and medical teams are likely frequent and may be fraught with difficult decisions. Indeed, particularly as treatment options are exhausted, there may be a need for conversations that switch focus from curative to palliative, and decisions regarding end-of-life care must be made. Research with parents regarding end-of-life decisions has identified a number of factors that may influence families' ability to make decisions regarding their child's end-of-life care, including trusting in and feeling supported by the medical team, having information about their child's status and time to process this information, observing changes in their child, valuing their child's preferences, maintaining religious faith, and ultimately doing what is needed to feel like a good parent (Hinds & Kelly, 2010; Hinds et al., 2009).

With these discussions of such a sensitive nature, there is likely a role for pediatric psychologists to help facilitate these conversations by guiding parents in making their wishes known and advocating for their child. Psychologists may also serve in a supportive role to other members of the medical care team, and their presence may help to reduce potential for avoidance of difficult discussions that could lead to a perception of abandonment by the patient and family. This is critically important, because absence of staff at the time of death is a significant predictor of parent distress, a fact that points to the "centrality of nonabandonment" as a guiding principle of end-of-life care (Solomon & Browning, 2005). Finally, psychologists may also have a role in helping parents speak with their children: to provide education and reassurance regarding the developmental understanding of the child and to encourage open and honest conversations that are simple, straightforward, and understandable to all parties.

Children's Involvement in Decision Making

Discussion of death with children calls for an appreciation of what children are likely to understand about death. Research on children's understanding of death has indicated four separate components of death concepts: non-functionality, irreversibility, universality, and causality (Cotton & Range, 1990; Speece & Brent, 1996). Nonfunctionality refers to the understanding that all life-defining bodily functions cease at death. Irreversibility is the understanding that once the physical body dies it cannot be made alive again. Universality refers to the understanding that all living things, including the self, must eventually die. Causality is the understanding that there are physical or biological events that lead to death. The literature suggests that each of these concepts emerges from separate developmental continuums. Speece and Brent (1996) suggest that by the age of 7, the majority of children have achieved a mature understanding of these concepts. Others have disputed this and suggest that, in addition to chronological age, understanding of death depends on the child's cognitive functioning and experiences with death; but there is a consensus that virtually all typically developing children will demonstrate understanding of these concepts no later than age 12 (Cotton & Range, 1990).

Although parents ultimately have the legal right to make decisions regarding the care of their children, it is recommended that the preferences of children and adolescents be considered. Research in the 1970s indicated that regardless of whether or not physicians or parents informed the child about his or her prognosis, the child was generally acutely aware of his or her dire situation, and a failure to openly acknowledge this contributed to the children's increasing isolation (Bluebond-Langner, 1978; Spinetta, 1974; Waechter, 1971). It was these studies that provided the basis for advocating more open communication with children in the context of life-threatening illness. However, it is often very difficult for parents and children to engage in these discussions, and both parties are often reluctant to broach the topic (Bluebond-Langner, Belasco, & Wander, 2010; Whitty-Rogers, Alex, MacDonald, Pierrynowski Gallant, & Austin, 2009). Ultimately, when deciding whether a child should be involved in decision making, the child's capacity to understand the options and consequences must be determined. Furthermore, parents may have preferences regarding what types of decisions they want their children involved in, with some questions deemed too burdensome or difficult (Bluebond-Langner et al., 2010; Whitty-Rogers et al., 2009).

Bluebond-Langner and colleagues (2010) outlined several factors that must be considered when involving a child in medical decision-making conversations, including child-specific factors such as age, experiences, view of illness, and potential actions to protect his or her parents, and parent-specific factors, such as their understanding of the illness and prognosis and their preferences regarding a child's role in the discussion and what the child should be told. Finally, the parent–child relationship is also particularly important to consider, especially with respect to typical decision-making practices in the family, remembering that children are likely to defer to their parents. Similarly, one also needs to consider social and cultural factors that may influence a family's preferences. Pediatric psychologists may play a particular role in helping to determine the influence of such factors on a child's participation in medical decision making. More specifically, they can help determine a child's cognitive and developmental capacity to understand, can assist parents in determining what decisions they are comfortable allowing their child to participate in, and/or can help a child express his or her wishes to his or her parents in a manner that respects the parent–child relationship. Ultimately, a balance must be found between the desire to include a child in such decisions and the rights of parents to decide what is best for their child.

In one of the few recent studies that directly assessed the viewpoint of the terminally ill child, Hinds and colleagues (2005) interviewed children and adolescents (age 10 years and up) with advanced cancer after an end-of-life decision had been made. They found that these children understood the implications of this end-of-life decision and were capable of participating and desired to participate in this decision process. The children's decisions were influenced primarily by their concern for others, particularly their parents, and were surprisingly altruistic in nature. Their findings confirm the understanding of children regarding the terminal nature of their illness and support the ability of children age 10 and up to participate in end-of-life decisions on their own behalf. In practice, however, children are often excluded from such discussions.

In a population-based study from Sweden, parents who had lost a child with cancer were queried about whether they had talked about death with their children (Kreicbergs, et al., 2004). Only 34% had spoken with their children about death. Interestingly, none of those who talked with their children about death expressed any regret about it, whereas 27% of those who had not spoken with their children about death regretted not having done so. Clearly, this is another area in which the input of pediatric psychologists can be critical: in assessing the child's understanding and readiness to engage in such discussions, in assuaging the reluctance of parents or medical staff to broach such difficult issues, and in facilitating discussions when indicated.

CASE EXAMPLES

To illustrate the psychologist's role in facilitating communication with pediatric patients at the end of life, we provide two brief case vignettes reflecting opposite ends of a continuum of patient readiness to discuss issues about death and dying.

Case Example 1

Maria was a 16-year-old with cystic fibrosis who was having increasing problems with panic attacks during a prolonged inpatient admission. The panic was triggered by disease-related breathing difficulties, and Maria verbalized a strong fear that she was about to die during these attacks. She frequently brought up her fear of dying with medical staff, who tried to reassure her that her condition was not that serious. The attending physician who ordered the psychology consultation emphasized that the patient was "not terminal" and requested help with anxiety reduction. In the initial meeting with the consultation–liaison (C-L) psychologist, Maria acknowledged immediately her high level of anxiety and her belief that she was likely to die soon. She did not feel reassured by medical staff, whom she felt were lying to protect her. As she talked about this, her anxiety escalated, and she became more agitated. The psychologist did not dispute her belief that she was failing but rather attempted to explore what the possibility of death meant to her. Maria began to focus on things she was afraid she might not get to do before she died. With further discussion of specific events that she did not want to miss (e.g., going to the prom; graduating from high school), she became more relaxed and animated. Eventually, we were able to use imagery of these events intentionally to induce a relaxation response.

In the subsequent meeting, Maria reported that she continued to have almost constant anxious thoughts about dying. This fear was addressed with psychoeducation and a paradoxical suggestion. Her problem was reframed from fear of death to a lack of control over the fear. In order to gain control, it was suggested that she stop attempting to avoid thinking about it but set aside a certain time each day to think about dying. This paradoxical intervention is likely to have a positive impact regardless of patient adherence. Maria subsequently reported having difficulty thinking about death on command at a specific time, but in response to the attempt, the frequency of her death-related thoughts were declining, and those thoughts were less anxious. At this point, the psychologist also needed to do some psychoeducation with the medical staff, many of whom, including the attending physician, were very concerned about the nature of these recommendations given their still firmly held belief that the patient was doing well. In fact, Maria remained in the hospital, and her physical state gradually declined. The psychologist continued to work with Maria several times per week, with treatment focused on two main approaches: (1) processing death-related thoughts and fears, giving Maria an opportunity to do this in session so that she could be free of these thoughts at other times, and (2) anxiety reduction with relaxation/imagery work. The imagery of Maria's choosing typically involved places and activities she hoped to do before she died and, paradoxically, had a profoundly relaxing effect.

Maria's parents were divorced. Maria had a close relationship with her mother, who was the primary caregiver. In a separate meeting with the psychologist, her mother shared that she was very worried about Maria's medical status, but she attempted to hide this from Maria in order to avoid increasing Maria's fear. The psychologist was able to clarify that Maria suspected this of her mother and of many of her medical caregivers as well. Her mother was encouraged to be more forthright in her discussions with Maria. Another of Maria's death-related fears was how her mother would be able to function if she died. This concern led to some conjoint sessions in which mother and daughter were able to more openly share their concerns with each other.

Despite the reassurances of the medical staff, Maria's medical status continued to decline. She was never discharged from the hospital, and she died 6 weeks after the initial psychology consultation. Her panic attacks improved initially, but as her condition worsened, her anxiety increased, and this was difficult to manage even with aggressive pharmacological and nonpharmacological interventions. From a purely objective standpoint, intervention for the presenting problem might be considered a treatment failure. However, by allowing the patient to express her fears and facilitating a more open communication about them, Maria was able to have some intimate end-of-life conversations with her mother that might otherwise not have occurred.

The previous case is somewhat atypical in the direct way that death issues remained consistently at the forefront of the work. More commonly, patients will tend to be avoidant of and unlikely to directly address such issues. A question, then, for the clinician is how much to push for direct discussion of issues of death, loss, and end-of-life decisions. This will depend on many factors, most notably the nature of the presenting problem, but also the patient's developmental status and his or her defensive posture, the family environment and family wishes, and the strength of the patient–therapist relationship. In most cases, it is prudent to respect the patients' defenses, but if one wishes to confront or to push for more direct discussion of the issue, there must be a well-established therapeutic alliance for this to be fruitful. Because breaching these difficult topics can be threatening for the clinician as well as the patient, it calls for a high level of therapist self-awareness and is a circumstance in which supervision or consultation with colleagues should always be considered.

Case Example 2: Carlos

Carlos was a 15-year-old Hispanic male with nasopharyngeal carcinoma who had already been receiving treatment for 6 months and had metastatic disease when a psychology consultation was ordered, after he had a transient episode of acute mental status changes. A neurological workup, including an electroencephalogram (EEG) and a brain magnetic resonance imaging (MRI), was negative. When seen by the psychologist the next day, Carlos was fully oriented and coherent but demonstrated a rather flat, subdued affect and acknowledged feeling significantly depressed. An etiology for the mental status changes was never confirmed, but the psychologist began following Carlos, focusing on his depressive symptoms. He was seen weekly when he returned for clinic visits and more frequently when he was an inpatient. This treatment lasted for the next 16 months until his death.

Already at the time of the initial consultation Carlos's prognosis was very poor, and his chance for long-term survival slim. However, Carlos did not bring this up, and it was not clear how well he appreciated his chances. His parents did not discuss this with him and were reluctant to discuss it themselves, but they did not object to medical staff, including the psychologist, having frank discussions with Carlos. In sessions over the next several months, the psychologist worked with Carlos on a number of illness-related concerns, particularly how these affected his family, school, and social lives. Nonpharmacological pain management was also a major focus. However, Carlos did not bring up end-of-life issues, nor express thoughts or worries that he might not survive, and the therapist's attempts to subtly or gently bring the discussion to this topic went nowhere. As the psychologist struggled with this, debating how, and how hard, to push, an opportunity was provided with the death of another patient who was a friend of Carlos's.

In a session after he had been informed of his friend's death, Carlos described how he had become close to three friends who had died from cancer. When the therapist suggested this must be frightening, Carlos denied this, stating, "No, it's not scary, it's just sad," with tears welling up. After providing some empathic support, the psychologist persisted, again suggesting that these events must make him worry about his own prognosis, and Carlos provided a clear answer, stating, "I don't know why, but ever since I was diagnosed, I never thought I would die from my disease." He went on to explain his thinking, related to his positive response to his first round of chemotherapy, and although some of it was magical, he ended with, "And I just knew I wasn't going to die from this." This was a clear time to respect the patient's defenses, and this striking communication informed the psychologist how best to respond to Carlos, which was to support him in his optimistic beliefs and future orientation, as this was the most adaptive coping style for him. Only much later, closer to the terminal phase and when he was more debilitated, did Carlos begin to acknowledge anxiety and the possibility that he would die. Even then, he did so rarely and tentatively, with statements such as, "I always thought I would be cured, but now my hopes are down." The psychologist's response in such moments was to accept Carlos's perspective with simple empathic statements, for example, "I'm sorry, it must be so hard," and not to attempt a more active processing of how he would like to handle final days, funerals, and so forth, because Carlos had made clear he could not tolerate such frank discussion. Fortunately, there were no crucial medical decisions that required Carlos's input, and the primary role of the psychologist in this case was provision of emotional support.

TOOLS FOR FACILITATING COMMUNICATION AND DECISIONS ABOUT END-OF-LIFE CARE

Although the ultimate goal of medical care is curative, when treatment options have been exhausted, it is necessary to change goals to focus on palliative and end-of-life care. With adult patients, end-of-life care is often carried out through such legal documents as living wills and durable powers of attorney. Unfortunately, access to similar legal documents is not widely available for children and adolescents, and there is significant variability across hospitals and illness types in how the need for such decisions is broached to the children and their families. However, tools are available that may help families to sift through the numerous decisions they need to make. These plans allow parents to put in writing decisions regarding medication usage, place of death (e.g. home, hospital, hospice), life support, and extraordinary measures. Although not all deaths are expected, when the opportunity to plan is available, it can remove pressure from families who are already anticipating the grief associated with losing a child and therefore may be unable to make their preferences known.

Wolff, Browne, and Whitehouse (2011) documented the creation of a *family-held personal resuscitation plan*, a document developed for the families of children with life-limiting neurodevelopmental conditions in the United Kingdom. The authors suggested that a typical hospital "do not resuscitate" order was not appropriate for their patients due to the potential number of hospitalizations and the lengthy deterioration period, and therefore they sought to develop a more comprehensive document. This document included information regarding the child's illness and reason for the plan, typical symptoms the child may show in an emergency situation, the family's wishes regarding potential interventions, and the contact information of important people, including the child's primary physician and family members (Wolff et al., 2011). The document is intended to remain with the child and to be provided to medical personnel who may be involved in the medical care of the child in a crisis situation; it is placed in the child's medical chart at his or her home hospital and registered with a national program in the United Kingdom.

In the United States, similar documents, known as *advance care plans*, are often used to help families and medical teams make decisions regarding care at the end of a child's life. The optimal time to initiate discussions regarding the creation of these documents is somewhat difficult to determine, but research suggests that they tend to be first initiated during an acute deterioration, with families not often interested in thinking about such decisions during times of stability (Edwards, Kun, Graham, & Keens, 2012). The advance care plan is typically considered a working document, with multiple discussions and revisions taking place as needed. Indeed, although the document may be first created during a time of relative stability, it can be adjusted over time as the child's condition changes or as families make decisions regarding their preferences.

Finally, tools and mechanisms are also available to guide a conversation with a child regarding end-of-life care and preferences. Booklets such as *My Wishes* (Aging with Dignity, 2006) help adults guide children through verbalizing their preferences. With questions or wishes that address subjects such as comfort, family, and placement, these booklets allow children the opportunity to make their own wishes known: whether to die at home or in a hospital, who they want to be around, and what they want their families and medical teams to know.

CONCLUSIONS

Infants and children who would have died quickly from illness several decades ago are now living longer with ongoing symptoms throughout the course of their illness. As a result of medical advances that have prolonged life in infants with congenital malformations and children with chronic illness, there is a growing need for palliative and end-of-life care for pediatric patients. Children at the end of life have a high burden of symptoms, both physical and psychological. Family members of children at the end of life also, as expected, experience significant distress, both during the child's illness and following his or her death. Because of the significant symptom burden and family distress, there is great need for interdisciplinary care teams to meet the physical and psychological needs of children at the end of life and their families. Psychologists are uniquely suited to provide an essential role as part of an interdisciplinary palliative care team or as consultants with children at the end of life.

Pediatric psychologists can serve an important role in assessing symptoms, including pain and emotional distress, while providing interventions to ameliorate these symptoms. Additionally, psychologists are well qualified to provide support to family members and caregivers who are witnessing the symptom burden in dying children while anticipating significant grief. Pediatric psychologists, as experts in child development, are essential members of the palliative care team with respect to recognizing the child's developmental understanding of death and dying, assessing the child's readiness to discuss such topics, and assisting parents and other team members in communicating openly with the child in developmentally appropriate ways. A psychologist may also serve the role of facilitator while assisting children and their families in communicating their needs and wishes to medical teams. As a member of a palliative care team or a consultant to the medical team, pediatric psychologists are well qualified to provide a wide spectrum of care for children at the end of life, from symptom assessment and management to communication facilitation.

REFERENCES

Aging with Dignity. (2006). *My wishes*. Tallahasse, FL: Aging with Dignity.

Bluebond-Langner, M. (1978). *The private worlds of dying children*. Princeton, NJ: Princeton University Press.

Bluebond-Langner, M., Belasco, J. B., & Wander, M. D. (2010). "I want to live until I don't want to live anymore": Involving children with life-threatening and life-shortening illnesses in decision making about care and treatment. *Nursing Clinics of North America, 45*, 239–343.

Committee on Bioethics and Committee on Hospital Care. (2000). Palliative care for children. *Pediatrics, 106*, 351–357.

Cotton, C. R., & Range, L. M. (1990). Children's death concepts: Relationship to cognitive functioning, age, experience with death, fear of death, and hopelessness. *Journal of Clinical Child Psychology, 19*, 123–127.

Dokken, D. L., Heller, K. S., Levetown, M., Rushton, C. H., Fleischman, A. R., Truog, R. D., et al.. (2002). *Quality domains, goals, and indicators of family-centered care of children living with life-threatening conditions*. Newton, MA: Education Development Center. Retrieved from *www.ippcweb.org/domains_eap.pdf*.

Drake, R., Frost, J., & Collins, J. J. (2003). The symptoms of dying children. *Journal of Pain and Symptom Management, 26*, 594–603.

Edwards, J. D., Kun, S. S., Graham, R. J., & Keens, T. G. (2012). End-of-life discussions and advance care planning for children on long-term assisted ventilation with life-limiting conditions. *Journal of Palliative Care, 28*, 21–27.

European Association for Palliative Care Taskforce for Palliative Care in Children. (2009). *Palliative care for infants, children, and young people: The facts.* Rome, Italy: Fondazione Maruzza Lefebvre D'Ovidio Onlus.

Friebert, S. (2009) . *NHPCO facts and figures: Pedatric palliative and hospice care in America.* Alexandra, VA: National Hospice and Palliative Care Organization.

Himelstein, B. P., Hilden, J. M., Boldt, A. M., & Weissman, D. (2004). Pediatric palliative care. *New England Journal of Medicine, 350*, 1752–1762.

Hinds, P. S., Drew, D., Oakes, L. L., Fouladi, M., Spunt, S. L., Church, C., et al. (2005). End-of-life care preferences of pediatric patients with cancer. *Journal of Clinical Oncology, 23*, 9146–9154.

Hinds, P. S., & Kelly, K. P. (2010). Helping parents make and survive end of life decisions for their seriously ill child. *Nursing Clinics of North America, 45*, 465–474.

Hinds, P. S., Oakes, L. L., Hicks, J., Powell, B., Srivastava, D. K., Spunt, S. L., et al. (2009). "Trying to be a good parent" as defined by interviews with parents who made Phase I, terminal care, and resuscitation decisions for their children. *Journal of Clinical Oncology, 27*, 5979–5985.

Kreicbergs, U., Valdimarsdottir, U., Onelov, E., Björk, O., Steineck, G., & Henter, J.-I. (2005). Care-related distress: A nationwide survey of parents who lost their child to cancer. *Journal of Clinical Oncology, 23*, 9162–9171.

Maurer, S. H., Hinds, P. S., Spunt, S. L., Furman, W. L., Kane, J. R., & Baker, J. N. (2010). Decision making by parents of children with incurable cancer who opt for enrollment on a phase I trial compared with choosing a do not resuscitate/terminal care option. *Journal of Clinical Oncology, 28*, 3292–3298.

Phipps S., & Noll, R. B. (2010). Do symptoms of anxiety in the terminally ill child affect long-term psychological well-being in bereaved parents? *Pediatric Blood and Cancer, 55*, 1245.

Solomon, M. Z., & Browning, D. (2005). Pediatric palliative care: Relationships matter and so does pain control. *Journal of Clinical Oncology, 23*, 9055–9057.

Speece, M. W., & Brent, S. B. (1996). The development of children's understanding of death: A review of three components of a death concept. In C. A. Corr & D. M. Corr (Eds.), *Handbook of childhood death and bereavement* (pp. 29–50). New York: Springer.

Spinetta, J. J. (1974). The dying child's awareness of death. *Psychological Bulletin, 4*, 256–260.

U.S. Department of Health and Human Services, Health Resources and Services Administration, Maternal and Child Health Bureau. (2011). *Child Health USA 2011.* Rockville, MD: Author.

Waechter, E. H. (1971). Children's awareness of fatal illness. *American Journal of Nursing, 71*, 1168–1172.

Whitty-Rogers, J., Alex, M., MacDonald, C., Pierrynowski Gallant, D., & Austin, W. (2009). Working with children in end-of-life decision making. *Nursing Ethics, 16*, 743–758.

Wolff, A., Browne, J., & Whitehouse, W. P. (2011). Personal resuscitation plans and end of life planning for children with disability and life-limiting/life-threatening conditions. *Archives of Disease in Childhood: Education and Practice Edition, 96,* 42–48.

Wolfe, J., Grier, H. E., Klar, N., Levin, S. B., Ellenbogen, J. M., Salem-Schatz, S., et al., (2000). Symptoms and suffering at the end of life in children with cancer. *New England Journal of Medicine, 342,* 326–333.

Index

An *f* following a page number indicates a figure; a *t* following a page number indicates a table.

Treatment (*continued*)
  characteristics of pediatric psychology practice, 8–10
  collaboration and consultation, 40–41
  elimination disorders and, 304–307
  evidence-based practice, 10, 39–40
  financial issues and, 49–53, 50*t*
  outcome measurement, 38–39
  referrals to community-based resources and, 86–87
  reintegration to school and home, 34–35
  seizure disorders and, 269–270
  settings for practice, 7–8
  strategies, 33–34
  traumatic brain injury and, 316, 320–321
  use of technology and, 142–144
Treatment adherence. *See also* Compliance
  HIV (human immunodeficiency virus), 218–220
  organ transplantation and, 287–290
Treatment planning
  diabetes, 237
  procedural pain and, 166–167
  reintegration to school and home, 117–118
  traumatic brain injury and, 317

U

Universal level of intervention, 258
Universal prevention, 129, 132. *See also* Prevention

V

Video modeling, 170

W

Weight issues, 247–254